THE BIOCHEMISTRY
OF MYASTHENIA GRAVIS
AND MUSCULAR DYSTROPHY

THE BIOCHEMISTRY
OF MYASTHENIA GRAVIS
AND MUSCULAR DYSTROPHY

Edited by

G.G. LUNT

Department of Biochemistry,
University of Bath,
Bath.

and

R.M. MARCHBANKS

Department of Biochemistry,
Institute of Psychiatry,
De Crespigny Park,
Denmark Hill,
London SE5 8AF.

1978

ACADEMIC PRESS
London . New York . San Francisco
A Subsidiary of Harcourt Brace Jovanovich, Publishers

ACADEMIC PRESS INC. (LONDON) LTD.
24/28 Oval Road,
London NW1

United States Edition published by
ACADEMIC PRESS INC.
111 Fifth Avenue
New York, New York 10003

Copyright © 1978 by
ACADEMIC PRESS INC. (LONDON) LTD.

37526

All Rights Reserved
No part of this book may be reproduced in any form by photostat, microfilm,
or any other means, without written permission from the publishers

Library of Congress Catalog Card Number: 77-85108
ISBN: 0-12-459650-9

Printed in Great Britain by
Whitstable Litho Ltd., Whitstable, Kent

Lanchester Polytechnic Library

Contributors

C.P. AHERN, Department of Pre-Clinical Veterinary Sciences and Department of Biochemistry, Trinity College, Dublin 2, Ireland.

L. ANGLISTER, Department of Neurobiology, Weizmann Institute of Science, Rehovot, Israel.

T. BARKAS, Department of Biochemistry, University of Bath, U.K.

E.A. BARNARD, Department of Biochemistry, Imperial College, London, S.W.7, U.K.

P.J. BARNARD, Department of Biochemistry, Imperial College, London, S.W.7, U.K.

D. BARTFIELD, Department of Chemical Immunology, The Weizmann Institute of Science, Rehovot, Israel.

K. BERGSTROM, Department of clinical chemistry, Karolinska Institutet, Karolinska sjukhuset, S-10401 Stockholm, Sweden.

W.G. BRADLEY, Tufts University, New England Medical Centre, 171 Hamilton Ave., Boston, Massachusetts, U.S.A. 02111.

C.J. BRANFORD WHITE, Department of Biology, Oxford Polytechnic, Headington, Oxford. OX3 0BP., U.K.

M.M. BURGER, Biozentrum der Universitat Basel, Klingelbergstr. 70, CH-4056 Basel, Switzerland.

W. BURKART, Biozentrum der Universitat Basel, Klingelbergstr, 70, CH-4056 Basel, Switzerland.

J.-P. CHANGEUX, Neurobiologie Moleculaire, Institut Pasteur, Paris, France.

F. CLEMENTI, Department of Pharmacology and CNR Center of Cytopharmacology, University of Milan, Italy.

B. CONTI-TRONCONI, Department of Pharmacology and CNR Center of Cytopharmacology, University of Milan, Italy.

F. CORNELIO, Department of Pharmacology and CNR Center of Cytopharmacology, University of Milan, Italy.

G.S. CRUICKSHANK, Department of Pharmacology, Royal Free Hospital School of Medicine, 8 Hunter Street, London WC1N 1BP, U.K.

P.A. DREYFUS, I.N.S.E.R.M. U 153 Groupe de Biologie et Pathologie Neuromusculaire Division Risler, La Salpetriere 47 bd de l'Hopital Paris (13è), France.

R. DUBS, Immunology Laboratory, Department of Internal Medicine, University Hospital, 8091 Zurich, Switzerland.

D.A. ELLIS, Midland Centre for Neurosurgery and Neurology, Smethwick, U.K.

A. FONTANA, Immunology Laboratory, Department of Internal Medicine, University Hospital, 8091 Zurich, Switzerland.

S. FUCHS, Department of Chemical Immunology, The Weizmann Institute of Science, Rehovot, Israel.

B.W. FULPIUS, Department of Biochemistry, University of Geneva, Sciences II, 1211 Geneva 4, Switzerland.

H. GAZIT, Department of Neurobiology, Weizmann Institute of Science, Rehovot, Israel.

H.H. GOEBEL, Division of Neuropathology, University of Gottingen, Göttingen, German Federal Republic.

C. GOTTI, Department of Pharmacology and CNR Center of Cytopharmacology, University of Milan, Italy.

P.J. GROB, Immunology Laboratory, Department of Internal Medicine, University Hospital, 8091 Zurich, Switzerland.

L. HAMMARSTROM, Division of Immunology, Wallenberglab, Lilla Frescati, S-104 05 Stockholm, Sweden.

P.S. HARPER, Departments of Child Health, Medicine & Medical Genetics, Welsh National School of Medicine, Cardiff.

R. HARRISON, Department of Biochemistry, University of Bath, U.K.

A.L. HARVEY, Department of Physiology and Pharmacology, University of Strathclyde, U.K.

E. HEILBRONN, Section of Biochemistry, National Defence Research Institute, S-172 04 Sundbyberg, Sweden.

K. HOWELLS, Department of Biology, Oxford Polytechnic, Headington, Oxford. OX3 0BP, U.K.

Y. ITO, Department of Biophysics, University College, London WC1E 6BT.

I. JIRMANOVÁ, Institute of Physiology, Czechoslovak Academy of Sciences, Prague.

H. JOCKUSCH, Biozentrum der Universitat Basel, Klingelbergstr. 70, CH-4056 Basel, Switzerland.

S.E. KITCHEN, Department of Pharmacology, Royal Free Hospital School of Medicine, 8 Hunter Street, London WC1N 1BP, U.K.

A.K. LEFVERT, Department of clinical chemistry, Karolinska Hospital, S-10405 Stockholm, Sweden.

M.H.R. LEWIS, Department of Biochemistry, Queen's University of Belfast, B17 1NN, U.K.

R. LIBELIUS, Department of Pharmacology, University of Lund, Sweden.

J. LINDSTROM, The Salk Institute for Biological Studies, P.O. Box 1809, San Diego, California, U.S.A. 92112.

I. LUNDQUIST, Department of Pharmacology, University of Lund, Sweden.

G.G. LUNT, Department of Biochemistry, University of Bath, U.K.

G. MATELL, Department of Medicine, South Hospital, S-100 64 Stockholm, Sweden.

C. MATTSSON, Section of Biochemistry, National Defence Research Institute, S-172 04 Sundbyberg, Sweden.

J.V. McLOUGHLIN, Department of Pre-Clinical Veterinary Sciences and Department of Biochemistry, Trinity College, Dublin 2, Ireland.

R. MILEDI, Department of Biophysics, University College, London WC1E 6BT.

P.C. MOLENAAR, Department of Pharmacology, Sylvius Laboratories, University of Leiden, Wassenaarseweg 72, Leiden, The Netherlands.

M. MORGUTTI, Instituto Neurologico 'Besta', Milan, Italy.

I. MOTHERSILL, Immunology Laboratory, Department of Internal Medicine, University Hospital, 8091 Zurich, Switzerland.

D. NADEAU, NIEHS/NIH, P.O. Box 12233, Research Triangle Park, N.C. 27709., U.S.A.

J.S. NEERUNJUN, Muscle Research Unit, Department of Pediatrics and Neonatal Medicine, Hammersmith Hospital, London W.12, U.K.

D. NEVO, Department of Chemical Immunology, The Weizmann Institute of Science, Rehovot, Israel.

J. NEWSOM DAVIS, Department of Neurology, Royal Free Hospital, London N.W.3 2QG.

A.C. PALMER, School of Veterinary Medicine, Cambridge, U.K.

R. PARSONS, Muscular Dystrophy Research Laboratory, Regional Neurological Centre, Newcastle upon Tyne NE4 6BE

R.J.T. PENNINGTON, Regional Neurological Centre, Newcastle upon Tyne, U.K.

A. PERSSON, Department of Clinical Neurophysiology, Huddinge Hospital, S-141 86 Huddinge, Sweden.

A.J. PINCHING, National Hospital for Nervous Diseases, Queen Sq., London, U.K.

R. PIRSKANEN, Department of clinical chemistry, Karolinska Institutet, Karolinska sjukhuset, S-10401 Stockholm, Sweden.

R. POLAK, Medical Biological Laboratory, T.N.O., Rijswijk-Z.H., The Netherlands.

E.B. SANDBORN, Départments d'Anatomie et de Pharmacologie, Faculté de Medecine, Université de Montréal, Montréal, Quebec, Canada H3C 3J7.

R. SAUTER, Immunology Laboratory, Department of Internal Medicine, University Hospital, 8091 Zurich, Switzerland.

J.R. SIBERT, Departments of Child Health, Medicine & Medical Genetics, Welsh National School of Medicine, Cardiff, U.K.

I. SILMAN, Department of Neurobiology, Weizmann Institute of Science, Rehovot, Israel.

J.A. SIMPSON, Institute of Neurological Sciences, Southern General Hospital, Glasgow, U.K.

E. SMITH, Division Immunology, Wallenberglab, Lilla Frescati, S-104 05 Stockholm, Sweden.

C.J. SOMERS, Department of Pre-Clinical Veterinary Sciences and Department of Biochemistry, Trinity College, Dublin 2, Ireland.

G. SPIEGEL, Department of Chemistry, Washington University, St. Louis, Missouri, U.S.A.

E. STAHLBERG, Department of Clinical Neurophysiology, Academic Hospital, S-750 14, Uppsala, Sweden.

H.R. STEPHENS, Muscle Research Centre, Department of Pediatrics and Neonatal Medicine, Hammersmith Hospital, Du Cane Road, London W12 0HS, U.K.

J.M. STRICKLAND, Pathology Department, Midland Centre for Neurosurgery and Neurology, Holly Lane, Smethwick, Warley, West Midlands B67 7JX, U.K.

R. TARRAB-HAZDAI, The Department of Chemical Immunology, The Weizmann Institute of Science, Rehovot, Israel.

V.I. TEICHBERG, Neurobiologie Moleculaire, Institut Pasteur, Paris, France.

S. THESLEFF, Department of Pharmacology, University of Lund, Sweden.

R.J. THOMPSON, Department of Medical Biochemistry, Welsh National School of Medicine, Cardiff, U.K.

J.E. TYE, Pathology Department, Midland Centre for Neurosurgery and Neurology, Holly Lane, Smethwick, Warley, West Midlands B67 7JX, U.K.

A. UDDGARD, Section of Biochemistry, National Defence Research Institute, S 172 04 Sundbyberg, Sweden.

W.B. VAN WINKLE, Department of Cell Biophysics, Baylor College of Medicine, Houston, Texas, U.S.A.

A. VINCENT, Department of Neurology, Royal Free Hospital, London N.W.3 2QG, U.K.

G. VRBOVÁ, Department of Anatomy and Embryology, University College London, Gower Street, London, WC1E 6BT.

R.R. WALLACE, Department of Biochemistry, Queen's University of Belfast, BT7 1NN, U.K.

J. WATKINS, Department of Biochemistry, Guy's Hospital Medical School, London SE1 9RT, U.K.

D.C. WATTS, Department of Biochemistry, Guy's Hospital Medical School, London SE1 9RT, U.K.

R.L. WATTS, Department of Biochemistry, Guy's Hospital Medical School, London SE1 9RT, U.K.

M.R. WEST, Muscular Dystrophy Research Laboratory, Regional Neurological Centre, Newcastle upon Tyne NE4 6BE, U.K.
P. WILSON, Department of Pre-Clinical Veterinary Sciences and Department of Biochemistry, Trinity College, Dublin 2, Ireland.
E. ZAIMIS, Department of Pharmacology, Royal Free Hospital School of Medicine, 8 Hunter Street, London WC1N 1BP, U.K.
D. ZURN, Department of Biochemistry, University of Geneva, Sciences II, 1211 Geneva 4, Switzerland.

Preface

The isolation and purification of the nicotinic post-synaptic receptor for acetylcholine carried out in the early 1970s by groups of biochemists in England, France and Argentina has had in the last two or three years direct and dramatic repercussions on the diagnosis, understanding and therapy of Myasthenia Gravis. The development of experimental models of Muscular Dystrophy in which the biochemical lesion and clinical features can be reproduced is likely to have an equally important effect on diagnosis and therapy of this group of muscular diseases. One of the aims of the workshops organized by the Neurochemical Group of the Biochemical Society is to stimulate the interests of investigators in areas of Neurobiology where scientific understanding has develop to such a level that it can readily be exploited in the interests of the patient. We believe that recent progress in the understanding of Myasthenia Gravis and Muscular Dystrophy has reached such a state; hence the workshop organized by the Neurochemical Group at Bath in March 1977 the proceedings of which are recorded here.

In organizing the workshop we invited some speakers to cover the broader aspects of nerve-muscle interactions, clinicians to describe illnesses resulting from malfunctions of the neuromuscular systems and specialists who were asked to review recent clinical and biochemical progress in particular disorders. Time and space did not permit a comprehensive coverage of the whole topic of neuromuscular disorders and the workshop tended to concentrate on certain subjects, such as the induction of experimental autoimmune myasthenia and the development of experimental models of muscular dystrophy. These topics represent the thrust of current interest and it is appropriate that they should predominate. In any rapidly expanding field of research there will be several groups engaged in work on closely related and overlapping themes. This book reflects that tendency and we have made no attempt to constrain it because we believe that comparison of the experiences and difficulties of different laboratories can be illuminating, particularly when the findings are very recent.

The workshop, and hence the book, were only made possible by generous donations from the following (in alphabetical order); Academic Press, Beechams Pharmaceuticals CIBA Laboratories, Muscular Dystrophy Group of Great Britain, The Patrick Trust and The Wellcome Trust.

We would like to thank these and the contributors for their help.

July 1977

G.G. LUNT

R.M. MARCHBANKS

Contents

Histopathology

Experimental models

Subject Index

Abbreviations

We have followed the conventions adopted by the Biochemical Journal (Instruction to Authors 1977) and used the list of abbreviations given there along with others of neurobiological interest that are allowed by the Journal of Neurochemistry. Those investigating the acetylcholine receptor and its immunology have generated a new set of abbreviations which we have attempted to standardise; these along with other common ones are listed below as well as at first mention in the text.

ACh	Acetylcholine
AChE	Acetylcholinesterase
AChR	Acetylcholine receptor
ATP, etc.	5′ pyrophosphates of adenosine etc.
ATP-ase	Adenosine triphosphatase
α-Bgtx	α-Bungarotoxin
CP	creatine phosphate
CPK	creatine phosphokinase
DEAE	Diethylaminoethyl
EAMG	Experimental autoimmune myasthenia gravis
ECG	Electrocardiogram
EMG	Electromyogram
e.p.p	end plate potential
HRP	Horseradish Peroxidase
HLA	Human leucocyte antigen
IgA, (G)	immunoglobulin A, (G) etc.
m.e.p.p	miniature end plate potential
MG	Myasthenia Gravis
RCM-AChR	reduced carboxymethylated acetylcholine receptor
REM	Rapid eye movement
SDH	Succinate dehydrogenase
SDS	Sodium dodecyl sulphate

Introduction

1 The influence of the motor nerve on the characteristic properties of skeletal muscle

G. VRBOVÁ

Department of Antomy and Embryology, University College London,
Gower Street, London. WC1E. 6BT.

Introduction

It is common experience that the nerve is essential for the maintenance of the functional and structural integrity of vertebrate skeletal muscle. Following damage to the peripheral nerve changes take place in the paralysed muscle, all of which can be reversed on reinnervation. This dependence of the structural integrity of the muscle on innervation led to the idea that the nerve exerts a special 'trophic' influence on the muscle it supplies (see Gutmann, 1962).

Experiments in which all the changes observed in muscle on cutting the peripheral nerve could be reproduced by cutting the ventral roots firmly established that it is the motor nerve fibres that exert this 'trophic' influence (Tower, 1937). All normal activity of a muscle is usually initiated by the motor nerve and following damage of the nerve this activity ceases. It therefore seemed probable that many of the changes that follow denervation might be attributable to the inactivity of the muscle. The question that is raised is whether there is a special 'trophic' influence of the nerve on muscle in addition to the main function of the motor nerve, which is of course to activate the muscle.

Different properties of skeletal muscles that are altered by denervation and said to be determined by the motor nerve, have been studied throughout the years. In this paper I would like to discuss two of these. The role of the motor nerve (a) in the control of the distribution of chemosensitivity along skeletal muscle fibres, and (b) in determining the mechanical and biochemical properties of skeletal muscle.

Control of chemosensitivity of skeletal muscle fibres

Differentiated skeletal muscle fibres are sensitive to acetylcholine (ACh) only at the endplate region. Immature muscle fibres respond to ACh along

3

their entire surface, and only some time after innervation has taken place does ACh sensitivity become restricted to the endplate region. Following denervation such a differentiated muscle fibre again becomes sensitive to ACh along its entire surface and on reinnervation this chemosensitive area becomes once more restricted to the endplate region (Ginetzinsky and Shamarina, 1942; Diamond and Miledi, 1962; Miledi, 1960a). From this it was suggested that the role of the motor nerve is, among other things, to reduce the chemosensitivity of the extrajunctional area, by exerting a special 'trophic' influence on the muscle fibre it supplies.

Miledi (1960a) suggested that a special substance is released from the nerve endings, independent of impulse activity, or transmitter release. These conclusions were based on the following findings: The presence of miniature endplate potentials (mepps) was taken as an indication of ACh release, and no correlation between the presence, or absence of mepps and chemosensitivity was found. Miledi (1960a and b) concluded that the transmitter has little to do with the control of chemosensitivity. Moreover, on reinnervation muscle fibres could be found where the frequency of mepps was still low, and transmission had not yet been established, yet the chemosensitive area was already restricted to the endplate region. (Miledi, 1960a).

A slightly different proposal was made by Thesleff (1960) who considered the spontaneous release of ACh to be responsible for maintaining the area outside the endplate region insensitive to ACh. Unlike the studies of Miledi in frog muscle, Thesleff (1960) found in mammalian muscle a correlation between the frequency of mepps and size of the chemosensitive area.

There is, however, a curious feature to both these suggestions, for they postulate a direct chemical influence of the nerve that is to have a desensitising influence on structures several cm away from the nerve terminals, while at the same time the area of contact is always extremely sensitive to the transmitter. How this part of the membrane could avoid the allegedly desensitising influence of the nerve on muscle has not been explained.

I would like to discuss evidence in favour of the hypothesis that the extra-junctional area of muscle fibres becomes insensitive to ACh as a result of the activity of the muscle itself. During development the sensitivity of skeletal muscle fibres to ACh outside the endplate region decreases with age (Diamond and Miledi, 1962; Brown, 1975). The size of the chemo-sensitive area is proportional to the strength of contractions elicited by ACh applied to the muscle, and this method has often been used to estimate the size of the chemosensitive area. The sensitivity to ACh of the soleus muscle of a rat was studied during development, and the smallest dose required to produce a contraction found. As expected, a much larger dose of ACh was needed when soleus muscles from four week old animals were studied, confirming that the sensitivity of ACh of this muscle decreases with age. When however the nerve to these muscles was cut during the first week of the animal's life this decrease of sensitivity of the soleus muscle did not take place, and Fig. 1a illustrates this point. Whether this decrease of chemosensitivity that has taken place during development is brought about by a special influence of the nerve on muscle, or by the activity imposed on the muscle was studied by Brown (1975). She found that electrical stimulation of denervated rabbit skeletal muscles reduced their sensitivity to depolarising drugs. The time course of this was similar to the reduction brought about by reinnervation of the muscles by their own motor nerve.

Another approach to the investigation of the role of activity for the reduction of chemosensitivity was applied by Gordon and Vrbová (1975). The motor system of chick embryos reaches maturity during embryonic development, so that at hatching the characteristic properties of chick muscles are to a large extent differentiated. If such embryos are temporarily paralysed by injecting hemicholinium into the yolk sac this decrease of sensitivity to ACh fails to develop, and the muscles so inactivated retain their high chemosensitivity (Fig. 1b), indicating that the decrease of chemo-sensitivity during development is brought about by muscle activity (Gordon and Vrbová, 1975).

In adult skeletal muscles normal activity of the muscle seems to be essential for the maintenance of low sensitivity of the extra-junctional area. It is now well established that when transmission is blocked, either by preventing transmitter release, or by blocking the postsynaptic mem-brane, the sensitivity of the muscle membrane to ACh outside the end-plate region increases (Thesleff, 1960; Berg and Hall, 1975). When muscles are inactivated by blocking conduction of action potentials along the motor nerve by enclosing the nerves into silastoseal cuffs containing local anaes-thetic, or by local application of tetrodotoxin, hypersensitivity is regularly noticed in muscles supplied by these nerves (Lømo and Rosenthal, 1972; Pestronk, *et al.* 1976). Thus even in the presence of the motor nerve, changes of chemosensitivity similar to denervation hypersensitivity can be produced by inactivity.

Another approach for testing the role of activity in the control of chemosensitivity of skeletal muscles is to replace by electrical stimulation of denervated muscle the activity usually imparted onto this muscle by its motor nerve. This method was used by Ginetzinski (1956), who concluded that electrical stimulation does not prevent the development of hyper-sensitivity of denervated cat muscles. This result differed from an earlier short report by Thomson (1952) who claimed to have reduced denervation hypersensitivity by direct electrical stimulation of skeletal muscles. At that time it was impossible to stimulate muscles for long periods of time, because

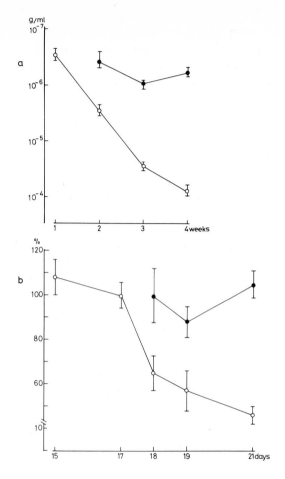

Fig. 1. The graphs show (a) the change of ACh sensitivity of control (○) and denervated (●) rat soleus muscles with age. The dose required to produce a threshold contraction increases with age in the control, and remains unaltered in the denervated muscles, (b) the changes of responses to 1 mg/ml of ACh of control (○) and hemicholinium treated (●) posterior latissimus dorsi muscles from chick embryos of different ages. The response is expressed as a per cent of maximal tetanic tension. Control PLD muscles become less sensitive to ACh with age, whereas muscles from treated embryos remain sensitive.

there were no implantable materials available. The availability of plastic materials that did not produce an inflammatory response when introduced into the body of animals has made it possible to stimulate their skeletal muscles for longer periods of time and in a more controlled way.

When electrodes were implanted into rats so as to stimulate their denervated muscles, the increase of sensitivity to ACh could be prevented (Jones and Vrbová, 1971) and Fig. 2 shows an example from such an experiment.

This finding was confirmed by Drachmann and Witzke (1972) and Lømo and Rosenthal (1972), and there is general agreement that up to three days after denervation hypersensitivity can be prevented by electrical stimulation. There was however a curious difference between the results of Lømo and Rosenthal and those of Jones and Vrbová (1974). While the former

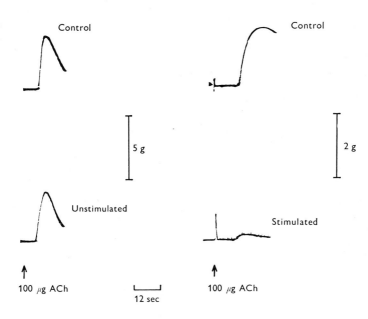

Fig. 2. Contractions of 48 hr denervated soleus muscles in response to ACh. Top tracings: denervated 'control' muscles, bottom left hand trace-electrodes implanted, but muscle left unstimulated, bottom right hand trace: electrodes implanted and muscles stimulated for 8 hours every day after operation.

authors claimed to have been able to reduce denervation hypersensitivity at any time after section of the nerve, the latter found it difficult, and near impossible to achieve this, when stimulation of muscles was started between the third and sixth days after denervation. This difference may be due to either a more vigorous stimulation regime of Lømo and Rosenthal (1972), or to the different ways in which increased sensitivity was recorded. Whatever the reason, the finding that the same type of activity that could entirely prevent the development of hypersensitivity during the first three days of denervation had virtually no effect when applied during the third and sixth day after denervation led Jones and Vrbová (1974) to consider the possibility that during this time another factor interferes with the effects of activity. There is indeed much evidence to suggest that other factors, in addition to lack of activity, are likely to contribute to the increased sensitivity of denervated muscles.

It was noticed that denervation changes occur earlier in muscles attached to a short stump of sectioned motor nerve than to a long stump (Luco and Eyzaguire, 1955; Gutmann, *et al.* 1955; Miledi and Slater, 1969; Harris and Thesleff, 1972), although the reduction in activity in both cases must be similar. Observations on the partially denervated frog sartorius muscle, also suggest that inactivity alone cannot account for all the changes that follow denervation (Miledi, 1960b). Muscle fibres of the frog sartorius are supplied by two nerve terminals from separate branches that form endplates on the same muscle fibres some distance apart from each other. When one branch was cut each muscle fibre would still be activated by the remaining terminal. Nevertheless, the part of the muscle fibre that was close to

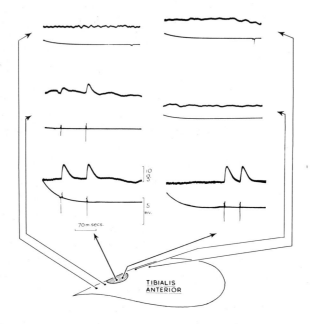

Fig. 3. Schematic representation of a rabbit tibialis anterior muscle. The shaded area represents the place where a section of the lateral popliteal nerve was implanted 5 days before the final experiment. Traces represent recordings of action potentials (top) and concentrations (bottom) taken when ACh at a concentration of 5×10^{-5} was released onto the indicated place on the muscle.

the denervated endplates became hypersensitive to ACh, while the inner-vated part of the muscle retained its normal low sensitivity (Miledi, 1960b). This result indicated that inactivity is not the only cause of denervation hypersensitivity, and that areas of high chemosensitivity can be induced on a normal, active muscle. This was further confirmed by the finding that injury to frog muscle fibres can induce an increase of sensitivity to ACh even in innervated muscle fibres (Katz and Miledi, 1964). On mammalian muscle fibres such an increased sensitivity can be induced merely by placing an isolated segment of nerve onto the surface of the muscle (Vrbová, 1967; Jones and Vrbová, 1974; Jones and Vyskočil, 1975). This increased sensitivity is most pronounced on the part of the muscle immediately beneath the degenerating piece of isolated nerve, and Fig. 3 illustrates this point. Thus by merely placing a piece of degenerating tissue on the surface of a normal innervated muscle, localized changes of ACh sensitivity of the muscle membrane can be produced.

It is interesting that the time course of the development of the increase of sensitivity of the muscle membrane to the transmitter is similar no matter how it is produced. Fig. 4 compares the development of hypersensitivity of the rat soleus muscle after section of the sciatic to that produced in the muscle by placing a foreign body on the surface of the muscle. The denervated soleus as well as the injured soleus become significantly more sensitive two days after the insult, and by three days maximum effect is reached in both types of experiments. Fig. 4 also illustrates that whereas denervation hypersensitivity persists, the increase in sensitivity of innervated muscles is transient, its disappearance probably being due to activity of the muscle fibre.

It is possible that in denervated muscle the presence of degenerating nerve terminals contributes to the early development of hypersensitivity, which in the absence of activity persists until reinnervation takes place. This could explain the later onset of hypersensitivity in muscles connected to a longer stump of nerve, since the onset of degeneration of nerve terminals depends on the length of the peripheral nerve stump (Miledi and Slater, 1969). It would also account for the finding that partially denervated muscle fibres become more sensitive near the denervated neuromuscular junction, and finally would be consistent with the finding that during the time when massive degeneration of the nerve terminals takes place in the muscle, i.e. after three days of denervation, activity is not very successful in preventing the increase of chemosensitivity. From this it was concluded that denervation hypersensitivity is caused by two factors: the presence of degenerating nerve terminals in the muscle, and inactivity of the muscle (Jones and Vrbová, 1974).

In normal muscle fibres the development and maintenance of the low ACh sensitivity of the extra-junctional area can be explained by the desensitizing effects of muscle activity; it is unnecessary to postulate that the nerve exerts a special 'trophic' influence that controls the chemosensitivity of the muscle fibre outside the endplate region.

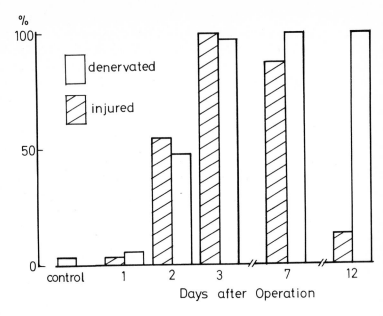

Fig. 4. The blocks represent the responses to 500 μg/ml of ACh expressed as a per cent maximum ACh response obtained, from denervated and 'injured' soleus muscles at different intervals after operation. The sensitivity of both denervated and 'injured' muscles increases up to the 7th days, but at 12 days the denervated muscle is still hypersensitive, whereas the sensitivity of the 'injured' muscle is returning to normal.

The role of the motor nerve in determining some mechanical and biochemical characteristics of mammalian skeletal muscle fibres

In mammals two distinct types of muscles with respect to the time course of their contraction and relaxation, as well as their biochemical properties, have been recognized: slow contracting muscles with high levels of oxidative and low levels of glycolytic anaerobic enzymes, and fast contracting muscles, with low levels of oxidative and high levels of glycolytic enzyme activities (Ranvier, 1874; Denny-Brown, 1929; Copper and Eccles, 1930).

Although more recent findings suggest that such a clear distinction is arbitrary, and moreover many additional differences in the composition of muscle fibres have been reported, the distinction into slow and fast muscles is certainly valid for particular leg muscles of mammals. These characteristic properties of slow and fast muscles are well matched to the functional requirements imposed upon them by their respective motor nerves. Motor nerves to the slow soleus muscles of the cat and rabbit fire at low rates of about 8 to 15 Hz, more or less continually; whereas motor nerves to fast muscles fire only occasionally and at higher frequencies (Denny-Brown, 1929; Eccles, Eccles and Lungberg, 1957). Since for co-ordinated movement it is important for the contraction to be smooth, the slow contraction and relaxation of the soleus is well adjusted to the slow firing rate, and the fast contraction of the fast leg muscles to the fast firing rate. The question as to how these contractile characteristics are determined is therefore of special interest.

The dependence of the muscle fibre on its neuron was most clearly demonstrated in experiments of Buller, Eccles and Eccles (1960). They sutured the motor nerve from the slow soleus muscle of the cat into the fast flexor digitorum longus and the nerve from this fast muscle into the soleus. Some time after this 'cross-innervation' the characteristic contractile speeds of the two muscles were examined and compared to those of the contralateral, unoperated side. The fast muscles now supplied by the slow nerve became slow contracting and the slow muscles supplied by a fast nerve became fast contracting. By this single series of experiments it was clearly established that the contractile properties characteristic of a given muscle are not inherent but are determined by the motor nerve.

It was later found that many other properties characteristic of a slow muscle came to resemble those of a fast muscle when it had become inner-vated by a nerve from the fast muscle, and vice-versa. So for example the enzyme pattern of the soleus muscle fibres changed from a homogeneously high oxidative, low anaerobic type to a heterogeneous population of muscle fibres resembling a fast muscle (Romanul and Van Der Meullen, 1967). The structure of contractile proteins is also different in slow and fast muscles. The myosin ATP-ase activity of soleus muscle is lower and that of fast muscle higher (Bárány, 1967), and this too changes after cross-innervation (Buller, *et al.* 1969). Many other biochemical features are also altered by cross-innervation; for example the ATP-ase activity of the sarcoplasmic reticulum also differs in slow and fast muscles and is transformed following cross-innervation. The myosin light chains are distinctly different in slow and fast muscles and after cross-innervation the light chains of the fast muscle will become to resemble those of the slow muscle and those of the slow muscle will become similar to those in fast muscles (Weeds *et al.,* 1974).

Not only does the structure of the thick filament and sarcoplasmic proteins change but that of the thin filament is also influenced by the alien innervation. As expected, when the soleus muscle of a rabbit is reinnervated by the lateral popliteal nerve which usually innervates fast muscle fibres, the contractile properties of the soleus muscle change, ie. it becomes a fast contracting and relaxing muscle. Fig. 5 shows that this change of contractile properties is accompanied by a transformation of the structure of troponin I, which is one of the three regulating proteins in skeletal muscles (Amphlett *et al.,* 1976).

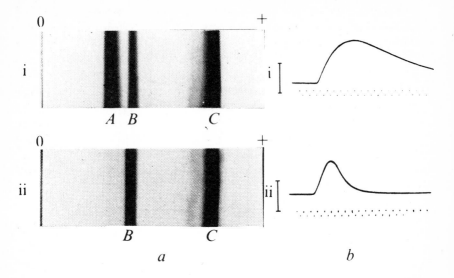

Fig. 5. Effect of cross innervation on the speed of contraction and the troponin I composition of rabbit soleus muscle, (a) Electrophoresis of troponin I (20μg), isolated by affinity chromatography from rabbit soleus muscle (rabbit 2, see Table 1), in the presence of troponin C(50μg) from rabbit white skeletal muscle. 6 M urea, 25 mM Tris-80 mM glycine, pH 8.6, 8% acrylamide. 0, Origin i, Control soleus; ii, soleus from the other leg of the same animal 26 weeks after cross innervation. A, slow troponin I-troponin C complex; B, fast troponin I-troponin C complex; C, troponin C. (b) Records of single isometric contractions of the soleus muscles used for troponin I preparations analysed in a. The distance between successive dots represents 100 g tension.

There are several possible explanations as to how the nerve exerts this influence over the muscle fibres it supplies. In their original paper, Buller, *et al.* (1960) suggested that the nerve exerts a special 'trophic' influence over the muscle fibres and that it is in this way that it determines what is to become of the muscle fibre. Another possible explanation of these results was put forward by A.F. Huxley and discussed by Buller, *et al.* (1960). Huxley suggested to Buller, *et al.* (1960) that the motor nerve maintains the slow time course of contraction of the soleus muscle fibres by imposing onto it a slow frequency activity, which may act as a 'vibratory stress' (see Buller, *et al.* (1960)). Buller *et al.* did not favour this interpretation, and it wasn't until later that evidence was provided to show the crucial importance of the activity of the muscle in determining its characteristic properties.

It is known from the work of Sperry (1944) that the activity pattern of motor nerves remains unaltered when they are transposed into different muscles. Thus, in the experimental situation of Buller, *et al.* (1960) the nerve from a fast muscle, now supplying a slow muscle, would activate the slow muscle by the same activity pattern as the original fast muscle, and the nerve from the slow muscle would carry on activating the fast muscle by the type of activity of the original slow muscle. From this it is clear that after crossing the motor nerves from one type of muscle to another, the activity pattern of each muscle would be changed. The effects produced by crossing the motor nerves could be explained by the altered activity the muscle was made to perform, without having to involve a special trophic influence.

A simple situation was sought that would alter radically the activity pattern of skeletal muscle without interfering with its innervation. Soleus motoneurones have a low threshold to stretch but are inexcitable by flexor reflex afferens. It might therefore be expected that the stretch reflex would be of greater importance for the activity of soleus than for that of muscles involved in other types of movement. When EMG activity was recorded from the soleus muscles of conscious, unrestrained rabbits, it was found that continuous activity could be recorded from this muscle, no matter whether the rabbit was walking, standing or just sitting quietly in its cage. Other muscles, like tibialis anterior were activated during movement of the animal or on pinching its foot. After cutting the tendons of these muscles, and thus preventing them from being stretched, the continuous activity of the soleus muscle can no longer be seen and only occasionally, activity of very small motor units can be detected (Fig. 6). Tenotomy of the

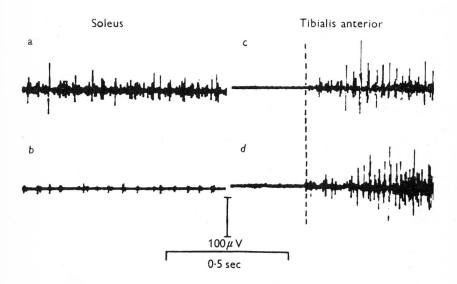

Fig. 6. EMG recorded with implanted electrodes from (a) control soleus, while the animal was standing; (b) the same muscle 1 day after tenotomy, when the position of the animal was changed; (c) control tibialis anterior when a flexor reflex was elicited at the interrupted line; (d) tibialis anterior 1 day after tenotomy while the animal was standing and when a flexor reflex was elicited at the interrupted line.

other calf muscles does not alter appreciably their phasic type of EMG activity as illustrated in Fig. 6 by the recording from the tibialis anterior before and after tenotomy (Vrbová, 1963a).

Thus tenotomy alters the activity pattern of soleus, but not that of tibialis anterior. When the contractile speeds of the tenotomized soleus muscle were examined some time after the operation it was found that the tenotomized soleus muscle had become fast contracting (Fig. 7). Thus in this experiment the innervation was unaltered and only the activity pattern of the soleus muscle was changed by tenotomy, nevertheless the contractile properties of the soleus muscle changed. The activity pattern of the tibialis anterior muscle was unaltered by tenotomy and correspondingly the contractile speeds remained unaffected (Vrbová, 1963b).

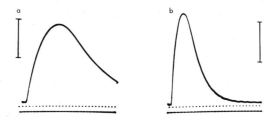

Fig. 7. Isometric contractions from a rabbit soleus muscle. (a) Control muscle; (b) two weeks tenotomized muscle. The intervals between the dots represent 10 ms. The vertical bar in (a) represents 100 and in.(b) 10 g.

In order to study the effects of activity at different frequencies on the contractile properties of muscle it was thought desirable to work with muscle that had no, or extremely little reflex activity of its own. As already mentioned, the tenotomized soleus, although quiescent, had some activity. If this residual activity was due to a supraspinal excitatory influence on soleus motoneurones, then cutting the spinal cord ought to abolish even this activity. Indeed, after section of the cord the tenotomized muscle is completely 'silent' whereas reflex activity can readily be elicited from the tibialis anterior muscle. The tenotomized soleus of a spinal rabbit became fast contracting, suggesting that its normal activity maintains the slow contractile speed. Electrodes were implanted close to the motor nerve of the 'silent' soleus muscle and electrical activity was imposed upon the muscle via these electrodes. When the muscle was stimulated at 5 or 10 Hz for eight hours a day over a period of two to three weeks the soleus muscle remained slow, when however higher frequencies of stimulation were used, 20 or 40 Hz, the soleus muscle became fast contracting. These results are summarized in Fig. 8, and clearly show that the contractile speed of the rabbit soleus is determined by the particular activity pattern of the muscle (Vrbová, 1966; Salmons and Vrbová, 1969).

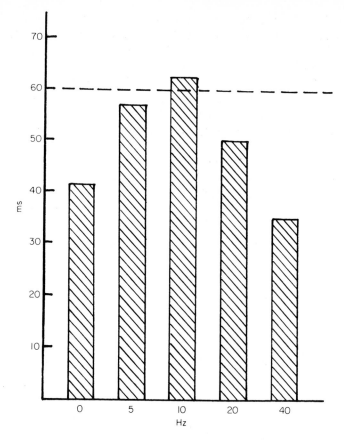

Fig. 8. The mean values of the time to peak (in ms) of tenotomized soleus muscles of spinal animals when subjected to different frequencies of stimulation. Interrupted line represents the mean time to peak of control soleus muscles from a separate group of animals.

Whether contractile properties of the fast muscles can also be influenced by activity was the next question. Since it is practically impossible to prevent reflex activity from reaching these muscles it was decided to superimpose a slow frequency activity onto the normal phasic activity of fast leg muscles. Electrodes were implanted so as to stimulate the motor nerves to tibialis anterior and extensor digitorum longus muscles of rabbits, and they were stimulated at 10 Hz. When the contractile characteristics of these stimulated muscles were examined two to four weeks after such stimulation it was found that these fast muscles had become slower contracting (Fig. 9). When stimulated for longer intervals such as two to three months their contractile speeds were similar to those of the fast soleus muscle. Thus even though the slow frequency activity was superimposed onto the normal activity of the muscle it had a dramatic, slowing effect (Salmons and Vrbová, 1969). From these results it is apparent that the nerve exerts its influence on the contractile properties by imposing a particular pattern of activity, and not by a special trophic influence.

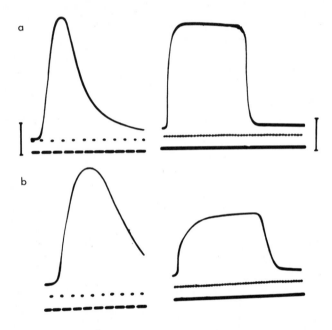

Fig. 9. Isometric contractions in response to a single stimulus and to repetitive stimulation (200 Hz) of a control (a) and 14 days stimulated; (b) tibialis anterior muscle of a rabbit. The intervals between successive dots represent 10 ms. The vertical bar on the left represents 50 and the bar on the right 500 g.

Not only the contractile speeds but the enzyme composition of fast muscles is also altered after long term electrical stimulation. The anaerobic muscles fibres of the tibialis anterior muscle and extensor digitorum longus muscles are transformed into predominantly aerobic ones, and this can be shown both by biochemical analysis of the muscles as well as by histochemical examinations (Pette *et al.*, 1973). The heterogeneous appearance of the muscles disappears, and all the muscle fibres become of a similar size and similar staining intensity for the oxidative enzyme succinate dehydrogenase (see Fig. 10). This is not so for myosin ATP-ase, for with regard to this enzyme the muscle fibres remain heterogeneous for a long time (Pette *et al.*, 1976). This may be due to the fact that the normal activity of the muscle is still present. If different activity patterns are applied to completely 'silent' muscles, like cat-tail muscles after they are deafferented and spinalized, the histochemical appearance of the muscles depended precisely on the

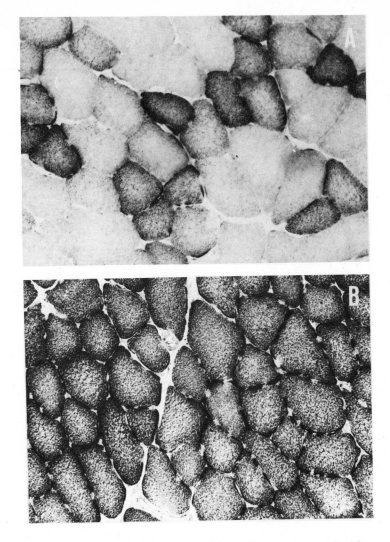

Fig. 10. Transverse sections of rabbit extensor digitorum longus muscles stained for succinic dehydrogenase. Control muscle (a), stimulated for 28 days (b). (x 190).

activity pattern. Slow, tonic type of activity made muscle fibres with high oxidative enzymes and low anaerobic enzymes, fast phasic activity produced muscle fibres with low oxidative and high anaerobic enzymes and high activity of myosin ATP-ase (Riley and Allin, 1973). Changes of the sarcoplasmic reticulum and its ability to bind Ca^{++} are also altered by the long-term electrical stimulation (Ramirez and Pette, 1974) as are the myosin light chains of fast muscles (Sreter *et al.*, 1973).

The mechanism by which the muscle fibre alters its biochemical composition and starts synthesizing a set of different proteins is poorly understood. Experiments where such changes are brought about by electrical stimulation seem to be a suitable model situation for studying this question. The time sequence of the development of particular changes may help to elucidate this problem, and an attempt was made to investigate the time sequence of the different changes induced by chronic electrical stimulation. The first apparent change in response to slow frequency activity is of course the well recognized functional hyperaemia. This is followed by a growth of capillaries. It was found that such increase in capillary density can be brought about only by electrical activity at slow frequencies, and not by stimulating the muscle at higher rates (Brown et al., 1976). The increase of capillary density is followed by an increase in the muscle oxidative enzyme capacity, and a decrease of enzymes concerned with anaerobic metabolism. Activities of membrane bound enzymes such as hexokinase and palmitoyl CoA synthetase that may be concerned with transport of 'substrates' in and out of the muscle fibres are already increased four days after electrical stimulation of fast muscles had started, and the increase of oxidative enzymes followed ten days later. Another change that can be detected is the change of ATP-ase activity of the sarcoplasmic reticulum (Ramirez, and Pette 1974). Finally, after a long time of continuous electrical stimulation the structure of the myosin light chains also changes. (Sreter et al., 1973). Fig. 11 illustrates the sequence of some of the changes within the muscle during its transformation from a fast type to a slow type. It seems as though the increased availability of oxygen produced by the denser capillary network may shorten the diffusion distance between the blood and working muscle cell, so that the muscle fibre will be working in an environment with a higher partial pressure of oxygen. It is possible that this induces the transformation from anaerobic to aerobic metabolism. How this is accomplished is unknown.

When muscles are stimulated continually for long periods of time, i.e., for 24 hours a day the variation of changes in contractile speeds is small and these muscles always become slower. Moreover, the myosin light chains are regularly transformed from the fast type to resemble those of the slow soleus muscle (Sreter et al., 1973). This complete transformation of a fast muscle activated for months, day and night by slow frequency activity is probably only possible because the animal entirely stops the normal usage of the stimulated muscles. That such a muscle is becoming very 'abnormal' is apparent from the loss of weight and decrease of its tetanic tension, which does not take place in muscles stimulated for only eight hours a day (Pette et al., 1976).

Since activity is considered to be the major regulatory influence in determining the functional and biochemical properties of skeletal muscle

m. tibialis anterior

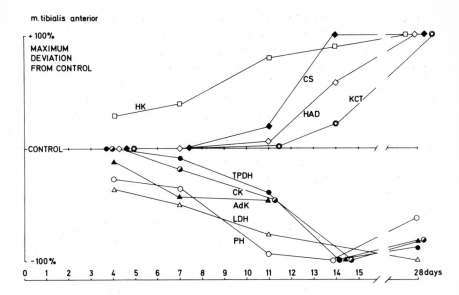

Fig. 11. Time course of development of changes in enzyme activity pattern of the tibidis anterior muscle stimulated for 8 hours a day for different periods of time. Values have been plotted for each enzyme as a percentage of maximum deviation. Abbreviations: AdK: Adenylate kinase; CK: Creatine kinase; CS: Citrate synthase; HAD: 3 Hydroxyacyl-CoA dehydrogenase; HK: Hexokinase; KCT: 3-Ketoacid-CoA transferase; LDH: Lactate dehydrogenase; PH: Glycogen phosphorylase; TPDH: Triosephosphate dehydrogenase.

fibres it is not surprising that the effects of the muscle's 'own' activity can be completely over-ridden only by the most strenuous regime. Thus the contractile and biochemical properties of skeletal muscles are determined by the activity pattern imposed upon the muscle by its motor nerve.

Conclusions

The mechanism by which the motor nerve exerts its influence on some properties of skeletal muscle were discussed.

(1) Evidence was presented to show that in normal innervated muscle the areas outside the endplate region are kept insensitive to ACh by the activity of the muscle imposed upon it by the motor nerve. Apart from activating the muscle, the motor nerve seems to have no other special role in the control of chemosensitivity of the extrajunctional area.

(2) The contractile and biochemical characteristics of skeletal muscle are determined by the particular pattern of activity that is imposed upon the muscle by its motor nerve. Each motor nerve fibre can in this way induce in the muscle fibres it supplies the development of those properties that will match the functional activity of its motoneurone.

References

Amphlett, G.W., Brown, M.D., Perry, S.V., Siska, H., and Vrbová, G. (1976). *Nature*, **257**, 602-604.

Bárány, M. (1967). *J. gen. Physiol.* **50**, (Suppl. part 2) 197-218.

Berg, D.K., and Hall, Z.W. (1975). *J. Physiol.* **244**, 659-676.

Brown, M.D. (1975). *Recent advances in myology. Proc. III Int. Cong. Muscle Disease.* pp.16-21, Ed. W.G. Bradley, D. Gardner-Medwin and J.N. Walton.

Brown, M.D., Cotter, M.A., Hudlická, O. and Vrbová, G. (1976). *Pflügers Arch.* **361**, 241-250.

Buller, A.J., Eccles, J.C., and Eccles, R.M. (1960). *J. Physiol.* **150**, 417-439.

Buller, A.J., Mommaerts, W.F.H.M., Seraydarian, K. (1969). *J. Physiol.* **205**, 581-597.

Cooper, S., and Eccles, J.C. (1930). *J. Physiol.* **69**, 377-385.

Denny-Brown, D. (1929). *Proc. Roy. Soc. B* **104**, 252-301.

Diamond, J., and Miledi, R. (1962). *J. Physiol.* **162**, 393-408.

Drachman, D.B., and Witzke, F. (1972). *Science* **176**, 514-516.

Eccles, J.C., Eccles, R.M., and Lundberg. A. (1957). *J. Physiol.* **137**, 22-50.

Ginetzinsky, A.G. (1956). *Acad. Sci. Georgian SSR.* pp.409-417. In honour of J. Beritash (In Russian).

Ginetzinsky, A.G., and Shamarina, N.M. (1942). *Usp. Sovr. Biol.* **15**, 283-294.

Gordon, T. and Vrobá, G. (1975). *Pflügers Arch.* **360**, 349-364.

Gutmann, E. (1962). *The denervated muscle.* (E. Gutmann, ed.) pp.13-56, Czechoslovak Academy of Science, Prague.

Gutmann, E., Vodička, Z., and Zelená, (1955). *Physiol. Bohemoslov.* **4**, 200-203.

Harris, J.B., and Thesleff, S. (1972). *Nature, New Biol.* **236**, 60-61.

Jones, R. and Vrbová, G. (1972). *J. Physiol.* **217**, 67-68 P.

Jones, R., and Vrbová, G. (1974). *J. Physiol.* **236**, 517-538.

Jones, R. and Vyskočil, L. (1975). *Brain Res.* **88**, 309-317.

Katz, B., and Miledi, R. (1964). *J. Physiol.* **170**, 389-396.

Lomo, T. and Rosenthal, J. (1972). *J. Physiol.* **2211**, 493-513.

Luco, J.V., and Eyzaguire, C. (1955). *J. Neurophysiol.* **18**, 65-73.

Miledi, R. (1960a). *J. Physiol.* **154**, 190-205.

Miledi, R. (1960b). *J. Physiol.* **151**, 1-23.

Miledi, R. and Slater, C.R. (1969). *J. Physiol.* **207**, 507-528.

Pestronk, A., Drachman, D.B. and Griffin, J. (1976). *Nature,* **260**, 352-358.

Pette, D., Smith, M.E., Staudte, H.W. and Vrbová, G. (1973). *Pflügers Arch.* **338**, 257-272.

Pette, D., Muller, W., Leisner, E. and Vrbová, G. (1976). *Pflügers Arch.* **364**, 103-112.

Ramirez, B.V., and Pette, D. (1974). *FEBS Lett.* **46**, 188-190.

Ranvier, L. (1874). *Arch. Physiol. norm. pathol.* **6**, 1-15.

Riley, D.A., and Allin, E.F. (1973). *Exp. Neurol.* **40**, 391-413.

Romanul, F.C.A., and Van Der Meullen J.P. (1967). *Arch.Neurol. (Chic.),* **13**, 263.

Salmons, S. and Vrbová, G. (1969). *J. Physiol.* **201**, 535-549.

Sperry, R.W. (1945). *Quart. Rev. Biol.* **20**, 311-370.

Sreter, F.A., Gergely, J., Salmons, S., and Romanul, F. (1973). *Nature, New. Biol.* **341**, 17-19.

Thesleff, S. (1960). *J. Physiol.* **151**, 598-607.

Thomson, J.D. (1952). *Am. J. Physiol.* **171**, 773.

Tower, S. (1973). *J. Comp. Neurol.* **67**, 241-269.

Vrbová, G. (1963a). *J. Physiol.* **166,** 241-250.
Vrbová, G. (1936b). *J. Physiol.* **169,** 513-526.
Vrbová, G. (1966). *J. Physiol.* **185,** 17-18 P.
Vrbová, G. (1967). *J. Physiol.* **191,** 20-21 P.
Weeds, A.G., Trentham, D.R., Kean, C.H.C., and Buller, A.J. (1974). *Nature,* **247,** 135-139.

2 The phosphorylation of the acetylcholine receptor:

VIVIAN ITZHAK TEICHBERG AND JEAN-PIERRE CHANGEUX.

Neurobiologie Moléculaire, Institut Pasteur, Paris, France.

Introduction

In the early phases of embryonic muscle development, the acetylcholine receptor (AChR) is distributed over the entire surface of the myotube (Fambrough and Rash, 1971). At this stage, its half-life in the membrane is around 20 hours (Devreotes and Fambrough, 1976; Merlie *et al.* 1976). Later, as a result of the early formation of nerve muscle contracts and the onset of muscle activity, AChR disappears from the extrasynaptic areas and becomes localized in the postsynaptic membrane under the nerve terminals (Hartzell and Fambrough, 1972). In the mature innervated muscle fibre, AChR is present only in the subsynaptic membrane in a stable form with a mean half-life of at least a week (Chang and Huang, 1975; Berg and Hall 1975). Thus two processes involving the AChR take place during synaptogenesis:

(1) A 'localization' that results in an increased concentration of AChR under the nerve terminals.

(2) A 'stabilization' that prolongs the life time of AChR in the membrane.

This situation is partially reversed upon denervation of the muscle fiber and AChR is rapidly synthesized and incorporated into the extrasynaptic membrane where its life time is similar to that of AChR in noninnervated embryonic muscle. However, AChR in the subsynaptic membrane is not affected throughout the process of denervation (Chang and Huang, 1975).

Recently, a biochemical model of selective stabilization of synapses has been presented (Changeux and Danchin, 1976) which accounts for these general phenomena. Among other postulates, it is proposed that the local accumulation and stabilization of the receptor protein under the nerve terminal during development may result, for instance, from a covalent modification which would immobilize the protein and make it resistant to degradation. The work that is presented here is an attempt to verify the above proposition.

Differences between extrasynaptic and subsynaptic AChR.

Our experimental approach has been first to study the biochemical nature of the differences between extrasynaptic and subsynaptic AChR. Physiological (Miledi, 1960; Beranek and Vyskosil, 1967), pharmacological (Chiu *et al.*, 1974) and biochemical (Brockes and Hall, 1975) differences have been reported between these two classes of receptor but these results have been questioned (Alper *et al.*, 1974; Colquhoun and Rang, 1976). In any event, these studies do not answer the question of whether separate genes code for the extra and subsynaptic receptors or alternatively whether the different classes of AChR could result from a covalent modification of a single protein species (as commonly found with regulatory or membrane bound proteins (Fischer *et al.*, 1970; Greengard, 1976). To approach this problem, we have used the electric organ of *Electrophorus electricus* for which autoradiographic data (Bourgeois *et al.*, 1973) indicate that AChR is present in both subsynaptic and extrasynaptic areas in almost equal amounts.

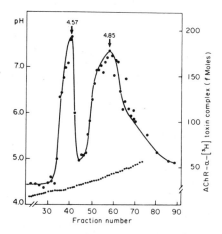

Fig. 1. Isoelectric focusing profile of a crude detergent extract from *Electrophorus electricus* electric organ.

The isoelectric focusing was carried out at 4°C for 12 h in a 80 ml electrofocusing glass column along a 52 ml sucrose gradient (44-16 %) containing 1 % pH 4-6 Ampholyte, 0.1 % Triton, 0.4 M urea in 10^{-4} M phenylmethylsulfonylfluoride, 0.014 M 2-mercaptoethanol, 0.02 % NaN$_3$.

The preparation of the crude detergent extract has been described: 118 pmole of [^{3}H]-toxin binding sites were applied to the column. 340 μl fractions were collected. The pH value of each fraction was determined at 4°C. Each fraction was then neutralized with 50 μl of 2 M Tris buffer pH 7.0.

AChR was assayed by incubation with [^{3}H] toxin and filtration throuch Millipore filters according to Meunier *et al.* (1974). The specific activity of the [^{3}H] toxin batch used was 30 Ci/mmol and 61% of the α-toxin molecules were pharmacologically active. The yield in toxin sites recovered was 56%.

From Teichberg and Changeux (1976).

In a study of the properties of AChR solubilized from extrasynaptic and subsynaptic areas of rat diaphragm, (Brockes and Hall, 1975) have reported differences in the behaviour of these receptors by isoelectric focusing. We have applied the same technique to crude detergent extracts of electric organ. Two forms of AChR were found (Fig. 1), with isoelectric points similar to those reported for the two receptor species from rat diaphragm and in proportions close to those found by autoradiography for extra and subsynaptic AChR (Teichberg and Changeux, 1976). In addition it could be shown that the two peaks (Fig. 1) represent distinct and stable forms of AChR.

In this experiment the fractions composing each toxin binding peak were pooled, dialysed against 0.1 % Triton X-100, concentrated on DEAE cellulose (Meunier *et al.*, 1974) and resubmitted to isoelectric focusing. Fig. 2 shows that each toxin binding peak refocuses as a single species. At this stage several plausible covalent modifications of the AChR were envisaged and tested separately. Among the covalent reactions that could

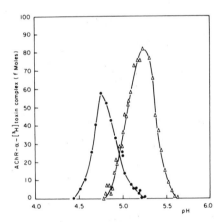

Fig. 2. Isoelectric focusing profiles of AChR forms. Acidic form of AChR (●–●) 13 pmoles of [³H] toxin binding sites. Alkaline form of AChR (Δ–Δ) 30 pmoles of [³H] toxin binding sites analysed under conditions as described Fig. 1. From Teichberg and Changeux (1976).

modify the isoelectric point of the molecule are those of phosphorylation, carbamylation, adenylation, glycosylation etc. (Segal, 1973). Because of the crucial role of phosphorylation reactions in the regulation of muscle metabolism (Cohen, 1976), a hypothetical phosphorylation of AChR was first considered. Assuming that the acidic form of AChR was phosphorylated, we looked for a method to dephosphorylate it. In this search, data on the dephosphorylation of phosphoglucomutase by the non-enzymatic action of NaF came to our attention (Layne and Najjar, 1973; Constantopoulos and Najjar, 1973).

We therefore incubated an aliquot of the crude detergent extract of electric organ for 30 minutes at 37°C in the presence of 0.1 M NaF. The extract was then dialysed for 24 h against 0.1 % Triton X-100 and submitted to isoelectric focusing: Fig. 3 shows the resulting profile of toxin binding activity. Unexpectedly, a peak of AChR with an isoelectric point of pH 4.58 was obtained with a broad shoulder extending to more basic pH. However, when the same experiment was carried out in the presence of 0.1 M NaCl instead of NaF, then, an entirely different profile was obtained (Fig. 4). Clearly, after treatment at 37°C only one of the two forms of the AChR remained: the acidic one with NaF, the more alkaline one with NaCl. Treatment at 37°C for 30 min without any salt did not modify the profile shown in Fig. 1.

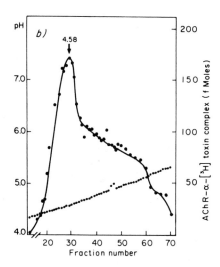

Fig. 3. Isoelectric focusing profile of crude detergent extract after 0.1 M NaF treatment at 37°C for 30 min and dialysis at 4°C against large volumes of PNM containing 0.1 % Triton X-100. 168 pmoles of [³H] toxin binding sites were applied. The yield in toxin binding sites after incubation at 37°C and dialysis was 76 % and the recovery in AChR after isoelectric focusing 54 %. From Teichberg and Changeux (1976).

Since a significant inactivation of AChR took place during the heat treatment and electrofocusing, two alternative interpretations could account for the observed results. Either, one of the two forms is selectively inactivated or an interconversion between the two forms takes place. However, it could be shown that the electrofocusing in itself did not cause a selective inactivation of one of the two forms, but it may still have taken place during the heat treatment. The following experiment ruled out the latter possibility. The crude detergent extract was first incubated in the presence of 0.1 M NaF under conditions which favour the acidic form. Then the extract was dialysed and heated again at 37°C but in the presence of 0.1 M NaCl. The profile obtained after this second treatment was, again, identical to that shown in Fig. 4. The alkaline peak which disappeared after the first treatment in NaF, reappeared after the second exposure to NaCl.

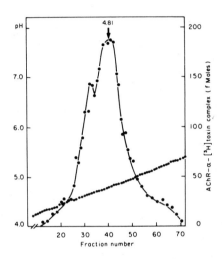

Fig. 4. Isoelectric focusing profile of crude detergent extract after 0.1 M NaCl treatment at 37°C for 30 min and dialysis at 4°C against large volumes of PNM containing 0.1 % Triton X-100. 198 pmoles of [³H] toxin binding sites were applied. The yield in toxin binding sites after incubation at 37°C and dialysis was 76 % and the recovery in AChR after the iso-electric focusing 49 %. From Teichberg and Changeux (1976).

These results are taken as a strong indication that the treatment of a crude extract of AChR at 37°C in the presence of NaCl or NaF leads to an interconversion between acidic and alkaline forms rather than to a selective inactivation of any one of these forms. It should be noticed however that in treating the crude membrane extract with NaF, the conversion of the alkaline peak into the acidic one was not always complete and a peak was often observed around pH 4.85. This was not the case after treatment of the crude membrane extract with NaCl which resulted always in a complete conversion into the AChR alkaline form. At this stage, the most likely interpretation of the data was that a catalytic interconversion of the two AChR species had taken place via reactions of phosphorylation-dephosphorylation catalysed by protein kinases and phosphoprotein phosphatases assumed to be present in the crude extract.

The inhibition of phosphoprotein phosphatases by NaF (Revel, 1963) rather than its non-enzymatic dephosphorylating action (Layne and Najjar, 1973; Constantopoulos and Najjar, 1973) would explain the differential effect of NaCl and NaF. In the presence of NaF and provided that the cofactors needed by the protein kinase are present in the crude membrane extract, AChR would be phosphorylated and therefore should focus at a more acid pH whereas in the presence of NaCl the phosphorylated AChR should be dephosphorylated by the phosphoprotein phosphatase and focus at a more basic pH. The reproductibility of the conversion of the acidic AChR into the alkaline species in contrast to the incomplete conversion observed in the presence of NaF could be explained by the stringent requirement of the protein kinase for cofactors that may not be present or active in each of our preparations.

The fact that a phosphorylation may indeed affect the isoelectric point of a protein has been demonstrated in the case of pig heart succinate thiokinase (Baccanari *et al.*, 1975). Phosphorylation of this enzyme (1 mole of phosphate per mole of enzyme of 77,000 M.wt) modifies its isoelectric point from pH 6.4 to pH 6.2. Interestingly, the non-phosphorylated form of succinate thiokinase is unstable (half-life of 140 minutes) whereas the phosphorylated form is stable.

Presence of protein kinases and phosphoprotein phosphatases in E. electricus electric organ.

Although this interpretation of the phosphorylation-dephosphorylation of AChR is attractive, it had to be substantiated by evidence for the existence of a phosphorylating system in the crude detergent extract of membrane fragments (Teichberg and Changeux, 1977). For this purpose, we submitted membrane fragments of electric organ to ultracentrifugation in sucrose gradients and analysed the various fractions obtained for the presence of AChR, protein kinase, phosphoprotein phosphatase as well as acetylcholinesterase and Na^+-K^+ ATPase.

The activity of the protein kinase was measured in the presence of NaF whereas the phosphoprotein phosphatase was determined by its opposing action to protein kinase in the absence of NaF. Fig. 5 shows the presence of a protein kinase in a membrane subpopulation migrating at a sucrose density higher than that of the AChR containing membranes labelled by *N. nigricollis* [^{3}H]-α-toxin. The phosphoprotein phosphatase as well as the Na^+-K^+ ouabain sensitive ATPase (data not shown) seem however to migrate at the same density as that of AChR. A very high activity of protein kinase is also present in membranes of a lower density (fractions 13-15) which are devoid of phosphoprotein phosphatase as well as of AChR whereas acetylcholinesterase migrates with membrane fragments of intermediate density.

From these data it appears that endogenous protein kinase and phosphoprotein phosphatase activities are indeed present in membrane

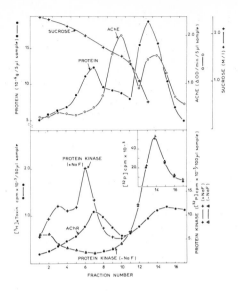

Fig. 5. Distribution of acetylcholine receptor AChR, acetylcholinesterase AChE, protein kinase (+ NaF), phosphoprotein phosphatase (Protein kinase-NaF) and total protein in a sucrose gradient after ultracentrifugation of a crude membrane preparation of *Electrophorus electricus* electric organ with [³H]-labelled α-toxin. The specific of fraction n°.7 was 80 nM of toxin binding sites per gram protein. The profile of migration of the Na⁺-K⁺ ouabain sensitive ATPase is identical under these conditions to that of AChR. From Teichberg and Changeux (1977).

fragments, but it is not yet clear whether these enzymes come originally from the excitable AChR-rich membrane and are redistributed during the preparation and isolation procedures. By analogy with acetylcholinesterase, which is known to be attached to the subsynaptic excitable membrane, it is possible that the phosphorylating system is bound to the excitable membrane without being an integral part of it. From our centrifugation studies, it seems however that the dephosphorylating system is more tightly bound to the AChR than is the phosphorylating system.

Since the interconversion between the two forms of AChR had been obtained in a detergent extract of membrane fragments, we also analysed this extract for the presence of protein kinase and phosphoprotein phosphatase. Table 1 shows the conditions needed for the incorporation of [³²P] phosphate groups into endogenous proteins from a crude Triton X-100 extract of membrane fragments. It can be also shown that the Km of the protein kinase activity for ATP is 4 μM. As seen in Table 1, NaF strongly stimulates the incorporation of [³²P] whereas adenosine 3′, 5′-monophosphate (cyclic AMP) has no effect. Such absence of stimulation by cyclic AMP seems to be a characteristic of muscle membrane kinases (Andrew *et al.*, 1975; Gordon *et al.*, 1977).

TABLE 1

Level of incorporation of [^{32}P] phosphate groups into endogenous proteins from a crude Triton X-100 extract of membrane fragments of *E. electricus*.

	Percentage of incorporation found in complete system
$-MnCl_2$	10
$-MnCl_2 + 10$ mM $MgCl_2$	82
$-NaF + 100$ mM NaCl	25
$+ 10^{-6}$ M cyclic AMP	98
$+ 10^{-6}$ M cyclic GMP	99
$+ 15$ mM ATP	1

The complete system contained:
100 mM Tris, pH 7.3, 10^{-3} M ouabain
 10 mM $MnCl_2$, 100 NaF
  4 μM γ-[^{32}P] ATP and
the incubation was carried out in a total volume of 100 μl at 22°C for 30 min. In a typical experiment, the total radioactivity from γ-[^{32}P] ATP was 6×10^5 cpm. The total radioactivity incorporated was 4.4×10^4 cpm, i.e., 7.3%. The blank (complete system + 15 mM ATP added at the beginning of the incubation) was 400 cpm.

Figure 6 illustrates the stimulation by increasing concentrations of NaF of the incorporation of [^{32}P]-phosphate groups into endogenous proteins from a crude Triton X-100 extract of membrane fragments. The concentration-effect curve has a slight sigmoid shape and half maximal stimulation occurs in the presence of 25 mM NaF, the maximal stimulation being

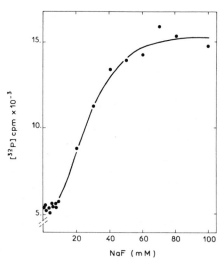

Fig. 6. Stimulation by NaF of the incorporation of [^{32}P]-phosphate in endogenous proteins of crude detergent extract. Assay System 38 mM Tris pH 7.3, 3.9×10^{-4} M ouabain, 7.8 mM $MnCl_2$. 1.31 M γ-[^{32}P] ATP (14.2 Ci/mM). The incubation mixture at each NaF concentration contains in 100 μl, 2.46×10^6 cpm of γ-[^{32}P] ATP. From Teichberg and Changeux (1977).

reached at 70 mM NaF. Clearly, a protein kinase is also present in the detergent extract of membrane fragments. The effect of NaF may result either from a direct effect of the protein kinase or from an inhibition of a phosphoprotein phosphatase (Revel, 1963).

To investigate this problem, the kinetics of [^{32}P]-incorporation into endogenous proteins from crude detergent extract were followed at 22°C in the presence of either 100 mM NaF or 100 mM NaCl (Fig. 7). In the presence of NaF, the incorporation of [^{32}P] is linear as a function of time for 3 min and reaches a plateau after 50 min. In the presence of NaCl however, a composite effect is observed. For this first 3 min, the incorporation is linear but then the level of incorporation slowly decreases and reaches a plateau corresponding to an incorporation of approximately 25 % of that

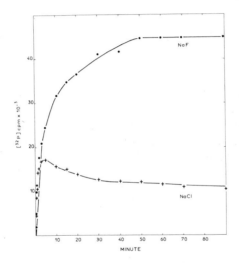

Fig. 7. Kinetics of incorporation of γ-[^{32}P] phosphate groups into endogenous proteins of crude detergent extract. In the presence of 100 mM NaF ●–●. In the presence of 100 mM NaCl (+–+). Assay System, 67 mM Tris, pH 7.3, 6.7 × 10^{-4} M ouabain, 10 mM MnCl$_2$, 10 μM γ-[^{32}P] ATP (13.7 Ci/mM). From Teichberg and Changeux (1977).

found in the presence of NaF. The most simple interpretation of this result is that a phosphoprotein phosphatase activity competes with that of the protein kinase. To document further the effect of salts on this phosphorylating system, we studied the protein kinase activity of membrane fragments in the presence or absence of NaCl or KCl. A possible role for K+ attracted our attention as Gordon *et al.* (1977) has reported a differential effect of Na+ and K+ on the level of phosphorylation of proteins in *Torpedo* membrane fragments. Figure 8 shows the level of phosphorylation of *Electrophorus* membrane proteins by the endogenous protein kinase as a function of increasing concentrations of NaCl and KCl. Figure 9 shows

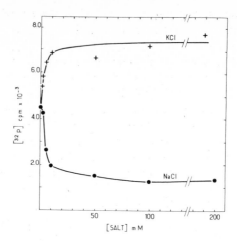

Fig. 8. Incorporation in the presence of NaCl and KCl of [^{32}P] phosphate groups from γ-[^{32}P] ATP into endogenous proteins of purified membrane fragments of *Electrophorus electricus* electric organ. Assay System, 10 mM Tris.HCl, pH 7.4, 1 mM MnCl$_2$, 0.75 μM ATP (3 C/mM) in the absence of ouabain, volume: 100 μl. Incubation time 1′ at 22°C. Reaction stopped by addition of 10 ml of 5 % perchloric acid and filtration over glass fiber disk.

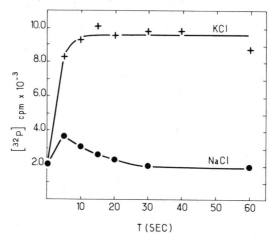

Fig. 9. Kinetics of incorporation of [^{32}P] phosphate groups from γ-[^{32}P] ATP into endogenous proteins of purified membrane fragments of *Electrophorus electricus* electric organ. The conditions were those described in Fig. 8. KCl and NaCl were at a concentration of 50 mM.

the kinetics of phosphorylation in the presence of NaCl and KCl. The biphasic curve observed clearly expresses the competition between protein phosphorylation and protein dephosphorylation which seems to be inhibited by K+. This selective inhibition of protein dephosphorylation by K+ (or its selective activation by Na+) leads to an overall increase in the net level of phosphorylation.

Because of the presence in the membrane fragments of a Na+-K+ ATPase, we repeated the experiments on the effect of Na+ and K+, this time in the presence of 1 mM ouabain. A more complex situation was observed although basically the results were similar to those observed in the absence of ouabain i.e. an inhibitory effect of K+ on the dephosphory- lation reaction. In any event, the level of phosphorylation of the membrane fragments appeared to be regulated by the same ions which are responsible *in vivo* for the ionic gradient across the excitable membrane.

Phosphorylation of the acetylcholine receptor protein

In order to strengthen our original assumption that the interconversion *in vitro* of the two AChR species was the result of phosphorylation- dephosphorylation reactions, it was essential at that stage to determine whether AChR could indeed serve as a substrate for the endogenous protein kinase. For this purpose, the polypeptides labelled in an incubation mixture of crude detergent extract with γ-[^{32}P]ATP were analysed by polyacrylamide gel electrophoresis in SDS. Figure 10 shows a typical

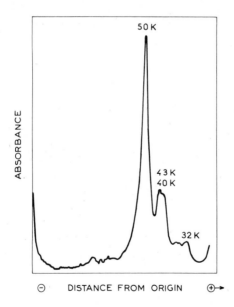

Fig. 10. Polyacrylamide gel electrophoresis in dodecyl sulfate of the products of phosphory- lation of crude detergent extract by an endogenous protein kinase. The incubation conditions were those described in Fig. 6 and the time of incubation was 30 min. From Teichberg and Changeux (1977).

autoradiograph obtained for a fraction of crude detergent extract labelled with $\gamma[^{32}P]$ATP. Four polypeptides of mol.wt 50.000, 43.000, 40.000 and 32.000 are the main substrates for the endogenous protein kinase. When such a fraction, after labelling with $\gamma[^{32}P]$ATP is passed through a column of erabutoxin B coupled to Sepharose 4B, eluted with 1 % SDS and further analysed by SDS-polyacrylamide gel electrophoresis and auto-radiography, an identical profile of radioactive polypeptides is also obtained. Although the purified AChR from *Electrophorus* is thought to be composed of polypeptides of mol.wt 48.000 ± 3.000 and 43.000 ± 3.000, with the appearance upon ageing of a polypeptide of mol.wt 35.000 (Meunier *et al.*, 1974) it was not possible to draw from this analogy any definite conclusion as to the AChR serving as a substrate for protein kinase.

To demonstrate the phosphorylation of AChR itself (Teichberg *et al.*, 1977), we decided to use crossed-immunoelectrophoresis to identify and separate the AChR from the bulk of the proteins and lipids present in the detergent extract. For this purpose, rabbit sera (anti-AChR) were raised against Triton X-100 extracted AChR purified from *E. electricus* membrane fragments by affinity chromatography. The anti-AChR antiserum was first assayed against an aliquot of detergent extract preincubated with $[^{125}I]\alpha$-bungarotoxin. Only one precipitation line was observed both by Coomassie blue staining and by autoradiography (Fig. 11 a & b). A fraction of crude detergent extract labelled with $\gamma[^{32}P]$ATP, and separated by gel filtration was then submitted to crossed-immunoelectrophoresis in a gel containing anti-AChR antibodies. Again only one precipitation line was seen both by

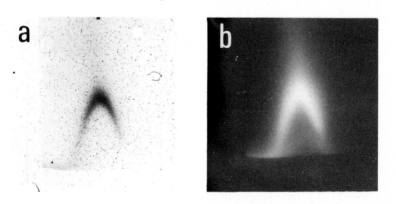

Fig. 11. Crossed immunoelectrophoresis of ^{125}I-α-bungarotoxin-AChR complex. (a) Coomassie blue staining of the precipitation line(s) between (a) anti-AChR antibodies and ^{125}I-α-bungarotoxin-AChR complex, (20 μl of detergent extract containing 1.8 pmoles AChR and 1.5 pmoles of ^{125}I-α-bungarotoxin (238 Ci/mM), were applied. Anti-AChR antiserum was at a density of 5 μl of serum/cm^2), and (b) autoradiograph of (a) after 24 hour exposure. From Teichberg, Sobel and Changeux (1977).

Coomassie blue staining and by autoradiography (Fig. 12 a & b). However a non-specific absorption of phosphorylated proteins on the AChR anti-AChR precipitate could have been the cause of the line seen by autoradiography (Fig. 12b). To test this possibility, a mixture of 'phosphorylated detergent extract' and bovine serum albumin was submitted to crossed-immunoelectrophoresis in a gel containing both anti-AChR and anti-bovine serum albumin antibodies. This time, two precipitation lines were stained by Coomassie blue: one corresponded to the AChR, the other to bovine serum albumin. However, only the line characteristic of the AChR was detected by autoradiography (Fig. 12 c & d) indicating without ambiguity that the AChR had been phosphorylated.

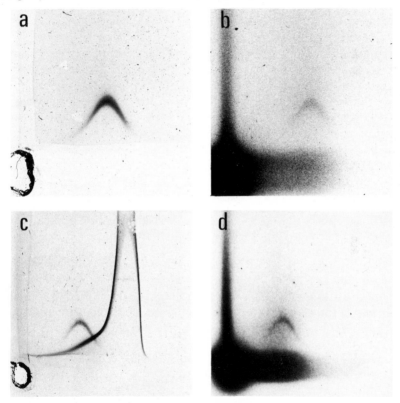

Fig. 12. Crossed-immunoelectrophoresis of (a) Anti-AChR antibodies and phosphorylated detergent extract. 1.1 pmoles of AChR in 18 μl were applied. Anti-AChR antiserum was at a density of 4.5 μl of serum/cm². (b) Autoradiograph of (a) after 24 hour exposure. (c) Anti-bovine serum albumin antibodies and bovine serum albumin (large peak) and Anti-AChR antibodies and phosphorylated extract. 1.3 pmoles of AChR and 15 pmoles bovine serum albumin were applied to 20 μl. Anti-AChR and anti-bovine serum albumin antisera were at a density respectively 3.3 μl and 0.55 μl of serum per cm². (d) Autoradiograph of (c) after 48 hour exposure. From Teichberg, Sobel and Changeux (1977).

To determine which polypeptide chains of the purified AChR had been phosphorylated, AChR anti-AChR precipitates obtained by crossed immunoelectrophoresis were cut out of agar coated plates, solubilized in 2 % SDS, 3 % mercaptoethanol, 0,062 M Tris at pH 6.8, and analysed by SDS polyacrylamide gel electrophoresis and autoradiography. Only one polypeptide of apparent molecular weight 48,000 could be clearly detected on the densitogram obtained after scanning of the autoradiograph (Fig. 13).

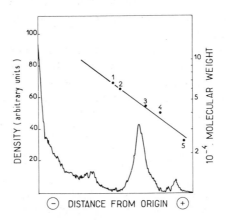

Fig. 13. Densitogram obtained from the autoradiograph of precipitates between anti-AChR antibodies and phosphorylated detergent extract after SDS polyacrylamide gel electrophoresis. The optical density was expressed in arbitrary units. The following proteins were used as markers for molecular weight determination: 1, Bovine serum albumin; 2, Catalase; 3, Albumin; 4, Aldolase; 5, Chymotrypsin. The band at 48.000 could not be detected by Coomassie blue staining. From Teichberg, Sobel and Changeux (1977).

As stated above, the AChR protein purified from *E. electricus* gives two (Meunier, *et al.*, 1974) or three (Karlin and Cowburn, 1973; Sobel— unpublished results) bands by polyacrylamide gel electrophoresis in SDS. Only one of them, corresponding to a polypeptide chain of apparent molecular weight 43,000 ± 3,000 is labelled by the two covalent affinity labels of the acetylcholine receptor site, [³H] maleimidobenzyl trimethylammonium (Karlin and Cowburn, 1973) or [³H] maleimidophenyl trimethylammonium (Sobel—unpublished results). Interestingly, it is not this chain which is phosphorylated *in vitro* but that of apparent molecular weight 48,000 ± 3,000.

Functional significance of the phosphorylation of the acetylcholine receptor protein: hypothesis

As the phosphorylation *in vitro* of AChR takes place under conditions close to those needed for the interconversion between the two forms of

AChR, one may relate these reactions to at least two different regulatory mechanisms.

(a) The 48,000 dalton polypeptide is the ionophore modulated by the AChR and its transport properties are regulated by phosphorylation-dephosphorylation reactions as proposed by Greengard (1976). It should be mentioned here that the phosphorylation-dephosphorylation of a 49,000 protein seems to take place in several systems: in brain synaptic membrane, (Ueda *et al.*, 1973), in mammalian smooth muscle (Casnellie and Greengard, 1974) and in toad bladder epithelium (Walton *et al.*, 1975) where it appears to be linked to Na^+ transport.

With *E. electricus* electric organ there is however no physiological evidence of any 'slow' change in permeability which might possibly be correlated with the activation of a protein kinase as has been suggested in the case of the superior cervical sympathetic ganglion (Greengard, 1976).

Moreover, the 'densensitization' reaction which takes place within seconds or minutes can be obtained *in vitro* in the absence of any source of energy (Weber *et al.*, 1975).

(b) In relation to the theory on selective stabilization of developing synapses (Changeux and Danchin, 1976), the phosphorylation of the AChR could be an element of the complex 'stablization reaction' postulated to cause the interconversion of the labile and mobile form of the AChR present in extra synaptic areas into its stable and immobile form in the mature subsynaptic membrane. If this reaction was indeed taking place in *E. electricus* electric organ despite the fact that it is not an embryonic system, then the phosphorylated 48,000 chain would not necessarily represent the ionophore but could for instance be involved in the aggregation of the receptor oligomer and (or) its protection against proteolysis.

Although phosphorylation reactions play a role both in stabilization (succinate thiokinase) and aggregation (phosphorylase system (Fosset *et al.*, 1971); tubulin (Shigekawa and Olsen, 1976)), of protein molecules, such a reaction may not be a sufficient but only a necessary step in the cascade of reactions that lead to the final stabilization of AChR in the mature synapse.

Mechanisms of subsynaptic phosphorylation

Whatever may be the exact physiological significance of the phosphorylation of AChR, one should keep in mind the fact that the two alternative interpretations proposed above are based on the assumption that only the subsynaptic AChR is phosphorylated. What are then the factors which may regulate this subsynaptic phosphorylation?

(a) The neurotransmitter released by the presynaptic nerve endings may regulate the phosphorylation of the receptor protein. For instance, in the postsynaptic membrane, it might act as an allosteric activator of a protein kinase or as an inhibitor of a phosphoprotein phosphatase, in either case at a site distinct from the acetylcholine binding site. Such a mechanism could account for the fact that the localization of AChR during development still takes place even in the presence of snake toxin bound irreversibly to the acetylcholine receptor site (Steinbach *et al.*, 1973).

(b) The receptor protein in its resting state might be a substrate for the protein kinase but may become phosphorylated only in the active or desensitized conformation stabilized by the neurotransmitter.

(c) An 'indirect' effect of the neurotransmitter might also be considered.

For instance, the local variations in ionic concentrations consequent to the permeability change triggered by acetylcholine might regulate the phosphorylation-dephosphorylation reactions. The effects of Na^+ and K^+ observed on these reactions could corroborate this interpretation.

(d) Our present knowledge of the synaptic components allows us to consider an other element, ATP, that could play a role, besides the neurotransmitter, in the phosphorylation of the subsynaptic AChR. The presynaptic ATP (Whittaker, 1974) released together with the neurotransmitter could be the preferential source of substrate for the protein kinase and as a consequence serve to phosphorylate the AChR.

Acknowledgements

This work was done during the tenure of a research fellowship of Muscular Dystrophy Associations of America to V.I.T. and was supported by funds from the Centre National de la Recherche Scientifique, the Délégation Générale à la Recherche scientifique et technique, the Collège de France and the Commissariat à l'Energie Atomique.

References

Alper, R., Lowy, J. and Schmidt, J. (1974). *FEBS Lett.* **48**, 130-134.

Andrew, C.G., Almon, R.R. and Appel, S.H. (1975). *J. Biol. Chem.* **250**, 3972-3980.

Baccanari, D.P., Kelly, C.J. and Sungman Cha (1975). In Isozymes, Molecular Structure I., ed. Clement L., Market A.P. p.807-822.

Beranek, R. and Vyskosil, F. (1967). *J. Physiol.* **188**, 53-66.

Berg, D. and Hall, Z.W. (1975). *J. Physiol.* **252**, 771-789.

Bourgeois, J.P., Popot, J.L., Ryter, A. and Changeux, J.P. (1973). *Brain Res.* **62**, 557-563.

Brockes, J.P. and Hall, Z.W. (1975). *Biochemistry* **14**, 2092-2099 and **14**, 2100-2106.

Casnellie, J.E. and Greengard, P. (1974). *Proc. Nat. Acad. Sci. USA* **71**, 1891-1895.

Chang, C.C. and Huang, M.C. (1975). *Nature* **253**, 643-644.

Changeux, J.P. and Danchin, A. (1976). *Nature* **264**, 705-712.

Chiu, T.H., Lapa, A.J., Barnard, E.A. and Albuquerque, E.X. (1974). *Exp. Neurol.* **43**, 399.

Cohen, P. (1976). *Trends Biochem. Sci.* **1**, 38-42.

Colquhoun, D. and Rang, H.P. (1976). *Molec. Pharmacol.* **12,** 519-535.
Constantopoulos, A. and Najjar, V.A. (1973). *Biochem. Biophys. Res. Comm.* **53,** 794-800.
Devreotes, P.N. and Fambrough, D.M. (1976). Cold Spring Harbour Symposia on Quantitative Biology, vol. XL, 237-251.
Fambrough, D.M. and Rash, J.E. (1971). *Devel. Biol.* **26,** 55.
Fischer, E.H., Heilmeyer, L.M.G. Jr. and Haschke, R.H. (1970). In 'Current Topics in Cellular Regulation', vol. 4.
Fosset, M., Muir, L.W., Nielsen, L.D. and Fischer, E.H. (1971). *Biochemistry* **10,** 4105-4113.
Gordon, A.S., Davis, C.G. and Diamond, I. (1977). *Proc. Nat. Acad. Sci. USA,* **74,** 263-267.
Greengard, P. (1976). *Nature* **260,** 101-108.
Hartzell, H.C. and Fambrough, D.M. (1972). *J. Gen. Physiol.* **60,** 248-262.
Karlin, A. and Cowburn, D.A. (1973). *Proc. Nat. Acad. Sci. USA,* **70,** 3636-3640.
Layne, P. and Najjar, V.A. (1973). *Fed. Proc.* **32,** 667.
Merlie, J.P., Changeux, J.P. and Gros, F. (1976). *Nature,* **264,** 74-76.
Meunier, J.C., Sealock, R., Olsen, R. and Changeux, J.P. (1974). *Eur. J. Biochem.* **45,** 371-394.
Miledi, R. (1960). *J. Physiol.* **151,** 1-23.
Revel, H.R. (1963). *Methods in Enzymology,* vol. VI, 211-214.
Segal, H.L. (1973). *Science,* **180,** 25-32.
Shigekawa, B.L. and Olsen, R.W. (1976). *Fed. Proc.* **1359.**
Steinbach, J.H., Harris, A.J., Patrick, J., Schubert, D. and Heinemann, S. (1973). *J. Gen. Physiol.* **62,** 255-270.
Teichberg, V.I. and Changeux, J.P. (1976). *FEBS Lett.* **67,** 264-268.
Teichberg, V.I. and Changeux, J.P. (1977). *FEBS Lett.* **74,** 71-76.
Teichberg, V.I., Sobel, A. and Changeux, J.P. (1977). *Nature,* **267,** 540-542.
Ueda, T., Maeno, H. and Greengard, P. (1973). *J. Biol. Chem.* **248,** 8295-8305.
Walton, K.G., De Lorenzo, R.J., Curran, P.F. and Greengard, P. (1975). *J. Gen. Physiol.* **65,** 153-177.
Weber, M., David-Pfeuty, M.T. and Changeux, J.P. (1975). *Proc. Nat. Acad. Sci. USA,* **72,** 3443-3448.
Whittaker, V.P. (1974). *Naturwissenschaften,* **60,** 280.

3 Neuromuscular disorders in man — clinical and pathological aspects

W.G. BRADLEY

Muscular Dystrophy Research Laboratories, Newcastle General Hospital, Newcastle upon Tyne

Introduction

Weakness in man may have many different causes in addition to diseases of the neuromuscular apparatus which are the main consideration of this chapter. These include psychiatric conditions and diseases of the central nervous system such as cerebrovascular disease and multiple sclerosis. The characteristic feature of diseases of the neuromuscular apparatus is the association of weakness, wasting, a reduction in tone and often a loss of tendon reflexes. Any part of the peripheral neuromuscular apparatus may be effected in such diseases, and a wide range of conditions are recognized effecting the spinal anterior horn motor nerve cell and its peripheral nerve axons, the neuromuscular junction and the skeletal muscles. Tables 1, 2 and 3 list some of the major human neuromuscular diseases. It is impossible in a chapter such as this to consider all the conditions in depth, and the aim is to provide an outline of the classification of the more important diseases, including the clinical and pathological features, paying particular attention to the muscular dystrophies. More detailed consideration may be found in a number of recent reviews (Dubowitz and Brooke, 1973; Pearson and Mostofi, 1973; Walton, 1974; Bradley, 1975; Bradley *et al.*, 1975).

The classification of disease

A disease is recognized as an entity if it has clearcut features which are restricted to that condition and not found in any other. Such diagnostic features may be clinical, physiological, biochemical or pathological. Let us look at four examples in human neuromuscular diseases. In myophosphorylase deficiency (McArdle's disease) the disease has relatively specific clinical features, but the entity is defined by the deficiency of myophosphorylase in the skeletal muscle. Pseudohypertrophic muscular dystrophy of the Duchenne type affects boys, is inherited in an X-linked manner, and has relatively specific pattern of muscle involvement. The serum creatine kinase activity is very greatly raised, and the muscle biopsy changes are

41

characteristic. Polymyositis is a condition with variable clinical features, but which has characteristic perivascular and interstitial inflammatory cell (mainly lymphocytic) infiltration of the skeletal muscle. In limb girdle muscular dystrophy the pattern of muscle involvement is somewhat variable, and in different individuals the upper or the lower limb girdle muscles may be the first to become involved. There is a relatively wide range of age of onset, and the muscle biopsy and electromyographic changes may show features of both myopathy and denervation.

Taking these four examples, it can be seen that the diagnosis has a varying degree of certainty. In myophosphorylase deficiency, the biochemical defect is known, and therefore the disease may be regarded as being fully characterized. Even in such an instance, further studies may yet necessitate a reconsideration of the classification. Thus recent evidence suggests that at least two different types of myophosphorylase deficiency occur, those with no detectable myophosphorylase protein, and those with a detectable protein of similar molecular weight, which is enzymically defective (Feit and Brooke, 1976). In Duchenne-type muscular dystrophy, though the constellation of clinical, genetic, biochemical and pathological features seems clearcut, the underlying biochemical defect remains to be indentified. It is therefore possible that several biochemically distinct entities exist among patients at present classified as having Duchenne muscular dystrophy. In polymyositis, though the clinical and biochemical features may be variable, the characterization of the disease is relatively

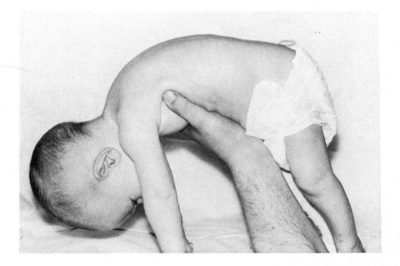

Fig. 1. A four month old baby with Werdnig-Hoffmann infantile spinal muscular atrophy showing gross hypotonia.

clearcut on the basis of the pathological changes. However inflammatory cell infiltration of muscle may be seen in other neuromuscular diseases, though it is usually of a less severe degree. It is likely that a number of different diseases exist in a group of patients diagnosed as having polymyositis, and also that an autoimmune polymyositic process complicates a number of other neuromuscular diseases (Papapetropoulos and Bradley, 1974). The variable clinical and pathological features of limb girdle muscular dystrophy make it very likely that there are several different disease entities included in this grouping.

It must therefore be recognized that the basis of the classification of any disease is of variable reliability, and an evolving matter. The classifications of today may become the jests of tomorrow! This is of importance in assessing the results of new research into such diseases. The classifications are however of importance for several reasons. They bring forth order from chaos. They allow reasonably well-based advice to be given to the patient on the genetic features of the disease and prognosis. In conditions in which some treatment is available, they allow directed therapy. The classifications however must not be regarded as sacrosanct.

Diseases of the Alpha-Motoneuron: The spinal muscular atrophies

The term spinal muscular atrophy is applied to a number of different diseases in which there is progressive denervation of the skeletal muscles due to progressive loss of α-motoneurons in the anterior horn of the spinal cord, without clinical sign of involvement of the central nervous system, and usually beginning in young life. In many cases the disease has an autosomal recessive mode of inheritance, though sporadic cases are common. In none is the cause of the α-motoneuron degeneration known.

Infantile spinal muscular atrophy (Werdnig-Hoffmann disease) is a relatively clearcut condition with onset in the first six months of life, and occasionally in the prenatal period as indicated by decreased fetal movements (Pearn and Wilson, 1973). The children are markedly hypotonic (Fig. 1). There is progressive severe denervation of all the muscles of the body (Fig. 2), including those of respiration and bulbar function, and all the children die by the age of two years, commonly from respiratory infections.

Juvenile spinal muscular atrophy presents at any age in the first and second decades, it is inherited in an autosomal recessive fashion, and is associated with progressive denervation of the muscles (Fig. 3). The pattern of muscular involvement may be selective, and similar to that seen in a muscular dystrophy, in which case the term pseudomyopathic spinal muscular atrophy is applied (Gardner-Medwin *et al.*, 1967; Meadows *et al.*,

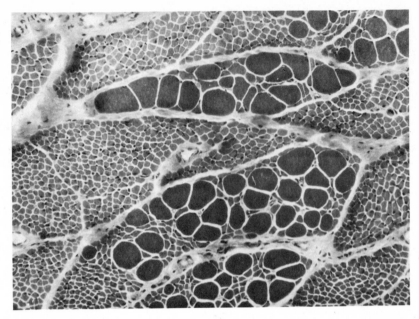

Fig. 2. Muscle biopsy from a baby with Werdnig-Hoffmann disease, showing a few groups of larger innervated muscle fibres in a sea of small denervated atrophied fibres. Haemotoxylin and Eosin. ×163.

1969). In other families, the pattern may be different, including distal involvement, diffuse involvement, or atypical and sometimes asymmetric involvement of muscles (Fig. 4). The prognosis of the condition is variable. The children may succumb during the first few years of life from a respiratory infection, or may suffer progressive paralysis with scoliosis but survive into the fourth or even fifth decade. In occasional cases the condition may appear to arrest. There is uncertainty concerning how many disease entities are represented in the group of patients with juvenile spinal muscular atrophy (Emery, 1971).

A number of other disease entities, in which there is progressive denervation of the skeletal muscles due to anterior horn cell degeneration, are recognized by the familial occurrence of a characteristic pattern of muscle involvement. These conditions include scapuloperoneal muscular atrophy, which is often X-linked, and in which the shoulder girdle muscles and the anterior tibial group of muscles are particularly involved (Thomas et al., 1972). Peroneal muscular atrophy of the pure neuronal type is also a spinal muscular atrophy, where the distribution of muscle involvement is distal, and effects the lower limbs with pes cavus and foot drop spreading to cause wasting of the small muscles of the hands. Some of these cases are autosomal recessively inherited, but many are sporadic (McLeod and Prineas,

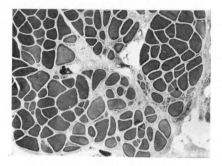 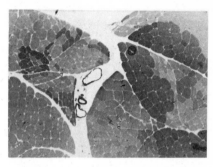

Fig. 3. (a) Muscle biopsy from an 8 year old boy with Kugelberg-Welander juvenile spinal muscular atrophy showing groups of atrophied denervated fibres, with many other fibres of more normal size. An occasional necrotic fibre is present, which is not uncommon in this condition. Haemotoxylin and Eosin. ×32. (b) Muscle biopsy from a 25 year old woman with Kugelberg-Welander disease, showing grouping of fibres of the same fibre type, indicating extensive reinnervation. Myosin ATPase. × 32.

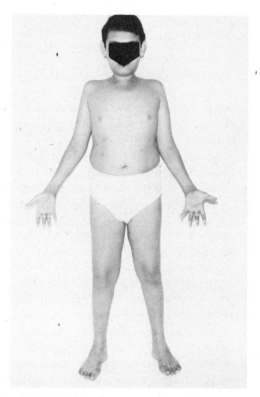

Fig. 4. A 12 year old boy with juvenile spinal muscular atrophy showing distal wasting of all four limbs and atrophy of both deltoid muscles.

Table 1 Diseases of the motor neuron

Inherited
  Infantile spinal muscular atrophy (Werdnig-Hoffmann disease) – autosomal recessive
  Juvenile spinal muscular atrophy (Kugelberg-Welander disease) – autosomal recessive
  Scapuloperoneal muscular atrophy – often X-linked
  Peroneal muscular atrophy, pure neuronal form – probably autosomal recessive

Others
  Acute anterior poliomyelitis
  Motor neuron disease

Peripheral Neuropathies (also involve sensory nerves)
  Toxic, for example lead
  Acute intermittent porphyria
  Inflammatory polyneuropathy (the Guillain-Barré-Strohl syndrome)

1971). There are several other types of peroneal muscular atrophy with a similar phenotypic presentation, but with a different pathological basis, including those due to hypertrophic neuropathy and those due to degeneration of both the sensory and motor neurons (Davis *et al.*, 1977).

Other anterior horn cell diseases

Acute anterior poliomyelitis is an illness caused by one of three strains of poliomyelitis virus, and rarely by other viruses. There is damage and acute death of many motoneurons in the spinal cord and brain stem, with resulting acute denervation of the skeletal muscles. The illness is associated with fever and muscle pains, and rapid paralysis. A variable degree of recovery can occur after the acute episode as surviving neurons branch to take over denervated muscle fibres.

Motor neuron disease or amyotrophic lateral sclerosis is a group of conditions with chronic progressive degeneration of the α-motoneuron in the spinal cord and brain stem, with in many cases an accompanying degeneration of the upper motoneuron in the corticospinal tracts. In rare instances the disease is inherited in a dominant fashion (Hirano *et al.*, 1967), but the vast majority of cases are sporadic. The disease can present at any age from young adulthood, but is commonest in the older age groups. Males are slightly more frequently involved than females. It is likely that many different diseases are included in this diagnostic title, for there are many different forms of presentation (Norris and Kurland, 1969). The typical cases of amyotrophic lateral sclerosis is a 60 year old man presenting with progressive wasting of the small muscles of the hands and a spastic paraparesis with increased reflexes and exterior plantar responses. The electromyogram shows the typical pattern of denervation with fibrillation potentials, giant polyphasic motor units, and a reduced interference pattern (see Bradley, 1974). The muscle has disseminated and grouped atrophic fibres, and may show fibre type grouping (Fig. 5). The progression of the disease is very variable, cases with bulbar involvement frequently dying from respiratory infections within two or three years, but some cases with pure progressive muscular atrophy of the lower motor neuron type surviving for 15 or 20 years. Though the small muscles of the hands are very frequently involved, any muscle in the body may be effected, and there is no specific pattern. The involvement may be very asymmetric and include some muscles and spare others.

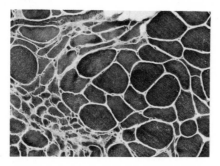

Fig. 5. Muscle biopsy from a 43 year old man with motor neuron disease showing groups of atrophied angulated fibres, and other areas of normal innervated fibres. Haemotoxylin and Eosin. × 82.

The aetiology of amyotrophic lateral sclerosis remains enigmatic. In large series of cases, there is an increased incidence of a previous attack of poliomyelitis, of gastrectomy, and of exposure to heavy metals including lead. It has therefore been suggested that some cases are due to chronic viral infections, vitamin or other deficiencies, or to toxic damage of the motor neurons. Therapeutic attempts to treat these possible aetiological factors have not to date produced any benefit.

The peripheral parts of the motoneuron may be damaged in a number of conditions falling into the category of peripheral neuropathies (Bradley, 1974). These usually involve both the sensory and motor fibres, with both sensory loss and weakness. A few peripheral neuropathies are purely motor, and the separation of these conditions from those affecting the anterior horn cell in the spinal cord is sometimes difficult, and may at times be artificial. A number of toxic agents, particularly lead, can produce a motor neuropathy, and it seems likely that the site of damage in these cases is the biochemical function of the anterior horn cell. The polyneuropathy associated with acute intermittent porphyria may affect any part of the peripheral nervous system, is often associated with sensory disturbance, but most classically produces a proximal muscle weakness of diffuse type. The condition is mainly associated with axonal degeneration in the affected nerves. Acute inflammatory polyneuropathy (the Guillain-Barré-Strohl syndrome) is an autoimmune disease effecting the peripheral nerves, and mainly producing inflammatory cell infiltration and segmental demyelination. It is likely that in many instances the inflammatory response is secondary to a preceding viral infection. Both porphyric neuropathy and acute inflammatory polyneuropathy show a tendency to recovery, though this is greater in the latter since axonal degeneration is much less prominent.

Diseases of the neuromuscular junction

Myasthenia gravis is the commonest human disorder of the neuromuscular junction, with the exception of the pharmacological blockade produced by anaesthetists using muscle relaxants. The clinical and biochemical features of myasthenia gravis are reviewed in this book by Professor Simpson (Chapter 4) and Dr. Vincent (Chapter 5) and will not be extensively considered here. The characteristic features of myasthenia gravis is muscle weakness with marked fatiguability, and the involvement of extraocular, bulbar and proximal upper limb musculature. The electrophysiological demonstration of a marked decrement with repetitive nerve stimulation, and the correction of the clinical and electrophysiological defect by anti-cholinesterase therapy are also the hallmark of the condition. Major advances in our understanding of this disease have occurred in recent years as a result of the isolation of the acetylcholine receptor. (Chapters 9 and 16).

The myasthenic syndrome is a condition first described by Eaton and Lambert (1957). The patients complain of mainly proximal muscle weakness and often fatiguability, but the diagnosis clinical and electrophysiological feature is the marked facilitation produced by repeated maximum effort or electrical stimulation. Areflexia is a common feature. The physiological basis of this condition appears to be an impairment of the release of acetylcholine quanta at the motor end plates (Elmqvist and Lambert, 1968). Guanidine, which increases the number of quanta of acetylcholine released with each nerve impulse, improves the symptoms. The onset is usually in the latter half of life, and in most of the patients there is an associated carcinoma, frequently of the lung.

Muscle weakness may be produced by pharmacological blockade of the neuromuscular junction, and a very large number of agents may be responsible. Pre-synaptic impairment of the release of acetylcholine from the nerve terminal is produced by botulinum toxin. Alpha-bungarotoxin and a number of other derivatives of snake venoms bind to the acetylcholine receptor of the motor end plate, as do curare-like drugs and antibiotics

Table 2 Diseases of the neuromuscular junction

Myasthenia gravis
The myasthenic syndrome
Pharmacological neuromuscular blockade
    Pre-synaptic blockade   −   Botulinum intoxication
    Post-synaptic blockade   −   bungarotoxin and other snake toxins
                     −   Curare-like drugs and the streptomycin group of antibiotics
                     −   Depolarizing blocking agents such as decamethonium

of the streptomycin group in high concentrations. A number of chemicals, including decamethonium, block the neuromuscular junction by depolarizing the end plate.

Diseases of skeletal muscle

A very large number of diseases damaging the skeletal muscle are recognized. These are most easily understood by grouping similar conditions as in Table 3.

Table 3 Diseases of skeletal muscle

Inherited diseases ('The Muscular Dystrophies')
    Severe pseudohypertrophic Duchenne muscular dystrophy − X-linked
    Benign pseudohypertrophic muscular dystrophy of Becker − X-linked
    Limb girdle muscular dystrophy − autosomal recessive
    Facioscapulohumeral muscular dystrophy − dominant
    Oculopharyngeal myopathy − dominant or recessive
    Distal myopathy − dominant

Myotonic diseases
    Dystrophia myotonica
    Myotonia congenita (Thomsen's disease) − autosomal recessive
    Myotonia congenita (Becker) − recessive
    Chondrodystrophic myotonia
    Myotonia with periodic paralysis

The periodic paralyses
    Familial periodic paralysis − hypokalaemic − dominant
    Adynamia episodica hereditaria − hyperkalaemic − dominant
    Normokalaemic periodic paralysis − dominant
    Paramyotonia congenita − dominant

Congenital myopathies
    Nemaline myopathy
    Central core disease
    Centronuclear myopathy
    Mitochondrial myopathies
    Finger print myopathy
    Reducing body myopathy
    Congenital muscular dystrophy

Polymyositis

Metabolic myopathies
    Glycogen Storage Diseases
        Myophosphorylase deficiency
        $\alpha 1,4$-glucosidase deficiency
    Lipid Storage Myopathies
        Carnitine deficiency
        Carnitine palmityltransferase deficiency

Endocrine myopathies
    Thyroid
    Adrenal
    Parathyroid

Deficiency myopathies
    Vitamin E deficiency
    Vitamin D deficiency

Toxic myopathies

The muscular dystrophies

The muscular dystrophies are a group of inherited diseases of skeletal muscle. The grouping has a historical basis, and a number of other inherited diseases of skeletal muscle have been identified since the grouping was defined, but are not usually termed 'muscular dystrophies'. The classification has however certain advantages. Early in the disease there is often specific involvement of certain muscle groups, sparing others until later, and the diseases are progressive.

The severe type of pseudohypertrophic muscular dystrophy of Duchenne. This is the most common of the muscular dystrophies. It shows a sex-linked recessive mode of inheritance, being restricted to boys (X^1Y) and rare cases of Turner's syndrome (X^1O), and inherited through the female line. In about a third of cases there is no known family history, and it seems that such cases are due to new spontaneous mutations. The incidence of the disease is approximately 30/100,000 male live births, and affects all races and parts of the world. In about 75% of definite female carriers of the disease the serum creatine kinase activity is above the upper limit of normal. However, in the remaining 25% the creatine kinase is normal, leading to the uncertainty which bedevils genetic counselling in this disease. Many attempts have been made to improve the reliability of detection of carriers by electromyography, muscle biopsy examination, the estimation of other enzymes, electrocardiography, etc. By and large these have only resulted in a small increment in certainty of detection of carriers (Gardner-Medwin, *et al.*, 1971).

The disease presents in boys, and impairment of motor development becomes obvious around about the age of three to five years, though frequently the child had delayed motor development in infancy (Fig. 6). Hypertrophy of the calves and sometimes of other muscles is a frequent finding, and at the time of presentation the child has weakness of the pelvic girdle musculature producing a waddling gait and difficulty in rising from the floor. Gradually the muscle weakness extends, and involves the pectoral girdle musculature. Muscles are selectively involved, with the biceps, brachioradialis, serrati and pectorals being particularly involved in the upper limbs with relative sparing of the deltoids and triceps muscles. Similarly in the lower limbs the hip flexors and extensors, the quadriceps and hamstring muscles are particularly involved with anterior tibial muscle weakness appearing relatively early as well. The muscle weakness increases, and about the age of 10 or 12 the child becomes unable to walk. Progressive kyphoscoliosis develops (Fig. 7) and respiratory impairment occurs. Before the era of antibiotics, many of the children died around the age of 12 or 14 from pneumonia. There is a cardiomyopathy in the great majority of patients with a characteristic ECG appearance. Symptoms of cardiac

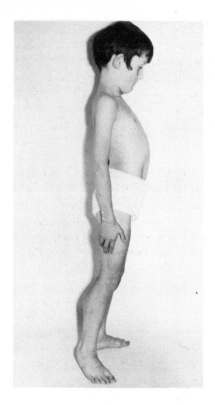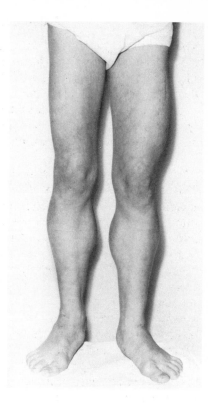

Fig. 6. A 5 year old boy with Duchenne muscular dystrophy showing (a) the increased lumbar lordosis and inability to place the heel flat on the ground and (b) pseudohypertrophy of the calves.

involvement with dysrhythmias and cardiac failure are fairly common in patients living into the late teens, and many patients die from cardiac problems. Survival beyond the age of 20 years is unusual. Mental retardation is present in about a third of patients, and the distribution of I.Q.s. is gaussian with the mean shifted to the left at approximately 85.

The pathological basis of the skeletal muscle degeneration has been the source of many studies over the years. At or soon after birth the skeletal muscle may be very little different from normal, though a proportion of the muscle fibres show overcontraction of myofibrils with hyaline fibre formation (Fig. 8) (Bradley *et al.*, 1972). There have been suggestions of abnormalities present in the muscle of the male fetus aborted from carriers of Duchenne dystrophy (Toop and Emery, 1974), though our own studies of such fetus have not confirmed these reports. Skeletal muscle degeneration with necrosis, phagocytosis and regeneration, together with marked clumping of the myofibrillary elements producing hyaline fibre formation,

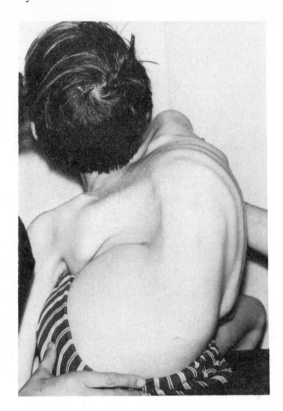

Fig. 7. A 15 year old boy with Duchenne muscular dystrophy showing the characteristic severe kyphoscoliosis.

is prominent within the first few months of life. Endomysial fibrosis occurs early, and by the time the boy is about six years there is already significant loss of muscle fibres with fibrous tissue and fat replacement. With increasing age this process increases, while the proportion of acute necrotising change decreases (Fig. 9). By the time of death, many of the skeletal muscles consist virtually entirely of fat and fibrous tissue, with only a few residual muscle fibres remaining (Fig. 10).

Biochemical changes occurring in this disease are fully reviewed in Chapter 18 by Dr. Pennington. The most striking abnormality in the blood is the very high level of creatine kinase, and to a lesser extent the high level of other muscle-derived enzymes including lactic dehydrogenase. The serum creatine kinase is raised even in the cord blood at birth in affected individuals (Bradley *et al.*, 1972a) and evidence is appearing that the level of creatine kinase may also be remarkably raised in the fetal blood as early as the 21st week of pregnancy (Stengel-Rutkowski *et al.*, 1976). Confirmation of this last observation may make it possible for affected male fetuses to be

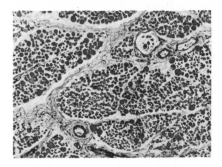

Fig. 8. Muscle biopsy of a 2 week old baby who later developed Duchenne muscular dystrophy showing the small muscle fibres characteristic of this age, and the scattered larger hyaline fibres. Haemotoxylin and Eosin. × 82.

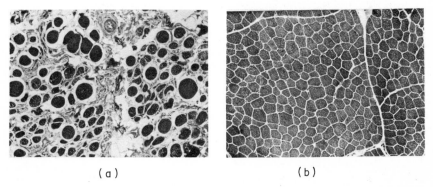

(a)   (b)

Fig. 9. Muscle biopsies of 8 year old boys (a) with Duchenne muscular dystrophy showing loss of fibres, fibrosis and hyaline fibres, in comparison with (b) a normal child. Haemotoxylin and Eosin. × 82.

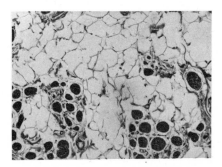

Fig. 10. Muscle at autopsy from 16 year old boy dying of Duchenne muscular dystrophy showing severe loss of fibres, with fat and fibrous tissue replacement. Haemotoxylin and Eosin. × 82.

recognized, and the pregnancy to be terminated. At present genetic counselling, and termination of all male pregnancies of carriers of Duchenne dystrophy is all that can be offered, and the ability to detect the affected male fetus would be a major advance.

The aetiology of Duchenne muscular dystrophy remains unknown at this stage. A number of theories which have received prominence in the last decade including the neurogenic theory and the vascular theory, appear unlikely to be true (Bradley, 1975; Bradley *et al.*, 1975). A search continues for the underlying biochemical defect, and in recent years membrane abnormalities both in the skeletal muscle and in other cells such as the erythrocyte have been reported (see review by Rowland, 1976). At present the abnormalities which have been reported do not appear to be of the fundamental defect, though work is developing rapidly in this field. An abnormality of the structural components of the cell membrane in Duchenne muscular dystrophy might best put together the wide range of reported changes. Mokri and Engel (1975) have suggested that the sarcolemmal membrane of individual fibres in Duchenne muscle has defects or holes. Our own observations have supported this report (Bradley and Fulthorpe, 1977). These defects might allow the entrance into the muscle fibre of excessive concentrations of calcium which would thereby produce excessive contraction and clumping of the myofilaments (hyaline fibres) (Cullen and Fulthorpe, 1974), poison mitochondria (Wrogemann and Pena, 1976), produce activation of a number of proteinases (Busch *et al.*, 1972), and thus lead to cell death and necrosis.

Unfortunately the investigation of the biochemical changes in skeletal muscle in many myopathic conditions, and in particular in Duchenne dystrophy is bedevilled by the complexity of secondary changes occurring in such muscle. In Duchenne dystropy for instance as can be seen from Fig. 9, in a five year old boy homogenates of the muscle contain derivatives not only of the intact skeletal muscle fibres themselves, but also of degenerating and regenerating muscle fibres, of phagocytes, excessive numbers of fibroblasts and other connective tissue cells, as well as other cells such as those of the blood vessels. The optimal system for investigating the underlying biochemical abnormality in the muscle in Duchenne dystrophy would therefore be fetal muscle prior to the development of the secondary changes. This approach is referred to by Dr. Ellis in Chapter 20.

The Becker type of pseudohypertrophic muscular dystrophy. Becker and Kiener (1955) first recognized the existence of an X-linked form of muscular dystrophy which was more benign than that described by Duchenne. The frequency of families with this condition is perhaps only a tenth of that with Duchenne muscular dystrophy. Though cases may often have somewhat delayed motor milestones early in life, the usual age of onset in

Becker muscular dystrophy is in the late first or second decade (Bradley *et al.*, 1977). Progress of the disease is considerably slower than in Duchenne dystrophy, and all patients are still able to walk at the age of 16, by which time all Duchenne patients have become confined to a wheelchair. Some patients with Becker muscular dystrophy may continue to be able to walk into the fifth decade. Cardiological abnormalities are considerably less common than in the Duchenne form, as is mental retardation.

The pattern of skeletal muscle involvement is very similar to that occurring in Duchenne dystrophy, being selective in involving the periscapular muscles, biceps and brachioradialis in the upper limbs, and the hip flexors and extensors, quadriceps and hamstrings in the lower limbs (Fig. 11). Pseudohypertrophy of the calves, and sometimes of other muscles is frequently found in Becker muscular dystrophy as well as in Duchenne dystrophy.

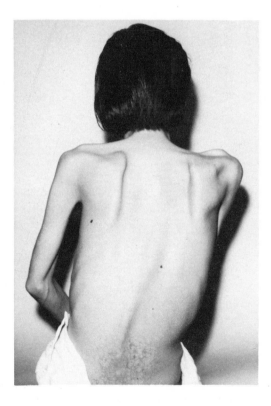

Fig. 11. A 21 year old man with Becker type dystrophy showing marked wasting of periscapular muscles, relative sparing of deltoids and triceps, and mild kyphosis.

The pathological changes in the muscle are still incompletely understood in this condition. The pathology is different from that in Duchenne dystrophy, though necrosis, phagocytosis and regeneration, fibrosis and fat replacement all occur to some extent. In some reports hyaline fibre formation and a picture somewhat reminiscent of Duchenne dystrophy have been encountered (Ringel *et al.*, 1977), while in others marked inflammatory cell infiltration a little suggestive of polymyositis has been prominent (Markand *et al.*, 1969). In our recent review of 25 cases from 8 families of X-linked benign muscular dystrophy, in addition to these changes a number of features reminiscent of chronic denervation of skeletal muscle was found (Fig. 12) (Bradley *et al.*, 1977). Becker's own cases have shown a rather similar picture (Chapter 25).

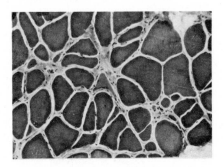

Fig. 12. Muscle biopsy of a 21 year old patient with Becker X-linked muscular dystrophy showing wide variation in fibre size, angulated atrophic fibres, nuclear clumps, split fibres, and a regenerating fibre in the middle of the picture. Haemotoxylin and Eosin. ×163.

Biochemical investigations have been less extensive than in Duchenne dystrophy. The serum creatine kinase activity is considerably raised, but to a lesser extent than in patients with Duchenne dystrophy of a similar age. Transmission of the disorder is by affected males through their carrier daughters to their grandsons, and the serum creatine kinase activity of definite carriers of Becker dystrophy is raised in only about 50% of cases (Emery *et al.*, 1967). Genetic counselling on this basis is therefore even less certain than in Duchenne dystrophy.

Genetic linkage data suggests that the two undoubtedly separate diseases of Becker and Duchenne muscular dystrophy have a different locus on the X chomosome, and are not allelic. It has however been suggested that these two loci were originally allelic, but that the translocation of the terminal part of the Y chromosome onto the X chromosome in the original development of the sex chromosomes allowed the gradual divergence of the actions of the abnormal genes, and thus of the character of the resulting diseases (Lyon, 1974).

Limb girdle muscular dystrophy syndromes. Since the end of the last century, there have been many descriptions of patients with weakness and wasting of proximal muscles beginning either in the upper or the lower limb girdle muscles at around the age of 20 or 30 years. In some instances these have been familial, and thus there may be an autosomal recessive mode of inheritance. Walton and Nattrass (1954) combined previous reports and their own experience of such cases under the term limb girdle muscular dystrophy. The condition may effect either sex, and most cases are sporadic. A detailed analysis of 30 such patients demonstrated that the pattern of muscle involvement is selective, with early involvement of similar muscles to those only involved in Becker and Duchenne dystrophy, but that there were frequent exceptions to this pattern (see Bradley, 1978). Pseudohypertrophy is sometimes seen. The incidence of this disease is about a sixth of that of Duchenne dystrophy, and the serum creatine kinase activity may be as high as 2,000 I.U., though lower values are more common.

Detailed electrophysiological and pathological investigations of these cases have indicated a polymorphism in this population. The investigations show features both of a myopathy similar to, though more indolent than that seen in Duchenne dystrophy, and a chronic denervation of the skeletal muscle. In some muscles and in some individuals one or other process seems to be predominant. The picture does not appear to show a clearcut separation of cases into one group which might be termed pseudomyopathic spinal muscular atrophy of the limb girdle type, and the other, myopathic limb girdle muscular dystrophy. Rather the picture appears to be a variable involvement both of skeletal muscle and of the motor nerves in different patients. Further studies of this group of patients are awaited with interest.

– *Facioscapulohumeral muscular dystrophy.* Patients with this condition commonly have a dominant family history of similar cases. Overall the condition is the most benign of the muscular dystrophies, with onset often delayed until the second to fifth decade, and many patients never having to take to a wheelchair. Many patients may live a normal span of years. The pattern of muscle involvement is characteristic, and different from that of the other muscular dystrophies so far described. Facial involvement is very early, as indicated by the fact that the patients have frequently never been able to whistle or blow up balloons. Complaints of facial muscle weakness are however extremely uncommon, and presentation is usually delayed until the onset of either upper limb proximal weakness or tripping due to weakness of the anterior tibial group of muscles. Examination at this stage shows a selective involvement of the facial, the periscapular and humeral muscles, and of the anterior tibial muscles. Atrophy of these muscles is frequently marked, while other muscles are to a very great extent spared and of normal bulk. In a few patients, however, there is a diffuse atrophy of all muscles, in addition to the marked involvement of the muscles described above.

The serum creatine kinase activity is usually raised, though the value is only about a third of that seen in patients with limb girdle dystrophy.

As in limb girdle dystrophy, detailed electrophysiological and pathological investigation of a large group of patients indicates hetergeneity in facioscapulohumeral dystrophy (see Bradley, 1978). Cases with mitochondrial myopathy (Fig. 13) (Hudson et al., 1972; Worsfold et al., 1973), spinal muscular atrophy (Fenichel et al., 1967) and inflammatory cell infiltration (Munsat et al., 1972) have been described. Our investigation of a large series of such patients showed that many have the combined features of chronic denervation and chronic myopathy of the skeletal muscle. In a few of the cases with inflammatory cell infiltrates clinical improvement may result from corticosteroid therapy (Papapetropoulos and Bradley, 1974) but in most cases a fall in serum creatine kinase activity without clinical change is all that results (Munsat and Bradley, 1977). Detailed biochemical investigations of the skeletal muscle in such patients have been few.

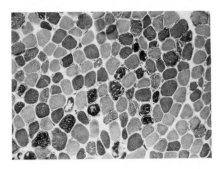

Fig. 13. Muscle biopsy of a 13 year old girl with dominantly inherited facioscapulohumeral muscular dystrophy due to a mitochondrial abnormality. Many fibres show excessive amounts of dark granular mitochondrial enzyme activity. Stained for NADH-diaphorase. ×163.

Ocular myopathy. A number of reports have appeared over the years of patients with progressive external ophthalmoplegia presenting with ptosis and sometimes diplopia, in whom skeletal muscle weakness particularly of the face, neck, limb girdle and arm muscles have been a feature (Fig. 14). Both dominantly inherited and sporadic cases have been reported. In some patients pharyngeal involvement had lead to the use of the term oculopharyngeal muscular dystrophy. In many of the patients there are other abnormalities, including retinitis pigmentosa, retardation of growth, cardiac abnormalities, cerebellar ataxia, neural deafness, spasticity, dementia and

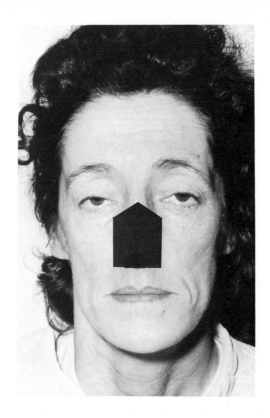

Fig. 14. A patient with ocular myopathy showing ptosis. The external ocular and facial muscles were also involved.

increased cerebrospinal fluid protein concentration (Kearns and Sayer, 1958; Drachman, 1968). It is therefore likely that a number of different diseases are present in this group, and perhaps the term muscular dystrophy should not be applied. The skeletal muscle, particularly when weak, shows a number of abnormalities of mitochondria in such cases. These abnormalities include subsarcolemmal aggregates of mitochondria, abnormally structured mitochondria including vacuolation, abnormalities of the arrangement of the cristae, and paracrystalline inclusions (Fig. 15) (Zintz, 1966; Olson *et al.*, 1972).

Distal muscular dystrophy. Patients with distal muscular wasting are usually found to have chronic denervation of the peripheral skeletal muscles, often the condition being one of the forms of peroneal muscular atrophy. However, in some instances, the skeletal muscle shows the changes of a myopathy, and no evidence of denervation can be found. Very detailed investigation however of such cases is required, and often the diagnosis

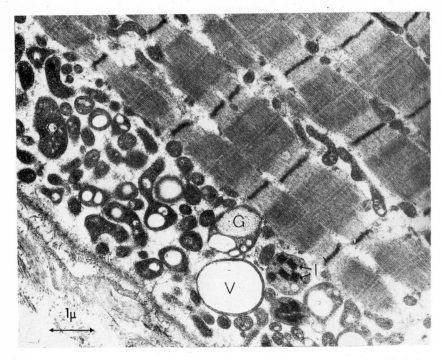

Fig. 15. Electron micrograph of muscle from a patient with ocular myopathy with bulbar muscle involvement showing bizarre abnormal mitochondria. V—vacuole probably in a mitochondrion. G—glycogen granules in a mitochondrion. I—paracrystalline inclusions in a mitochondrion.

cannot be established before a full autopsy examination (Sumner *et al.*, 1971). Distal muscular dystrophy appears to be much commoner in Sweden where Welander (1951) has reported a large number of patients, the inheritance being dominant.

The myotonic disorders

Myotonia is the delayed relaxation of a muscle after contraction, with the accompanying electromyographic characteristic of sustained waxing and waning high frequency discharges. In most instances the myotonia is worse in the cold, and is relieved by warming the muscles or by repetitive action. Physiological investigations of patients with these diseases, and experimental models including the inherited myotonia of the goat, and myotonia induced by agents blocking the synthesis of cholesterol such as diazacholesterol, have suggested that the underlying defect of the membrane is a reduced chloride conductance (Barchi, 1975). This results in a spontaneous tendency for the resting membrane potential to fall to the critical level for the firing of an action potential, followed by the temporary repolarization to normal levels. Treatment with quinine, procaineamide, phenytoin or corticosteroids is usually effective in decreasing the extent of the myotonia. A number of rather dissimilar diseases can be grouped together as the myotonic disorders on the basis of the presence of myotonia.

Autosomal dominant myotonia congenita (Thomsen). Thomsen's disease appears to be a pure form of myotonia, with no tendency for the development of a myopathy. Symptoms usually are present from birth, and the disease is inherited in an autosomal dominant manner (Thomasen, 1948). The typical symptom is that sudden attempts at major muscle contraction produce 'freezing', the patient being unable to move because of the repetitive discharge of the activated muscles, that is because of myotonia. The exacerbation by cold may prevent a patient being able to relax his grip on a cold bar, such as that of a bus. All skeletal muscles may be involved, and the muscles and the individual fibres of those muscles are generally somewhat larger than normal.

Autosomal recessive myotonia congenita (Becker). Becker (1973) drew attention to a recessively inherited form of myotonia congenita which appeared to be several times more frequent than Thomsen's disease. Sporadic cases were common. The onset of symptoms is usually delayed until childhood or early adult life, and there is gradual spread of myotonia from the legs to the arms and later to the face. Muscle hypertrophy may be pronounced, and muscle weakness gradually develops probably due to a low grade myopathic process.

Dystrophia myotonica. This condition, which is inherited in an autosomal dominant fashion and is a relatively common condition, combines some of the features of a muscular dystrophy with the presence of myotonia. The latter may be the presenting complaint, but the dystrophic process and other associated features are the main problems of the disease. Many of the organs of the body may be involved in addition to the skeletal muscle. There may be mild progressive dementia, cataracts, gonadal atrophy and frontal balding. The disease may present at any age, and may be of very variable severity. Most frequently the onset of muscle weakness is in early adult life. There is a characteristic facies with ptosis and facial myopathy as well as mild proximal and sometimes distal muscle weakness and myotonia. Cases may however present as floppy babies at birth, with feeding defects, and in such instances almost invariably the mother also bears the gene for dystrophia myotonica (Dyken and Harper, 1973). The disease may not present until late life, and this is sometimes as a result of the development of the characteristic cataract. The patients bearing the gene may however live for a normal span of years without any symptom whatsoever. The cause of this variability of manifestation is not known, but a major role of modifier genes and of environmental influence are that most likely possibilities.

The skeletal muscle may show a number of abnormalities ranging from peripheral sarcoplasmic masses, to ringbinden, chains of nuclei and type 1 fibre atrophy. Necrosis and phagocytosis is relatively uncommon, and the muscle spindles show bizarre splitting of the intrafusal fibres (Swash, 1972). Biochemical changes in this disease are frequent, and there is a moderate increase in serum creatine kinase activity. A decrease in levels of a number of hormones is related to the glandular atrophy, but there is an increased secretion of insulin in response to a glucose load in a proportion of patients. Reduced levels of immunoglobulins, and in particular of IgG, appear to be due to an increased catabolism of these proteins. A number of abnormalities of membranes, including those of the erythrocyte have been demonstrated (Roses and Appel, 1974, 1975; Butterfield et al., 1976).

Other forms of myotonia. Myotonia occurs in a number of other conditions which are all relatively rare. It may be associated with periodic paralysis (see below). Paramyotonia congenita is an autosomal dominant condition in which myotonia occurs paroxysmally, often produced by cold and sometimes associated with periodic attacks of weakness. Myotonia has been reported in association with a number of unusual skeletal deformities, and the term chondrodystrophic myotonia has been applied (Aberfeld et al., 1970).

The periodic paralyses

In a number of dominantly inherited conditions periodic attacks of weakness of the skeletal muscles are the main feature. The commonest of these is hypokalaemic periodic paralysis, in which low serum levels of potassium are found during the attack. In this condition, attacks are frequently precipitated by heavy carbohydrate meals, and by resting after exercise. The attacks may be severe, though rarely are respiratory or bulbar muscles involved. The skeletal muscle fibres show dilatation of the sarcoplasmic reticulum and vacuolation in the attack (Engel, 1970), and in a few patients, a progressive vascular myopathy may develop. The attacks usually only last for a few hours. A very similar syndrome can occur in association with hyperthyroidism, particularly in the Chinese population.

Adynamia episodica hereditaria (hyperkalaemic periodic paralysis) is a rather similar dominantly inherited disease in which the serum potassium levels are raised during the attack. Characteristically the attacks are rather briefer than those seen in familial periodic paralysis, and may be precipitated either by starvation, or by rest after exercise. Myotonia is rather commoner than in the hypokalaemic form, though it may be seen in all of the conditions. Adynamia episodica hereditaria is commoner is Scandinavian populations, and though the attacks are usually short, weakness lasting for months or years may also be seen (Bradley, 1969).

A third condition in which periodic attacks occur in an autosomal dominantly inherited fashion have also been described in which the serum potassium level does not alter during the attack. This has been termed the normokalaemic form. The possibility exists that it is simply a variant of the hyperkalaemic variety.

The basis of the periodic attacks of weakness is not fully understood. In both the hyper- and hypokalaemic forms of the condition, the resting membrane potential of the skeletal muscle during the attack is significantly lowered, and evidence suggests that this is due to an increase in sodium permeability (Creutzfeldt *et al.*, 1963; McComas *et al.*, 1968; Hoffmann and Smith, 1970). This would partially inactivate the sodium carrier mechanism necessary for the generation of the action potential, and thereby lead to the clinical paralysis. However the basis for the changes in serum levels of potassium has not been elucidated. In both conditions there appears to be an inflow of water and sodium into the skeletal muscle, with associated dilatation of the longitudinal and transverse tubular elements of the sarcoplasmic reticulum.

The congenital myopathies

A number of conditions have been grouped under this title on the basis that they frequently present in infancy or in the early years of life, and in a number of instances have evidence of an inherited trait. This is usually suggestive of an autosomal recessive inheritance, but some instances of possibly dominant inheritance with incomplete penetrance have been described. To a large extent the recognition of these conditions have been based upon apparently characteristic pathological changes in the skeletal muscle (Dubowitz and Brooke, 1973) though similar changes may sometimes be seen less extensively in a wide range of conditions.

Thus nemaline or rod body myopathy is associated with the accumulation, mainly in the subsarcolemmal areas, of paracrystalline rod-like structures (Heffernan *et al.*, 1968; Kulakowski *et al.*, 1973). There is morphological evidence to suggest that these are derived from abnormal Z-line material, though the biochemical characterization of the protein of these rods has not been fully completed (Engel and Gomez, 1967; Stromer *et al.*, 1976). The patients usually have a Marfanoid appearance, with a long face, a high arched palate, long spidery fingers, and generally thin atrophic muscle.

Centronuclear myopathy is again a condition probably inherited in an autosomal recessive fashion. It presents with ptosis and progressive external ophthalmoplegia, and an associated generalized weakness and wasting of the skeletal muscles, more particularly of the limb girdles (Bradley *et al.*, 1970). The muscle fibres are generally atrophied, with chains of central nuclei and other degenerative features. Other rather similar conditions, though sometimes not associated with external ophthalmoplegia, have been reported in which there was type 1 atrophy or hypotrophy with central nuclei, the type 2 fibres being relatively normal.

Central core disease is another condition which may present in infancy or later life, usually with a relatively nonspecific picture of muscle weakness, and in this instance frequently a dominant mode of inheritance (Dubowitz and Roy, 1970). Histologically the muscle is characterized by amorphous looking central areas within the muscle fibres composed of compact somewhat disorganized myofibrils. The central cores are devoid of oxidative enzymes and phosphorylase, and are presumably nonfunctioning. The cores seem particularly to affect type 1 fibres.

A number of different clinical neuromuscular syndromes associated with mitochondrial abnormalities in the skeletal muscle have been reported. These include the ocular myopathy syndromes referred to above, the picture of facioscapulohumeral muscular dystrophy with mitochondrial abnormalities (Hudgson et al., 1972), and a number of other syndromes of the infantile and juvenile onset of muscle weakness. In addition a very characteristic form of mitochondrial myopathy was first described by Luft et al. (1962), a further patient being described by Afifi et al. (1972). In this condition the skeletal muscle mitochondria are uncoupled, that is their oxidative activity continues uninfluenced by the levels of ADP and ATP. The characteristic feature of these rare patients is that they show gross hypermetabolism, though thyroid function is entirely normal. Mitochondrial abnormalities similar to those seen in the ocular myopathy syndromes have been reported in these patients. It is likely that all the myopathies with mitochondrial abnormalities will prove a fruitful field for biochemical study of cytochromes, and other respiratory chain intermediates (Spiro et al., 1970), and of carnitine and its related enzymes.

A number of other rare congenital myopathies have been characterized by the finding of apparently specific pathological changes, including the presence of reducing bodies, and of fingerprint bodies. Though these abnormalities have since also been reported in other conditions, their frequency and number appear to indicate the specific nature of these syndromes.

Congenital muscular dystrophy must also be mentioned in this context (Donner et al., 1975). Patients usually present with impaired motor function, hypotonia and feeding difficulties at birth, or sometimes with marked contractures and joint deformities, to which the term arthrogryposis multiplex congenita is applied. Many cases of the latter condition however are associated with conditions causing intrauterine denervation of skeletal muscle. Children with congenital muscular dystrophy may show a nonprogressive or slowly progressive picture of muscle weakness, wasting and contractures. The pathological changes in the muscle include marked fibrosis, and a number of degenerative changes including necrosis and phagocytosis of the skeletal muscle fibres. The biochemical basis of this disease group, and its inheritance is not clear.

Polymyositis

Skeletal muscle may be damaged by an autoimmune inflammatory process in a group of conditions to which the term polymyositis is applied. Inflammatory cells, particularly lymphocytes and occasional plasmacytes with macrophages and fibroblasts invade the skeletal muscle, occurring both in the interstitial tissue, and particularly around small blood vessels (Fig. 16). The process is very patchy, both within any one muscle, and in the overall muscles of the body. Patients are often aware of pain and tenderness of the muscles, as well as progressive muscle weakness and wasting. The proximal muscles of the limbs, including those of the neck are mainly involved, and dysphagia due to bulbar muscle involvement is not infrequent (DeVere and Bradley, 1975). Tendon reflexes are generally preserved, and may even by exaggerated in the early stages. An inflammatory cardiomyopathy with congestive cardiac failure may also develop.

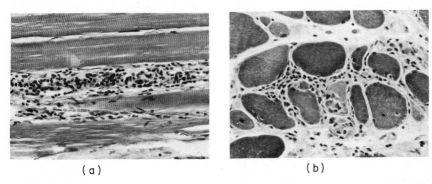

(a)   (b)

Fig. 16. Muscle biopsies in polymyositis. (a) An interstitial predominantly lymphocytic infiltrate with adjacent normal fibres. Haemotoxylin and Eosin. × 163. (b) A number of necrotic fibres undergoing phagocytosis. Haemotoxylin and Eosin. × 325.

The skeletal muscle fibres themselves show acute necrotising change with phagocytosis and regeneration. In addition there may be type 2 fibre atrophy, and perifascicular atrophy, the basis of which is not clear. In chronic cases, loss of muscle fibres with marked fibrosis, and some fat replacement occurs. The skeletal muscle damage leads to a marked rise in serum creatine kinase activity. Electromyography shows increased insertional activity, and pseudomyotonic discharges, as well as the changes of myopathy with low amplitude short duration polyphasic potentials and an early recruitment of a full low amplitude interference pattern.

The disease may occur at any age, though is more frequent in the later years of life. It may occur without any other evidence of a vasculitis or involvement of any other tissue, or may be associated with either a clearcut collagen-vascular disease such as rheumatoid arthritis, scleroderma or systemic lupus erythematosus, or with minor evidence of collagen-vascular disease such as a raised erythrocyte sedimentation rate and positive anti-nuclear factor. Polymyositis may also occur in combination with malignant disease such as a carcinoma of the bronchus, ovary or breast. In some patients, a characteristic skin rash of the face and hands develops, and the term dermatomyositis is given to this variant. Dermatomyositis is more commonly associated with carcinoma, particularly in male and older patients.

Since there are probably several different disease entities, it is likely that there are several different aetiological bases for polymyositis. The reason why the body reacts against its own skeletal muscle fibre, activating lymphocytes and antibodies to induce muscle fibre death is not known. A similar process occurs in all the autoimmune diseases. Activation of such a process by the presence of a carcinoma may also occur. It has been suggested that certain viruses enter the muscle fibres, to reproduce there and become the source of the antigen against which the lymphocytes react. Virus-like particles have been reported from time to time in electron microscopy studies of the muscle in polymyositis, though attempts to isolate the virus have met with almost universal failure.

Polymyositis is a treatable condition, which in the majority of patients appears to burn itself out after a number of years. Immunosuppressive therapy with high doses of corticosteroids with or without cytotoxic agents such as azathioprine appears to be the treatment of choice (DeVere and Bradley, 1975). In childhood the prognosis is almost universally good, but in the older age group recovery may be incomplete, and disease activity may occasionally persist for many years requiring continuation of therapy.

The important point about polymyositis is that it is a relatively frequent disease, the incidence probably exceeding that of Duchenne muscular dystrophy by an order of magnitude. It may present in very many different ways, sometimes simulating muscular dystrophy. Since it is a treatable disease, a high index of suspicion is required of clinicians responsible for the care of these patients.

Metabolic myopathies

Under this heading may be grouped a number of diseases in which a clue exists to the underlying metabolic cause of the myopathy. The division is rather arbitrary, for it must be hoped that eventually all diseases, including the muscular dystrophies, will come into this category. At present the clinical significance of these diseases is that in certain instances they are associated with known metabolic abnormalities, for which it may be possible to design an effective treatment. As this review has demonstrated, there are few neuromuscular diseases for which there is an effective treatment, and it is important that these rare instances do not escape detection.

Glycogen storage diseases. There is a considerable number of glycogen storage diseases, several of which affect the skeletal muscle (Huijing, 1975). The myopathies due to myophosphorylase and α-1,4-glucosidase are the commonest. Myophosphorylase deficiency (McArdle's disease: type V glycogenosis) prevents the splitting of glucose-1-phosphate from glycogen, and therefore blocks the anaerobic pathways of glycolysis. The muscle must therefore rely entirely upon aerobic metabolism, and during severe muscle exercise, particularly associated with ischaemia, the muscle becomes very anoxic and painful. Glycogen accumulates within the sarcoplasm (Fig. 17), though the degree of accumulation is not as high as that seen in α-1,4-glucosidase deficiency. The patients usually present in late juvenile or early adult life with muscle cramps on exertion, and sometimes with post-exercise myoglobinuria due to rhabdomyolysis (Rowland *et al.,* 1963). The diagnostic test is of a lack of the normal rise of venous lactate induced by ischaemic exercise, and the absence of myophosphorylase activity in the skeletal muscle biopsy which can be demonstrated by both histochemistry and biochemistry. Despite the apparently central site of the defect in the metabolic pathways relating to glycogen, patients rarely are severely incapacitated by the condition, and usually live a normal number of years.

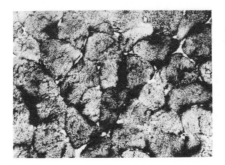

Fig. 17. Muscle biopsy of a patient with myophosphorylase deficiency showing subsarcolemmal glycogen accumulations (dark areas). Celloidin-coated, periodate Schiff-stained. ×163.

Deficiency of the lysosomal enzyme, α-1,4-glucosidase, results in massive glycogen accumulation within the skeletal muscle, even though it is not generally thought that this lysosomal enzyme plays a major role in the metabolic turnover of glycogen. The accumulation is predominantly within lysosomes, though sarcoplasmic glycogen is also abnormally increased. In this, as in other lysosomal storage diseases, it seems either that the lysosomal enzymes must play a larger part than generally believed in the metabolic turnover of compounds within the cell, or that there is some increase in a hitherto unrecognized synthetic enzyme capacity. Two forms of α1,4-glucosidase deficiency are recognized, the more common infantile form (Pompe's disease, type II glycogenosis) in which glycogen accumulates in most of the cells of the body including the heart, liver, neurons and skeletal muscle (Fig. 18). Infants with this disease present with rapidly progressive congestive cardiomyopathy and muscle weakness, and usually die within the first few months of life (Hudgson and Fulthorpe, 1975). The adult form of the disease is apparently associated with an identical degree of loss of enzyme activity in the skeletal muscle, but the degree of metabolic

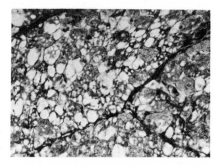

Fig. 18. Muscle biopsy of 4 month old child with Pompe's disease showing gross disruption of fibres due to glycogen accumulation, most of which has dissolved out in this non-celloidin-coated periodate Schiff-stained preparation. × 163.

impairment and of glycogen accumulation is considerably less (Fig. 19). The probable reason for the later onset in the adult form is the presence of normal levels of neutral maltase in the skeletal muscle, compared to the low levels in the infantile form (Angelini and Engel, 1972). Patients present in late juvenile or adult age, and the picture may not be dissimilar from a limb girdle muscular dystrophy (Engel and Dale, 1968).

Lipid storage diseases. An increasing number of patients with a myopathy associated with abnormal metabolism of lipids in skeletal muscle is being recognized. A.G. Engel and colleagues have played a large part in elucidating the role of carnitine in one group of patients. Carnitine is required for the transfer of long-chain fatty acids through the mitochondrial membrane prior to omega-oxidation. Transfer to and from the long chain fatty acid-coenzyme A complex is catalysed by carnitine-palmityl-transferase.

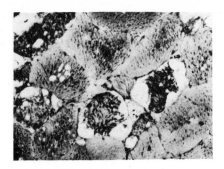

Fig. 19. Muscle biopsy from a 34 year old woman with adult acid maltase deficiency, showing the fewer fibres are involved and the accumulation of glycogen less massive than in the infantile form. Non-celloidin-coated, periodate Schiff. × 163.

Deficiency either of carnitine or of the transferase will impair the oxidation of fatty acids.

Bradley *et al.* (1969, 1972) described a young woman with a relapsing-remitting proximal myopathy, which was not responsive to corticosteroid therapy. Later studies have demonstrated a low muscle carnitine and normal serum carnitine level in the serum (Bradley *et al.*, 1978). The patient reported by Engel and Siekert (1972) was clinically similar, except that corticosteroids improved the weakness, and that the serum and muscle carnitine levels were reduced (Engel and Angelini, 1973; Engel, *et al.*, 1974). Reports of other cases support the conclusion that there is no clinical difference between those with normal and those with low serum carnitine levels (Karpati *et al.*, 1975; Van Dyke *et al.*, 1975). Possibly different conditions with skeletal muscle lipid storage myopathy include cases with lipid storage in leucocytes and Schwann cells, low muscle but normal serum carnitine levels (Markesbery *et al.*, 1974) and those with systemic lipid deposition with deficient carnitine-palmityl-transferase activity in liver leading to low serum and muscle carnitine levels (Jerusalem *et al.*, 1975; Boudin *et al.*, 1976).

A different syndrome with skeletal muscle transferase deficiency can now be clinically recognized. The characteristic feature is muscle pains and cramps some time after exercise, with myoglobinuria. W.K. Engel *et al.* (1970) described identical twin sisters with this syndrome. The biochemical defect was first indentified in a pair of brothers with a similar presentation (Bank *et al.*, 1975).

The optimal treatment differs in the two main groups of conditions. In skeletal muscle carnitine-palmityl-transferase deficiency treatment with a high carbohydrate diet prior to exercise, and with frequent meals may be adequate. In the more severe skeletal muscle carnitine deficiency, treatment with oral carnitine and a diet rich in medium chain fatty acids is beneficial (Engel *et al.*, 1974).

Endocrine myopathies

Skeletal muscle weakness is frequently seen in conditions associated with a deficiency of some of the endocrine glands, or with an excessive activity of those glands or the administration of hormonal derivatives. Hypothyroidism is associated with slowed muscle contraction and sometimes cramps, and there may also be muscle weakness with hypertrophy. Hyperthyroidism is associated with clinical proximal muscle weakness in about a quarter of patients, and almost all thyrotoxic patients have electrophysiological evidence of skeletal muscle impairment (Walton and Bradley, 1971). Hypercorticism, whether from an adrenal cortical adenoma, or treatment with adrenocorticosteroids for prolonged periods may produce a severe proximal myopathy, often associated with type 2 fibre atrophy. The clinical importance of these diseases is that recognition of the cause of the myopathy allows effective treatment.

Deficiency myopathies

Deficiency of vitamin E in animals produces a profound necrotizing myopathy, though so far this deficiency has not been recognized as a cause of muscle disease in man (Blaxter, 1974). Vitamin D deficiency, usually in the presence of osteomalacia, and due to a number of different causes including dietary fads, malabsorption, chronic renal failure and the administration of anticonvulsant drugs, may be associated with a painful proximal myopathy (Smith and Stern, 1969; Pierides *et al.*, 1976). Muscle weakness is the predominant sign, with little or no wasting. The disease appears to be specifically due to a deficiency of vitamin D, and therapy with this vitamin is rapidly curative.

Toxic myopathies

A number of different agents, including therapeutically administered drugs, snake toxins, etc. may produce a toxic myopathy, sometimes with profound rhabdomyolysis and consequent renal failure. These conditions are however rare.

Conclusions

This review has demonstrated the very wide range of different diseases producing impairment of the neuromuscular system in man. An equally extensive list of diseases could be presented for animals. In few of the conditions is the underlying biochemical basis known, and similarly in few is there an effective treatment. A considerable amount can be done for patients with what is sometimes called symptomatic treatment. This involves physiotherapy to maintain the weak muscles in as fit a condition as possible, advice on ways of circumventing muscle weakness, and help in the adaptation of occupation, hobbies and all the everyday features of life such as the home, the car, and work. A number of appliances including braces, supports, as well as wheelchair and specially built automobiles may totally revolutionize the patient's way of life. In only a few however is there a specific treatment which can cure the patient's disease and return him to a normal life. The prognostic and genetic advice which the clinician can give about the disease may be of great importance to the patient. It enables him to plan his life, change his work if necessary, and decide whether there is a risk of passing the disease on to his children.

It is hoped that the clear understanding of the classification and character of these diseases will lead to a greater impetus to discover the underlying biochemical cause of each condition. Only in that way will it be possible to expand the list of diseases for which there is a specific therapy.

References

Aberfeld, D.C., Namba, T., Vye, M.V. and Grob, D. (1970). *Arch. Neurol. (Chic.)*, **22**, 455-462.

Afifi, A.K., Ibrahim, Z.M., Bergman, R.A., Abu Hay dai, N., Mire, J., Bahuth, N. and Kaylani, F. (1972). *J. neurol. Sci.*, **15**, 271-289.

Angelini, C. and Engel, A.G. (1972). *Arch. Neurol. (Chic.)*, **26**, 344-349.

Bank, W.J., DiMauro, S., Bonilla, E., Capuzzi, D.M. and Rowland, L.P. (1975). *New. Engl. J. Med.*, **292**, 443-449.

Barchi, R.L. (1975). *Arch. Neurol. (Chic.)*, **32**, 175-180.

Becker, P.E. (1975). *In* 'New Developments in E.M.G. and Clinical Neurophysiology'. (J. Desmedt, ed.), Vol. I, pp.407-412, Karger, Basel.

Becker, P.E. and Keiner, F. (1955). *Arch. Psychiat. Nervenkr.*, **193**, 427-448.

Blaxter, K.L. (1974). *In* 'Disorders of Voluntary Muscle'. (J.N. Walton, ed.), 3rd edition, pp.908-916, Churchill Livingstone, Edinburgh.

Boudin, G., Mikol, J., Gillard, A. and Engel, A.G. (1976). *J. neurol. Sci.*, **30**, 313-325.

Bradley, W.G. (1969). *Brain*, **92**, 345-378.

Bradley, W.G. (1974). 'Disorders of Peripheral Nerves', Blackwell, Oxford.

Bradley, W.G. (1975). *In* 'Recent Advances in Clinical Neurology', (W.B. Mathews, ed.), Churchill Livingstone, Edinburgh.

Bradley, W.G. (1978). *In* 'Handbook of Clinical Neurology', (P.J. Vinken and G.W. Bruyn, eds.) 'Diseases of Muscle'. In press.

Bradley, W.G., Fawcett, P., Jones, M.Z. and Roberts, D.F. (1977). In preparation.

Bradley, W.G. and Fulthorpe, J.J. (1977). *Neurol (Minneap)*. In press.

Bradley, W.G., Hudgson, P., Gardner-Medwin, D. and Walton, J.N. (1969). *Lancet*, 495-498.

Bradley, W.G., Price, D.L. and Watanabe, C.K. (1970). *J. Neurol. Neurosurg. Psychiat.*, **33**, 687-693.

Bradley, W.G., Hudgson, P., Larson, P.F., Papapetropoulos, T.A. and Jenkison, M. (1972a). *J. Neurol. Neurosurg. Psychiat.*, **35**, 451-455.

Bradley, W.G., Jenkison, M., Park, D.C., Hudgson, P., Gardner-Medwin, D., Pennington, R.J.T. and Walton, J.N. (1972b). *J. neurol. Sci.*, **16**, 137-154.
Bradley, W.G., Gardner-Medwin, D. and Walton, J.N. (1975). 'Recent Advances in Myology'. Proceedings of the IIIrd International Congress on Muscle Diseases. Excerpta Medica, Amsterdam.
Bradley, W.G., Tomlinson, B.E. and Hardy, M. (1978) *J. neurol. Sci.* In press.
Busch, W.A., Stromer, M.H., Goll, D.E. and Suzuki, A. (1972). *J. Cell Biol.*, **52**, 367-381.
Butterfield, D.A., Roses, A.D., Appel, S.H. and Chesnut, D.B. (1976). *Arch. Biochem. Biophys.*, **177**, 226-234.
Creutzfeldt, O.D., Abbott, B.D., Fowler, W.M. and Pearson, C.M. (1963). *Electroenceph. Clin. Neurophys.*, **15**, 508-519.
Cullen, M.J. and Fulthorpe, J.J. (1975). *J. neurol. Sci.*, **24**, 179-200.
Davis, C.J.F., Bradley, W.G. and Madrid, R. (1977). In preparation.
DeVere, R. and Bradley, W.G. (1975). *Brain*, **98**, 637-666.
Donner, M., Rapola, J. and Somer, H. (1975). *Neuropadiat.*, **6**, 239-258.
Drachman, D.A. (1968). *Arch. Neurol. (Chic.)*, **18**, 654-674.
Dubowitz, V. and Brooke, M.H. (1973). 'Muscle Biopsy: A Modern Approach'. Saunders, London.
Dubowitz, V. and Roy, S. (1970). *Brain*, **93**, 133-146.
Dyken, P.R. and Harper, P.S. (1973). *Neurol. (Minneap.)*, 465-473.
Eaton, L.M. and Lambert, E.H. (1957). *J. Amer. med. Ass.*, **163**, 1117-1124.
Elmqvist, D. and Lambert, E.H. (1968). *Proc. Mayo Clin.*, **43**, 689-713.
Emery, A.E.H. (1971). *J. med. Gen.*, **8**, 481-495.
Emery, A.E.H., Clack, E.R., Simon, S. and Taylor, J.L. (1967). *Brit. med. J.*, **ii**, 418-420.
Engel, A.G. (1970). *Proc. Mayo Clin.*, **45**, 774-814.
Engel, A.G. and Angelini, C. (1973). *Science*, **173**, 899-902.
Engel, A.G. and Dale, A.J.D. (1968). *Proc. Mayo Clin.*, **43**, 233-279.
Engel, A.G. and Gomez, M.R. (1967). *J. Neuropath. exp. Neurol.*, **26**, 601-619.
Engel, A.G. and Siekert, R.G. (1972). *Arch. Neurol.*, **27**, 174-181.
Engel, W.K., Vick, N.A., Glueck, C.J. and Levy, R.I. (1970). *New Engl. J. Med.*, **282**, 697-704.
Engel, A.G., Angelini, C. and Nelson, R.A. (1974). *In* 'Exploratory Concepts in Muscular Dystrophy'. (A.T. Milhorat, ed.). Excerpta Medica, Int. Congr. Series, 333, pp.601-617.
Feit, H. and Brooke, M.H. (1976). *Neurol. (Minneap.)*, **26**, 963-967.
Fenichel, G.M., Dettbarn, W.-D. and Newman, T.M. (1974). *Arch. Neurol. (Chic.)*, **17**, 257-260.
Gardner-Medwin, D., Hudgson, P. and Walton, J.N. (1967). *J. neurol. Sci.*, **5**, 121-158.
Gardner-Medwin, D., Pennington, R.J.T. and Walton, J.N. (1971). *J. neurol. Sci.*, **14**, 459-474.
Heffernan, L.P., Rewcastle, N.B. and Humphrey, J.G. (1968). *Arch. Neurol. (Chic.)*, **18**, 529-542.
Hirano, A., Kurland, L.T. and Sayer, G.P. (1967). *Arch. Neurol. (Chic.)*, **16**, 232-243.
Hofmann, W.W. and Smith, R.A. (1970). *Brain*, **93**, 445-474.
Hudgson, P., Bradley, W.G. and Jenkinson, M. (1972). *J. neurol. Sci.*, **16**, 137-154.
Hudgson, P. and Fulthorpe, J.J. (1975). *J. Path.*, **116**, 139-147.
Huijing, F. (1975). *Physiol. Rev.*, **55**, 609-658.
Jerusalem, F., Spiess, H. and Baumgartner, G. (1975). *J. neurol. Sci.*, **24**, 273-282.

Karpati, G., Carpenter, S., Engel, A.G., Watters, G., Allen, J., Rothman, S., Klassan, G. and Mamer, O.A. (1975). *Neurol. (Minneap.)*, **25**, 16-24.

Kearns, T.P. and Sayre, G.P. (1958). *Arch. Ophthal.*, **60**, 280-289.

Kulakowski, S., Flamand-Durand, J., Malaisse-Lagae, F., Chevallay, M. and Fardeau, M. (1973). *Arch. Franc. Ped.*, **30**, 505-526.

Luft, R.D., Ikkos, G., Palmieri, L., Ernster, L. and Afzelius, B. (1962). *J. clin. Invest.*, **41**, 1776-1804.

Lyon, M.F. (1974). *Nature (Lond.)*, **250**, 651-653.

McComas, A.J., Mrozek, K. and Bradley, W.G. (1968). *J. Neurol. Neurosurg. Psychiat.*, **31**, 448-452.

McLeod, J.G. and Prineas, J.W. (1971). *Brain*, **94**, 703-714.

Markand, O.N., North, R.R., D'Agostino, A.N. and Daly, D.D. (1969). *Neurol. (Minneap.)*, **19**, 617-633.

Markesbery, W.R., McQuillen, M.P., Procopia, P.G., Harrison, A.R. and Engel, A.G. (1974). *Arch. Neurol. (Chic.)*, **31**, 320-324.

Meadows, J.C., Marsden, C.D. and Harriman, D.G.F. (1969). *J. neurol. Sci.*, **9**, 527-550, and 551-566.

Mokri, B. and Engel, A.G. (1975). *Neurol. (Minneap.)*, **25**, 1111-1120.

Munsat, T.L. and Bradley, W.G. (1977). *Neurol. (Minneap.)*, **27**, 96-97.

Munsat, T.L., Piper, D., Cancilla, P. and Mednick, J. (1972). *Neurol. (Minneap.)*, **22**, 335-347.

Norris, F.H. and Kurland, L.T. (eds.) (1969) 'Motor Neuron Disease', Grune and Stratton, New York.

Olson, W., Engel, W.K., Walsh, G.O. and Einauglar, R. (1972). *Acta neuropath. (Berl.)*, **24**, 214-221.

Papapetropoulos, T.A. and Bradley, W.G. (1974). Excerpta Medica Int. Congress Series No. 334, Abstr. No. 211.

Pearn, J.H. and Wilson, J. (1973). *Arch. Dis. Child.*, **48**, 425-430.

Pearson, C.M. and Mostofi, F.K. (1973). *The striated muscle*. Williams and Wilkins, Baltimore.

Pierides, A.M., Ellis, H.A., Ward, M., Simpson, W., Peart, K.M., Alvarez-Ude, F., Uldall, P.R. and Kerr, D.N.A. (1976). *Brit. med. J.*, **i**, 190-193.

Ringel, S.P., Carrol, J.E. and Schold, S.C. (1977) *Arch Neurol (Chic).*, **34**, 408-416.

Roses, A.D. and Appel, S.H. (1974). *Nature (Lond.)*, **250**, 245-247.

Roses, A.D. and Appel, S.H. (1975). *J. Membrane Biol.*, **20**, 51-58.

Rowland, L.P. (1976). *Arch. Neurol. (Chic.)*, **33**, 315-321.

Rowland, L.P., Fahn, S. and Schotland, D.L. (1963). *Arch. Neurol., (Chic.)*, **9**, 325-342.

Smith, R. and Stern, G. (1969). *J. neurol. Sci.*, **8**, 511-520.

Spiro, A.J., Moore, C.L., Prineas, J.W., Strasberg, P.M. and Rapin, I. (1970). *Arch. Neurol. (Chic.)*, **23**, 103-112.

Stengel-Rutkowski, L., Scheuerbrandt, G. and Pongrantz, D. (1976). 9th Information documentation. German Research Foundation, Munich.

Stromer, M.H., Tabatabai, L.B., Robson, R.M., Goll, D.E. and Zeece, M.G. (1976). *Exper. Neurol.*, **50**, 402-421.

Sumner, D., Crawford, M.D.A. and Harriman, D.G.F. (1971). *Brain*, **94**, 51-60.

Swash, M. (1972). *Brain*, **95**, 357-368.

Thomas, P.K., Calne, D.B. and Elliott, C.F. (1972). *J. Neurol. Neurosurg. Psychiat.*, **35**, 208-215.

Thomasen, E. (1948). *Myotonia*. Munksgaard, Copenhagen.

Toop, J. and Emery, A.E.H. (1974). *Clin. Genet.*, **5**, 230-233.

Van Dyke, D.H., Griggs, R.C., Markesbery, W. and DiMauro, S. (1975). *Neurol.*

(Minneap.), **25,** 154-159.

Walton, J.N. (ed.) (1974) 'Disorders of Voluntary Muscle'. Churchill Livingstone Edinburgh.

Walton, J.N. and Bradley, W.G. (1971). *Postgrad. Med.*, **50,** 118-121.

Walton, J.N. and Nattrass, F.J. (1954). *Brain*, **77,** 169-231.

Welander, L. (1951). *Acta Neurol. Scand., Suppl.* 265.

Worsfold, M., Park, D.C. and Pennington, R.J.T. (1973). *J. neurol. Sci.*, **19,** 261-274.

Wrogemann, K. and Pena, S.D.J. (1976). *Lancet*, **i,** 672-673.

Zintz, R. (1966). *In* 'Progressive Muskeldystrophie, Myotonia, Myasthenie', (E. Kuhn, ed.), Springer, Berlin.

Myasthenia Gravis

4 Myasthenia gravis: a clinical approach to pathogenesis

JOHN A. SIMPSON

Institute of Neurological Sciences, Southern General Hospital, Glasgow

In teaching the logic of clinical diagnosis to medical students it is valuable to group the data obtained from questioning and examining patients as answers to three questions 'Where, What, and Why?' – more formally, the localization, the pathology, and the aetiology of the disease process. The scientifically trained student will also ask 'How does the lesion produce the functional defect?' Concentration on the last question has, paradoxically, retarded understanding of myasthenia gravis.

Where is the lesion?

Myasthenia is a term to describe muscular weakness which increases with maintained or repeated contraction of skeletal muscle and is reduced by rest. The contraction may be voluntary, reflex or electrically provoked, but only if the electrical stimulus is applied to the motor nerve. The response to direct stimulation of the muscle fibre is normal, and the propagated action potential of the motor nerve fibre is also normal. It is therefore a reasonable conclusion that the disorder is at the neuromuscular junction, a conclusion supported by the therapeutic finding that anticholinesterase drugs such as neostigmine decrease the weakness whereas sensitivity to D-tubocurarine is increased.

A myasthenic disorder may be found in a number of diseases involving lower motor neurones or muscle (Simpson, 1966a). It is a sign of loss of the safety factor for transmission which is normally present and which can be reduced in several ways. The disease entity termed Myasthenia Gravis is characterized by a severe defect of neuromuscular transmission without clinical evidence of a motor neurone disease or of a myopathy in the usual sense. (There is a little evidence of dysfunction of the contractile mechanism but it is not the primary disorder). There is recent evidence from single fibre electromyography and the new methods for endplate receptor microscopy that the disease process may involve all motor endplates in skeletal muscle but the disorder is more severe, or involves more endplates, in certain muscles. This gives rise to a characteristic distribution though the exact pattern differs from patient to patient. The (statistical) order of appearance and the severity of clinical weakness are shown in Fig. 1 (Simpson, 1960). Thus the typical patient has drooping eyelids, double vision, weakness of face and jaw muscles, then of the neck and proximal muscles of the upper limbs, spreading ultimately to the muscles of respiration and swallowing − a combination dangerous to life (Fig. 2). The distribution is rarely symmetrical and the weakness varies remarkably. In one week the right eyelid may droop and in the next it may be the left. Weakness is increased by emotional stress or by exercising the appropriate muscle, and relieved by rest. Complete remission for weeks, months or years may occur. Atrophy of muscle is found in 10% of cases but is not an early feature and virtually confined to certain muscles, not within the distribution of any particular peripheral nerve. Furthermore the muscle stretch reflexes are retained and often unusually brisk. With rare exceptions sensation is not affected. Power is temporarily restored by anticholinesterase drugs.

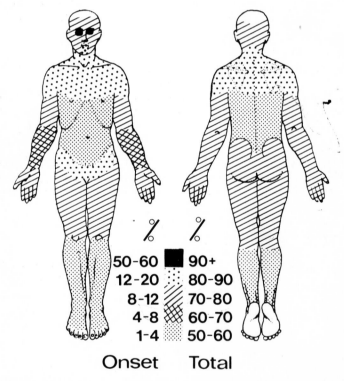

Fig. 1. The left of the key shows the percentage of various muscle groups involved at the onset, and the right of the key the percentage involved at some time during the course of myasthenia gravis. Note the early onset and frequent involvement of extra-ocular muscles and orbiculares oculi, then bulbar, neck and shoulder girdle muscles.

All these features lead to the conclusion that the disease causes a defect of transmission at the neuromuscular junctions which is disproportionate in certain muscles. On the other hand the function of other cholinergic synapses in the central nervous system and the peripheral autonomic nervous sytem is apparently normal.

How does the functional deficit occur?

From the time the disease myasthenia gravis was identified by Erb and Goldflam a century ago, the main interest has been in the mechanism of the muscular weakness. It is unnecessary to review the theories, all of which are essentially pharmacological analogues or models based on topical interests, an approach which led to bitter arguments between supporters of presynaptic, postsynaptic and 'myasthenic toxin' theories. Critical analysis leads to the conclusion that there is a disorder of all three types (Simpson, 1969) though recent developments have concentrated attention on the lesion of the receptors and on the antibody 'myasthenic toxin' so long denied since I first suggested it in 1960. The fatal flaw in all the models has been the failure to recognize that the pharmacology of the normal neuromuscular junction does not apply to one which is morpho- logically abnormal (Simpson, 1971). Having reiterated this warning, I leave further discussion on the mechanism of transmission failure to other speakers in this Symposium, with the observation that concentration on the proximate mechanism was responsible for failure to appreciate the true nature of the disease. The clues were already in the literature of the early 20th century. They disappeared after 1934 when it was confirmed that acetylcholine is a neuromuscular transmitter and this concentrated all attention on biochemical models of myasthenia gravis. The fallacies immediately become obvious if we proceed to the other elementary questions taught to the clinical student.

What is the pathology of the lesion?

The physician at the bedside makes a conclusion about the hidden pathology of disease by reading the 'pathological clock'. In this stage of the diagnostic logic the details of localization take second place to the natural history of the illness (how it has evolved) which is then related to the time course of the major categories of pathological processes. In addition the physician looks for the tissue specificity of the disease. Does it involve a number of organs or is it confined to one (or a few) cell lines, which would suggest a biochemical disorder?

Since the early descriptions of myasthenia gravis it has been recognized that severe illness may be followed by complete remission and then by later relapses. I have pointed out that it is unusual to have more than one or two complete remissions and that these are more likely to occur during the first 5-10 years of the illness. Later remissions are usually less complete and the disease then enters a stage of relative stability, still responsive to anticholinesterase medication but with less danger to life but, conversely, with less potential for improvement by the operation of thymectomy. Finally there may be a stage of permanent weakness with little response to anticholinesterases (Fig. 3, Simpson, 1974). In this stage atrophy may occur, especially in the extraocular muscles, the tongue (Fig. 2) and the triceps humeri muscles. Previously termed 'myasthenic myopathy', modern histochemical studies indicate that the atrophy of stage 3 is of denervation type (Fenichel and Shy, 1963). There is increasing evidence that the pathological process may be arrested or reversed, even at stage 3, by long-term administration of corticosteroids.

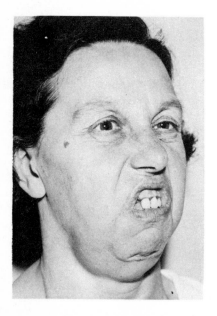 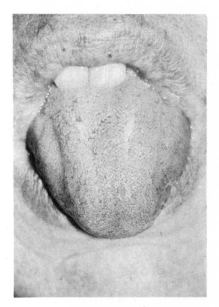

Fig. 2. (a) A myasthenic patient showing her teeth. Note the vertical snarl, left ptosis and paresis of left external rectus oculi. (b) Same patient. Early stage of the triple grooved tongue.

In 1960 I pointed out that this natural history (early relapses and remissions with progressively irreversible change) has resemblances to allergic disease and connective tissue diseases (notably systemic lupus erythematosus) which were then beginning to be recognized as immunological in nature. At the same time (Simpson, 1960) I drew attention to previously unrecognized correlations with a number of disorders of other organs – 'rheumatoid' arthritis, pernicious anaemia, sarcoidosis and other lymphoproliferative disease, and diabetes mellitus. At the same time it was pointed out that the known linkage between myasthenia gravis and thyrotoxicosis was only part of the story. Myasthenia gravis is linked (in the same individual and also in siblings) with all non-malignant diseases of the thyroid and there is no necessary temporal sequence, making it unlikely that myasthenia is *caused* by thyrotoxicosis as had been suggested by many earlier authors. In a Honyman-Gillespie Lecture in Edinburgh on 28 April 1960 in which I made the first complete proposal that myasthenia gravis was an autoimmune disease, I showed a section of thyroid gland as possible Hashimoto's disease. This was omitted from the published version as the pathologists were undecided, but I later published it (Simpson, 1966b) and also a confirmed case of Hashimoto's disease (and incidentally vitiligo) in myasthenia gravis after thymectomy (Simpson, 1964). Reviewing the relationship between myasthenia gravis and disorders of the thyroid gland (Simpson, 1960, 1968) it is apparent that they are genetically-linked diseases with a related immunopathology. More recently other 'autoimmune' diseases have been recognized in myasthenics such as Sjögren's disease (Downes *et al.*, 1966; Simpson, 1966b), pemphigus vulgaris (Wolf *et al.*, 1966; Vetters *et al.*, 1973) and ulcerative colitis (Alarćon-Segovia *et al.*, 1963).

It was the natural history and the related non-muscular diseases that suggested to me that myasthenia gravis was a disease of the same type as systemic lupus erythematosus which is sometimes associated with myasthenia (Harvey *et al.*, 1954). Lymphorrhages in muscles had been described for many years in myasthenic patients but were considered non-specific by Russell (1953) because of their prevalence in other diseases. Most of those listed by Russell would now be regarded as having immunological abnormalities. It was also believed that there were no histological abnormalities at the neuromuscular junction until Coërs and Desmedt (1959) demonstrated consistent morphological changes, a finding recently extended by electronmicroscopy. This review does not require a full account of these changes. It is enough to point out that (i) they are sufficient to account for loss of the safety factor of transmission and certain abnormal responses to drugs in myasthenics (Simpson, 1969, 1971) and (ii) they withdraw validity from pharmacological 'models' of myasthenia (Simpson, 1971), (iii) the changes indicate cycles of degeneration and active but abnormal regeneration of motor nerve terminals as well as of endplates of muscle. This is important as the variability of the clinical state could indicate a balance between a degenerative lesion (possibly immunological) and a restorative one.

So the tentative answer to the question 'what is the lesion?' is that the symptoms and signs can be accounted for by an active lesion on both sides of the neuromuscular junction, but also in other organs, with a natural history which suggests an immunological disease.

Why has it occured?

The question of aetiology is the crucial one for designing therapy and providing a prognosis. At this point in the diagnostic logic the clinician should ask four questions: (i) is the disease of the presenting organ(s) secondary to abnormal function of another organ? (ii) does it occur randomly or is it age or sex linked? (iii) is the primary organ damage determined genetically or by an environmental factor − or both? (iv) is the disease transmissible to other human or animal subjects?

The primary defect. It has been recognized since the beginning of the century that 10-15% of myasthenic patients have a tumour of the thymus gland of the mixed epithelial lymphocytic type. In others the organ was considered to be 'hypertrophic'. In fact the glands removed from myasthenic patients are rarely larger than normal and the change of size with age is within normal limits. Castleman and Norris (1949) pointed out that the significant abnormality is the unusual number of 'germinal centres' in the cortex and medulla of the thymus, even in those cases with a thymoma. Furthermore, the early conflict of opinion regarding the therapeutic value of thymectomy was resolved when it was shown (Simpson, 1958) that the best results obtained from removal of the non-tumour gland, and especially if this was removed during Stage 1 (Fig. 3). However, myasthenia may relapse years after thymectomy or may even occur for the first time after removal of the gland (for other indications), and there is no correlation between the therapeutic benefit from thymectomy and the number of

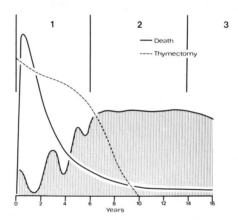

Fig. 3. The three stages of myasthenia gravis. The time scale is an average one. In the active stage (1) there are major relapses and remissions, most of the mortality, but also best response to thymectomy. In the inactive stage (2) there are fewer deaths or severe relapses but also fewer remissions and less response to thymectomy. In the burned out stage (3) there is no response to thymectomy and resistance to anticholinesterase drugs but improvement may occur spontaneously or with steroids.

germinal centres in the gland (Vetters and Simpson, 1974). These facts make it impossible to accept that the gland produces a neuromuscular blocking substance as in earlier theories and more recently advocated by Goldstein (1968, for review). Although it was then regarded as an endocrine gland, Simpson (1960) was impressed with its lymphoid structure and suggested a cellular and humoral mediated immunological function leading to structural damage of neuromuscular junctions and production of antibodies against AChR protein and other tissues. As this hypothesis preceded the paper by Miller (1961) which established the immunological role of the thymus, it is necessary to examine the reason for postulating a receptor-blocking antibody *(vide infra)*. The immunological work of the next 10 years established that immunological reactivity could persist after removal of the thymus and this aspect will not be pursued in this paper.

Age and sex distributions: Myasthenia gravis occurs in every race. Estimates of prevalence range from 1 in 50,000 to 1 in 10,000 of the population. There is a distinct difference between the tumour and non-tumour types. If the age at onset of symptoms is charted for those without a thymoma (Fig. 4), both sexes show a modal age of 20 years with 4.5 females to 1 male in the under 30's, changing to an equal incidence or slight male preponderance in later life − a distribution found in systemic lupus erythematosus and other connective tissue disease. Patients with a thymoma, on the other hand, have a modal age of 45 years and account for 30% of cases starting over the age of 40 years. There is no significant sex difference for the latter group. Whatever 'causes' myasthenia gravis, young women are more susceptible, but the relative insusceptibility of later life is lost if a thymoma occurs.

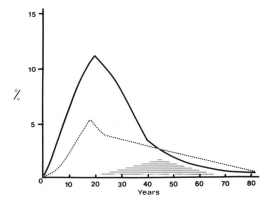

Fig. 4. Age at first symptoms of myasthenia gravis (percent of total cases). The solid line indicates age of onset for females without thymoma, the dotted line the onset age for males without thymoma. The hatched area indicates the ages of onset of cases of both sexes with a thymoma.

Genetic or environmental factors? Cases of myasthenia gravis in more than one generation of a family are rare. Less rare are same generation cases starting in early childhood (Congenital Myasthenia). If these are excluded, because some workers do not accept that they have 'true' myasthenia gravis, the existence of a genetic mechanism is considered to be not definitely established (Herrmann, 1966; Jacob *et al.*, 1969). However, I have drawn attention to the possibility of alternative gene expression (as thyroid disease or non-myasthenic autoimmune disease), a concept given limited support by the study of Bundey (1972). Recently it has become clear that there is an association between myasthenia gravis and at least one of the human histocompatibility antigens HLA-B8, though this is not an essential precursor of myasthenia gravis (for review, see Dick *et al.*, 1975). Eddleston and Williams (1974) suggest that the HLA-B8 antigen may be a marker of defective suppressor T-cell function. Genetic factors probably constitute risk factors for autoimmune diseases but the relative scarcity of familial cases indicates that the causation is multifactorial. We have no evidence for the nature of manifesting factors, but this is now the most important aspect of research.

Is the disease transmissible? The possibility of a 'curare-like substance' in the blood stream has been considered for a century and, in the last half of that era, that it could be formed in the thymus. There has never been acceptable evidence of transfer of the disease from one adult human to another by plasma or serum, and Nastuk *et al.* (1959) discredited all claims to cause block of neuromuscular transmission *in vitro*. Nevertheless there is one important fact which must be accounted for in any theory of myasthenia gravis. A myasthenic mother commonly (1 in 7 live births) has a baby which is myasthenic for the first few weeks of life and then recovers. The duration of this effect and the apparent restriction of passive transfer to her own child suggested to me that the neuromuscular block could be due to an antibody raised by the mother against her own ACh receptors and active only against those of her genetically similar offspring (Simpson, 1960). It could not be the 'thymin' postulated by Goldstein as this neonatal type of myasthenia still occurs after thymectomy. For many years it was impossible to test the hypothesis because the postulated antibody could not be detected and isolated, or else the test preparations were too insensitive to detect the presence of blocking substances in the serum of myasthenic patients. Using the more sensitive indicators now available (reduction in amplitude of miniature endplate potentials, or reduction in number of acetylcholine receptors at neuromuscular junctions), it is now claimed that serum IgG from myasthenic patients induces characteristic changes in the muscle endplates of mice when passively transferred (Toyka *et al.*, 1975, 1977). Though we have not been able to reproduce this work (Rees *et al.*, 1977) it looks very convincing. It is exactly the mechanism I postulated in 1960. Is it immunological?

The immunological status of myasthenia gravis

It would need another chapter to do justice to this aspect. But for the present purposes some short conclusions will be sufficient to concentrate attention on the essentials which remain for the research of the '80s. (i) It is now fully accepted that there is clinical overlap between myasthenia gravis and many diseases now recognized as 'autoimmune' (Simpson 1960, 1964, 1977). (ii) For 16 years we have known that myasthenic patients produce antibodies against skeletal muscle, thyroid, rheumatoid factor, anti-nuclear factor and other tissues (Strauss *et al.*, 1960; van der Geld *at al.*, 1963). Only recently, with new techniques described elsewhere in this book (Chapter 9), is it confirmed that the blood of myasthenics has a high titre of anti-AChR globulin (Almon *et al.*, 1974; Lindstrom *et al.*, 1976). (iii) There is some evidence of cell-mediated immunity against muscle and thymus (Behan *et al.*, 1975). (iv) An experimental model of myasthenia gravis can be produced in a wide range of mammals immunized with AChR protein from the eel electroplax (Patrick and Lindstrom, 1973; Engel *et al.*, 1976). These are, of course, exciting events. Placed in a long term conspectus they show (a) that the proposed immunological lesion of neuromuscular junctions is reasonable and likely, and (b) that it is part of a breakdown of immunological tolerance involving a number of tissues. Some alterations in plasma proteins (Simpson, 1966c) and particularly a low level of serum IgA (which is T-cell dependent) in some myasthenics (Simpson *et al.*, 1976; Behan *et al.*, 1976) point to an immunodeficiency type of autoimmune disease with defective T-cell function. This could be genetic or secondary to neoplasia or other disorder of the thymus.

Conclusions

It has not been possible in the available space to give a full discussion of many important aspects. For that reason the bibliography of this chapter refers to personal and other papers with fuller discussion of controversial points, or to the first description of significant findings. At the time of this review I feel reasonably certain that we have the answers to Where, What, and How? The 'Why' question remains the important one. What is the link between genes, thymus and autoimmunity? Is there a trigger that fires a pre-loaded gun? Is it a virus, hormonal, even psychosomatic? These are now the important questions in myasthenic research. For decades it was side tracked into arguments about neuromuscular transmission and then about antibodies which are epiphenomena. Now that we can mimic the end stage of the immunological lesion it would be tragic if we are again side tracked from the only questions that will lead to prevention or cure of myasthenia gravis.

References
Alarćon-Segovia, D., Galbraith, R.F., Malnado, J.E. and Howard, F.M. (1963). *Lancet,* **ii,** 662-665.
Almon, R.R., Andrew, C.G. and Appel, S.H. (1974). *Science,* **186,** 55-57.
Behan, P.O., Simpson, J.A. and Behan, W.M.H. (1976). *Lancet,* **ii,** 593-594.
Behan, W.M.H., Behan, P.O. and Simpson, J.A. (1975). *J. Neurol. Neurosurg. Psychiat.,* **38,** 1039-1047.
Bundey, S. (1972). *J. Neurol. Neurosurg. Psychiat.,* **35,** 41-51.
Castleman, B. and Norris, E.H. (1949). *Medicine (Baltimore),* **28,** 27-58.
Coërs, C. and Desmedt, J.E. (1959). *Acta neurol. Belg.,* **59,** 539-561.
Dick, H.M., Behan, P.O., Simpson, J.A. and Durward, W.F. (1975). *J. Immunogenet.,* **1,** 401-412.
Downes, J.M., Greenwood, B.M. and Wray, S.H. (1966). *Quart. J. Med.,* **35,** 85-105.
Eddleston, A.L.W.F. and Williams, R. (1974). *Lancet,* **ii,**1543-1545.
Engel, A.G., Tsujihata, M., Lambert, E.H., Lindstrom, J.M. and Lennon, V.A. (1976). *J. Neuropathol. exp. Neurol.,* **35,** 569-587.
Fenichel, G.M. and Shy, G.M. (1963). *Arch. Neurol. (Chic.),* **9,** 237-243.
Goldstein, G. (1968). *Lancet,* **ii,** 119-124.
Harvey, A.M., Shulman, L.E., Tumulty, P.A., Conley, C.L. and Schoenrich, E.H. (1954). *Medicine (Baltimore),* **33,** 291-437.
Herrmann, C. (1966). *Neurology (Minneap.),* **16,** 75-85.
Jacob, A., Clack, E.R. and Emery, A.E.H. (1968). *J. Med. Genet.,* **5,** 257-261.
Lindstrom, J.M., Lennon, V.A., Seybold, M.E. and Whittingham, S. (1976). *Ann. N.Y. Acad. Sci.,* **274,** 254-274.
Miller, J.F.A.P. (1961). *Lancet,* **ii,** 748-749.
Nastuk, W.L., Strauss, A.J.L. and Osserman, K.E. (1959). *Amer. J. Med.,* **26,** 394-409.
Patrick, J. and Lindstrom, J. (1973). *Science,* **180,** 871-872.
Rees, D., Behan, P.O., Behan, W.H. and Simpson, J.A. (1977). *In* 'Seventh Symposium on Current Research in Muscular Dystrophy'. Abstract 16. Muscular Dystrophy Group of Great Britain.
Russell, D.S. (1953). *J. Path. Bact.,* **65,** 279-289.
Simpson, J.A. (1958). *Brain,* **81,** 112-144.
Simpson, J.A. (1960). *Scot. med. J.,* **5,** 419-436.
Simpson, J.A. (1964). *J. Neurol. Neurosurg. Psychiat.,* **27,** 485-492.
Simpson, J.A. (1966a). *Proc. roy. Soc. Med.,* **59,** 993-998.
Simpson, J.A. (1966b). *Ann. N.Y. Acad. Sci.,* **135,** 506-516.
Simpson, J.A. (1966c). *In* 'Progressive Muskeldystrophie, Myotonie, Myasthenie' (E. Kuhn, ed), pp.339-349. Springer-Verlag, Berlin.
Simpson, J.A. (1968). *In* 'Research in Muscular Dystrophy. Proceedings of the 4th Symposium' (Members of the Research Committee of the Muscular Dystrophy Group, eds), pp.31-41. Pitman Medical Publishing Co. Ltd., London.
Simpson, J.A. (1969). *In* 'The Biological Basis of Medicine − 3' (E.E. Bittar and N. Bittar, eds), pp.345-387. Academic Press, London and New York.
Simpson, J.A. (1971). *Ann. N.Y. Acad. Sci.,* **183,** 241-247.
Simpson, J.A. (1974). *In* 'Neurology. Proceedings of the X International Congress of Neurology, Barcelona, Spain, 1973'. (A. Subirana and J.M. Espadaler, eds), pp.399-411. Excerpta Medica, Amsterdam.
Simpson, J.A. (1977). *Scot. Med. J.,* **22,** 201-210.
Simpson, J.A., Behan, P.O. and Dick, H. (1976). *Ann. N.Y. Acad. Sci.,* **274,** 382-389.

Strauss, A.J.L., Seegal, B.C., Hsu, K.C., Burkholder, P.M., Nastuk, W.L. and Osserman, K.E. (1960). *Proc. Soc. exp. Biol. Med.*, **105**, 184-191.

Toyka, K.V., Drachman, D.B., Pestronk, A. and Kao, I. (1975). *Science*, **190**, 397-399.

Toyka, K.V., Drachman, D.B., Griffin, D.E., Pestronk, A., Winkelstein, J.A., Fischbeck, K.H. and Kao, I. (1977). *New. Engl. J. Med.*, **296**, 125-131.

Van Der Geld, H., Feltkamp, T.E.W., Van Loghem, T.J., Oosterhuis, H.J.G.H. and Biemond, A. (1963). *Lancet*, **ii,** 373-375.

Vetters, J.M. and Simpson, J.A. (1974). *J. Neurol. Neurosurg. Psychiat.*, **37,** 1139-1145.

Vetters, J.M., Saikia, N.K., Wood, J. and Simpson, J.A. (1973). *Brit. J. Dermatol.*, **88,** 437-441.

Wolf, S.M., Rowland, L.P., Schotland, D.L., McKinney, A.S., Hoefer, P.F.A. and Aranow, H. (1966). *Ann. N.Y. Acad. Sci.*, **135,** 517-534.

5 Neuromuscular transmission in myasthenia gravis and the significance of anti-acetylcholine receptor antibodies

Y. ITO · R. MILEDI · P.C. MOLENAAR · J. NEWSOM DAVIS*
R. POLAK† AND ANGELA VINCENT

Dept. of Biophysics, University College London WC1E 6BT.

Introduction

Weakness in myasthenia gravis (MG) has been attributed to a defect in neuromuscular transmission ever since Mary Walker noticed the similarity between patients suffering from this illness and animals treated with curare (1934). Early observations suggested the presence of a circulating 'curare-like' blocking substance, but the results of applying serum to nerve-muscle preparations, both *in vivo* and *in vitro*, were often conflicting, and confused in some instances by the presence of cytolytic activity in the serum (for review see Osserman, 1969).

In support of a postsynaptic defect Grob *et al.* (1956) found similarities between the electromyographical responses in MG and in lightly curarized normal subjects, and their results (Johns *et al.*, 1956) using intra-arterial acetylcholine (ACh) injection suggested an abnormal response of the post-synaptic acetylcholine receptors (AChR) to ACh. On the other hand Desmedt (1958) found striking similarities between the post-tetanic be-haviour of muscle responses in MG and in cats treated with hemicholinium — a drug which blocks ACh synthesis. This observation was not borne out, however, when results of the first intracellular recordings from MG and control human muscle (Elmqvist *et al.*, 1960, 1964; Dahlbäck *et al.*, 1961) were published. These suggested a defect in ACh packaging, or the release of a false transmitter, but did not support the concept of a block in ACh synthesis.

In the last few years interest has swung again to the postsynaptic side. Morphological changes at the neuromuscular junction in MG are large-ly postsynaptic (Santa *et al.*, 1972); postsynaptic acetylcholine recep-tors are reduced in numbers at the endplate (Fambrough *et al.*, 1973; Green *et al.*, 1975a); and the introduction of an animal model in which immuniza-tion against purified AChR results in clinical, morphological and physio-

* Dept. of Neurology, Royal Free Hospital, London N.W.3 2QG.
† Medical Biological Laboratory, T.N.O., Rijswijk-Z.H., The Netherlands.

logical changes characteristic of MG (See Chapters 9 and 16; Green *et al.*, 1975b) suggests the possibility of a similar autoimmune reaction against the postsynaptic membrane in the human disease.

Neuromuscular transmission

Electrophysiology

According to the quantal hypothesis acetylcholine is released from the motor nerve terminal in packets or quanta (Katz, 1969), diffuses across the synaptic cleft and binds to acetylcholine receptors which are an integral part of the postsynaptic membrane. This interaction results in the opening of ion channels permeable to small cations, sodium ions enter the muscle fibre and cause it to become depolarized. The depolarization is brief and can be recorded by an intracellular electrode (see Fig. 1). When a nerve impulse reaches the nerve terminal about 100 packets of ACh are released more or less simultaneously and the resulting depolarization, the endplate potential or e.p.p., rises above the threshold of the muscle fibre and initiates an action potential, which propagates along the fibre and results in contraction of the myofibrils. In the absence of nerve impulses small depolarizations (miniature e.p.p.s or m.e.p.p.) can be recorded which are due to the spontaneous release of single quanta of ACh. Their amplitude in various vertebrate species is around 1 mV but depends on several factors such as the input resistance and membrane potential of the fibre.

Healthy human muscle: There has been relatively little electrophysiology performed on isolated human muscle because of the difficulty in obtaining

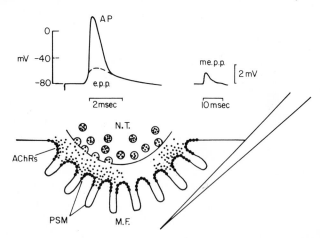

Fig. 1. Diagramatical representation of a neuromuscular junction. NT, nerve terminal; M.F., muscle fibre; PSM, postsynaptic membrane; AChR, acetylcholine receptor; e.p.p., endplate potential; m.e.p.p., miniature e.p.p.; A.P., action potential.

suitable material. Arm or leg muscle, as used for histochemistry, is not ideal because the muscle fibres are several centimetres long and it is difficult to remove intact fibres. Fortunately transmission in normal human muscle seems to be essentially similar to that in other mammals (Elmqvist *et al.*, 1960). Most work has been done on intercostal muscle biopsies taken during thoracotomy from patients with pulmonary or cardiac disease. The electrical properties of the fibres are somewhat similar to those of rat muscle, and the amplitude of m.e.p.p. is about 0.8 mV. M.e.p.p. frequency however was only about 0.2 per second rather than 1 per second as in the rat (Elmqvist *et al.*, 1960). Nerve stimulation resulted in the release of about 60 quanta of ACh (Elmqvist *et al.*, 1964), and as in other mammals repetitive stimulation caused a run down in the amplitude of e.p.p. due to a reduction in the number of quanta released.

Myasthenia gravis: Elmqvist *et al.* (1964) described two major differences between control human muscle and muscle from patients with MG. The first was the reduced amplitude of the m.e.p.p. which were about 20% of control values. Secondly there was failure of transmission at many endplates — the e.p.p. was simply not large enough to rise above threshold — and at other endplates failure of transmission resulted after only a few stimuli at low frequency. This was not due to any change in the threshold or in the quantum content, i.e. the number of quanta released per impulse. Moreover, during continuous stimulation there was no further reduction in e.p.p. or m.e.p.p. size as occurs during treatment with hemicholinium (Elmqvist *et al.*, 1965). They also obtained an estimate of the total number of releasable quanta by stimulation in the presence of hemicholinium to block all further synthesis of transmitter, and concluded that there was no appreciable difference from control values. Their data indicated that the effectiveness of each quantum was reduced and suggested either a presynaptic defect in the packaging or release of ACh, or a defect in the postsynaptic sensitivity to released ACh. Since depolarization achieved by bath-applied carbachol was the same in both control muscle and that from patients with MG they concluded that the defect was most likely to be presynaptic (Elmqvist *et al.*, 1964). They also suggested the possibility of a 'false' transmitter which could be packaged and released, but would be unable to initiate depolarization.

Albuquerque *et al.* (1976b) have recently published data from 5 patients with MG and found a less marked reduction in m.e.p.p. amplitude (to about 35%). On the other hand they found some muscle fibres where they were unable to record any postsynaptic activity, either spontaneous or evoked, in spite of being satisfied that they had located the endplate. They have also made a more detailed evaluation of ACh sensitivity. Depolarization of the muscle fibre can be achieved artifically by application of ACh through an iontophoretic pipette. The technique of iontophoresis has enaabled physiologists to map the distribution of AChR in normal and experimental muscle (e.g. Miledi, 1960). Albuquerque *et al.* have found that the ACh sensitivity is significantly reduced at the endplate area of MG muscle. Furthermore, this reduction was greatest at endplates where no e.p.p. could be found. On the other hand they found no change in the area of ACh sensitivity at the endplate, and particularly noticed the complete lack of extra-junctional sensitivity which would have suggested denervation of the fibres (see Axelsson and Thesleff, 1959; Miledi, 1960).

We have correlated m.e.p.p. amplitude with alpha-bungarotoxin binding (see below) in biopsies from MG and control patients (Ito *et al.*, 1977a). The muscle was taken through the thymectomy incision and was therefore parasternal intercostal rather than lateral intercostal. M.e.p.p. amplitude was found to vary from patient to patient but in each of them the mean amplitude was reduced. Many of our recordings were done in the presence of prostigmine, which by preventing ACh hydrolysis increases the amplitude and duration of depolarization as shown in Fig. 2(a). M.e.p.p. from MG biopsies (Fig. 2(b) and (c)) are markedly reduced even in the presence of prostigmine. Fig. 3(a) illustrates the amplitude distribution of m.e.p.p. in a typical control and an MG fibre, showing in this case an overall reduction

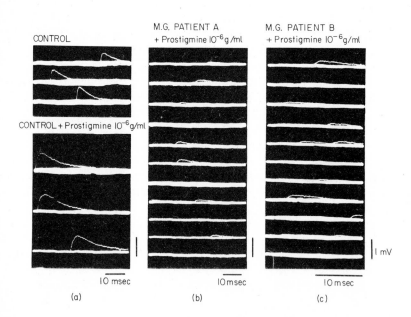

Fig. 2. M.e.p.p. recorded intracellularly from control and MG endplates: (a) control m.e.p.p. in normal solution (top) and with 10^{-6} g/ml prostigmine (bottom) show the increase in amplitude and time-course which is observed in the presence of an anticholinesterase. (b) and (c), m.e.p.p. from 2 different MG biopsies show a marked reduction in amplitude even in the presence of prostigmine. Vertical bar, 1 mV; Horizontal bars, 10 msec.

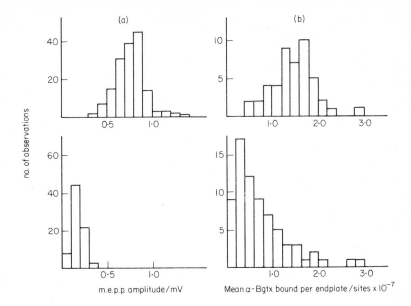

Fig. 3. M.e.p.p. amplitude distribution and alpha-bungarotoxin binding distribution in control and muscle from patients with MG: (a) amplitude histograms from 1 typical control fibre (resting potential −79 mV) in normal ringer (top), and from 1 typical MG fibre (−71 mV) in prostigmine ringer (bottom). (b) histograms of the average no. of specific α-Bgtx binding sites per endplate in bundles of muscle fibres taken from 6 controls (top) and 11 patients with MG (bottom). (In each case the binding to a similar length of muscle fibres without endplates has been subtracted). Note the shift to lower values in MG. Ordinates: no. of observations. Abscissa: (a) m.e.p.p. amplitude /mV. (b) average α-Bgtx bound per endplate/ sites $\times$ 10^{-7}.

to about 25%, and the mean values from each patient are given in Table 1. We, too, have found no evidence of denervation hypersensitivity in MG.

Acetylcholine in human muscle:

Previous studies of ACh content and ACh release from motor terminals have been few and limited mainly to measurements in which biological assays were used (e.g. Krjnević and Mitchell, 1961). We have measured ACh directly using mass fragmentography − a recently developed chemical method which has the advantage of being specific and highly sensitive (Jenden et al., 1973; Polak and Molenaar, 1974).

Values for the ACh content of human muscle are shown in Table 1. In eight out of nine patients with MG there was a significant increase in the ACh content of muscle bundles extracted 15 mins − 3 hours after biopsy. In spite of this neither the resting release nor the release in the presence of 50 mM K^+ was different in four and five biopsies respectively (Ito et al., 1976). An important additional finding in this study was the absence of a false transmitter. Mass fragmentography allows the recognition of many

TABLE 1
SUMMARY OF DATA FROM 9 PATIENTS WITH MG

CLASSIFICATION			M.E.P.P. AMP[1] (mV) Prostigmine 10^{-6}g/ml		α-BgTX BINDING[2] (sites × 10^{-7} per end-plate)	ACh CONTENT (picomoles per gram wet wt.)	END PLATE LENGTH (sarcomeres)
Age	Grade	AntiChE	+	−			
28	IV	+	0.59 ± .13		0.70 ± .20	719	16.9 ± 2.3
22	IIB	+	0.73 ± .13		2.39 ± .23	498	13.6 ± 2.7
18	IIB	+	0.37 ± .12	0.26 ± .10	0.64 ± .18	360	15.9 ± 5.8
27	IIB	+	0.19 ± .04		0.51 ± .11	95	13.3 ± 3.9
54	IV	+	0.26 ± .10		0.61 ± .22	335	9.9 ± 1.7
18	III	+	0.23 ± .06		0.51 ± .16	284	15.2 ± 5.8
54	IV	−	0.44 ± .16		0.79 ± .13	293	13.3 ± 3.9
36	IIB	±	0.33 ± .08		0.24 ± .24	709	15.7 ± 5.6
48	IIB	−	0.24 ± 0.3	0.17 ± .01	0.38 ± .03	279	8.4 ± 1.6
MEAN ± S.D.			0.38 ± .18	0.22 ± .06	0.75 ± .64	396 ± 207	13.6 ± 2.8
CONTROLS MEAN ± S.D.			0.97 ± 0.10	0.68 ± .03	1.55 ± .34	184 ± 46	7.6 + 0.4

1. Mean ± S.E.M. from 4-14 fibres; corrected to −80 mV.
2. Mean ± S.E.M. from 3-8 bundles of muscle fibres.

different choline esters which appear as distinct peaks on the chromatograms. There was no evidence of any choline ester besides ACh in these muscle biopsies.

Morphology of the neuromuscular junction

Light microscopy: Cöers and Desmedt (1959) have examined the neuromuscular junction in muscle from patients with MG by a number of techniques including vital staining with methylene blue which stains the unmyelinated nerve terminals, and cholinesterase staining which demonstrates the subneural apparatus. On the basis of their results Cöers (1975) has suggested two main classes of endplates in MG: 1. dysplastic or elongated endplates found mostly in young female patients and 2. dystrophic endplates with distal branching of motor axons forming expanded arborizations. They also found in older patients an increase in the terminal innervation ratio − that is the number of muscle fibres innervated by each nerve fibre − and this was sometimes associated with changes in the muscle fibres themselves suggesting a denervation process. We have measured the length of cholinesterase-stained endplates in our biopsies and the results (expressed as the number of adjacent sarcomeres) are found in Table 1. In all but one patient the mean endplate length was increased. The exception was a woman who had not had anticholinesterase treatment, but one other untreated patient did have elongated endplates.

Electron microscopy: Ultrastructural studies of the neuromuscular junction in disease need to take account of the wide variation found in sections of normal endplates, particularly after different methods of fixation. Early workers reported marked abnormalities of the endplate in MG but only Engel and his colleagues have applied histometric techniques to quantifying their findings. They found no significant change in the size or number per unit area of synaptic vesicles (Santa *et al.*, 1972), changes which might have given support to a presynaptic defect. In contrast the length of postsynaptic membrane on cross-section was reduced to 40% and there was also a reduction in the area of the presynaptic nerve terminal. Many endplates looked immature with a reduction in the number and depth of postsynaptic folds, and widening of the synaptic cleft. These abnormalities resembled those seen in developing neuromuscular junctions and may represent simultaneous processes of degeneration and repair. Similar changes were found by Albuquerque *et al.* (1976b) who also noticed 'fuzzy-coated' vesicular remnants of degenerating folds and the presence of various types of leucocytes at the affected endplates.

Alpha-bungarotoxin binding

The technique of acetylcholine iontophoresis does not allow a quantitative analysis of acetylcholine receptors, for this a more biochemical approach was required. This was provided by the discovery of a polypeptide in the venom of Bungarus multicinctus, the Formosan banded krait, which blocks neuromuscular transmission by binding specifically to the AChR in an essentially irreversible manner. (Chang and Lee, 1963, Miledi and Potter, 1971). This toxin is easily purified and can be labelled radioactively to high specific activity with very little reduction in its activity. Since this discovery many groups have used the labelled toxin to map and assay AChR in intact muscle, muscle homogenates and during purification (see Barnard *et al.*, 1975; Karlin, 1974). The number of binding sites is proportional, if not equal, to the number of acetylcholine receptors and their distribution corresponds to the distribution of ACh sensitivity as determined by iontophoresis.

Fambrough *et al.* (1973) determined the binding of alpha-bungarotoxin (α-Bgtx) to endplates in deltoid muscle from patients with MG and found that the amount of AChR was reduced to about 20% of control values. We have also looked at α-Bgtx binding and found that the number of receptors per endplate in intercostal muscle is somewhat less than in deltoid, the average values being 1.6×10^7 rather than the 3.9×10^7 sites per endplate found by Fambrough *et al.* (1973). This probably reflects the smaller diameter and endplate area of these fibres whose average length is approximately 1.1 cm. All but one of the nine biopsies from MG patients showed significantly reduced numbers of toxin binding sites at the endplate (Table 1). Fig. 3(b) shows binding histograms from MG and control muscle and demonstrates an overall reduction in endplate binding to about 40% in MG.

The one patient with raised values also had the largest m.e.p.p. and there was a significant positive correlation (P< .05) between toxin binding sites and m.e.p.p. amplitude for data from patients and controls taken together (see Fig. 4).

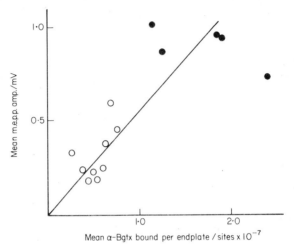

Fig. 4. Mean m.e.p.p. amplitudes (in the presence of 1μg/ml prostigmine) plotted against mean α-Bgtx binding per endplate from the same biopsies. O MG and ● Controls. The correlation coefficient is 0.78, P< 0.05. Ordinate: m.e.p.p. amplitude /mV. Abscissa: average α-Bgtx bound per endplate/sites ×10⁻⁷.

The reduction in binding could be due to a difference in the characteristics of the binding site rather than to fewer functioning AChR. We have therefore investigated the kinetics of α-Bgtx binding. Analysis of binding to intact muscle is subject to large variation and we were limited in the number of bundles we could study from each biopsy. Nevertheless, our results, show little difference between control and MG muscle. The time taken to saturate the endplate binding sites is shown in Fig. 5a where the results have been expressed as a percentage of the values derived from the longest incubation time. Control and MG muscle appear to saturate by about one hour in the presence of toxin at a concentration of 1 microgram/ml. It was also important to look at the reversibility of toxin binding. A considerable loss of endplate bound toxin occurred during the first few hours after the incubation and amounted to about 60% of the total (Fig. 5b). This was evident in both controls and MG muscles and was therefore not related to the pathological state. 80% of the endplate binding at short wash-out times could be inhibited by carbachol, so it seems that there may be two classes of pharmacologically specific binding sites, one of which is slowly reversible. These studies indicate that the reduction in number of toxin binding sites in MG is due mainly to a reduction in the amount of AChR and not to a change in the affinity of the toxin for the AChR.

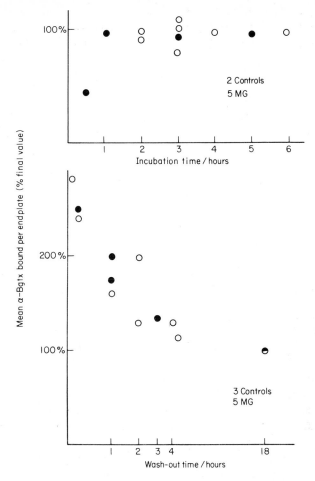

Fig. 5. Kinetics of α-Bgtx binding to MG (O) and control (●) muscle: (a) as a function of incubation time; (b) as a function of wash-out time. Endplate specific binding (see legend to Fig. 3) is expressed as a percentage of the final values: Ordinates: average α-Bgtx bound per endplate; Abscissa: (a) incubation time/hours; (b) wash-out time/hours.

Anticholinesterase treatment

Anticholinesterase treatment affects neuromuscular transmission in experimental animals. Neostigmine treated rats (0.8 mg/kg for 40-140 days) showed morphological changes at the endplates similar to those found in MG (Engel *et al.*, 1973), and also a 30% reduction in m.e.p.p. amplitude, although the quantum content was the same in controls and treated animals. In a previous study Roberts and Thesleff (1969) (2 mg/kg for 7 days) found a reduction in the quantum content of endplate potentials, as well as a reduction in m.e.p.p. amplitude. Using a similar regime Chang *et al.* (1973) found a reduction in ACh release from treated diaphragms though no change in the ACh content of muscle. There was, however, a 40% reduction in the number of α-BgTX binding sites per muscle, as also found by Fambrough *et al.* (1973).

Anticholinesterase treatment could contribute to the changes observed in some MG patients, but fortunately most reports include one or two cases which have not been treated. For instance Engel *et al.* (1976) have found the typical morphological changes in four untreated patients, and we have found small m.e.p.ps, reduced toxin binding and increased ACh content in two untreated cases (see Table 1).

Discussion

Fig. 6 summarizes the main experimental findings in MG. Any theory concerning the cause of the neuromuscular defect must take these into account and, particularly, must explain the origin of the small m.e.p.ps. Fig. 7 schematically illustrates some of the possibilities.

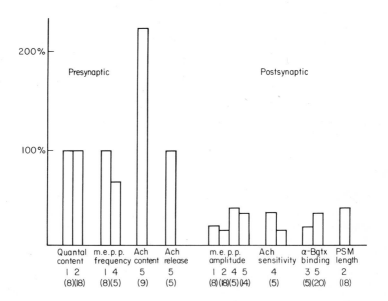

Fig. 6. Summary of the main experimental findings in MG. All results are expressed as a percentage of control values cited by the relevant authors (no. of biopsies in brackets). N.B. PSM length-postsynaptic membrane length as measured in cross sections of neuromuscular junctions. 1. Elmqvist *et al.* 1964. 2. Santa *et al.* 1972. 3. Fambrough *et al.* 1973. 4. Albuquerque *et al.* 1976b. 5. Ito *et al.* 1976 and 1978a.

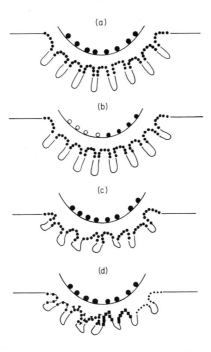

Fig. 7. Schematic illustration of some possible explanations for reduced m.e.p.p. amplitude in MG. (a) Normal endplate with highly folded postsynaptic membrane and a high density of AChR restricted to the tops of the folds. (b) Reduced ACh in each quantum could be due to reduction in quantum size. (●) or the presence of a false transmitter (○). (c) Morphological changes could be partly responsible for reduced m.e.p.p. amplitude (i.e. widened synaptic cleft) and reduced α-Bgtx binding (reduced postsynaptic membrane). (d) Defect in the postsynaptic membrane or in the density or characteristics of the AChR: ●−●−● defect in AChR membrane insertion, ■-■-■-■abnormal AChR, ●●●●● abnormal ion channel, ●●●●● normal AChR but partly blocked by circulating factor.

Presynaptic changes

Apart from a reduction in the nerve terminal area the only specifically presynaptic change (Fig. 7b) so far detected is the increase in ACh content. It is not clear how much of this is to be found in the nerve terminal but experiments with frog muscle suggest that the greater part is intraneural since only about 30% of the ACh remains after degeneration of the nerve (Miledi *et al.*, 1977). The same problem applies to the interpretation of ACh release data. The resting release from muscle is about two orders of magnitude higher than can be explained solely on the basis of spontaneous quantal release, although recent evidence suggests that molecular leakage of acetylcholine from the nerve terminals may make a substantial contribution (Katz and Miledi, 1977). K+ stimulated release is probably a reasonable indication of the events occurring when the nerve ending is depolarized by nerve impulses (K^+ causes a massive increase in the frequency of m.e.p.p.) but it is still only a rough guide. Unequivocal proof that the ACh quantum is normal in MG must await a satisfactory method for measuring nerve evoked release in human muscle biopsies.

Morphological changes

Interpretation of the physiological and biochemical data in MG is complicated by the presence of quite substantial morphological changes (Fig. 7c). Simpson (1969) has suggested that an altered geometry of the synaptic cleft might account for the reduction in m.e.p.p. amplitude and other changes in the postsynaptic response. If normal quanta of ACh have to diffuse further the peak depolarization will be smaller, particularly in the presence of a normal acetylcholinesterase. Two factors argue against such a morphological change as the cause of reduced m.e.p.p. size; first the time to peak of m.e.p.p. and e.p.p. (Elmqvist *et al.*, 1964; Ito *et al.*, 1978a) are similar to those in control endplates, and secondly the increase in amplitude and time course of m.e.p.p. after cholinesterase inhibition is also similar. This latter observation also makes it unlikely that an overactive cholinesterase is responsible for diminishing the effect of each quantum.

Postsynaptic changes

If the reduction in m.e.p.p. is not due primarily either to a defect in ACh release or to the morphological changes, we have to consider changes in the postsynaptic membrane itself. There are several possibilities (Fig. 7d). Small m.e.p.p. could be due to an alteration in the characteristics of the AChR or its associated ion channel. There is, however, little evidence to suggest that the AChR is abnormal in MG, at least in so far as α-Bgtx binds normally to it, and its binding is inhibited by curare and acetylcholine as in control muscle. Moreover preliminary analysis of ACh induced membrane noise fluctuations (see Katz and Miledi, 1976) indicate that the properties of the postsynaptic ion channel are not markedly different from those of control muscle (Katz, Miledi and Newsom Davis, unpublished observations).

Could the reduction in postsynaptic membrane length per nerve terminal be sufficient to account for the reduction in toxin binding sites in MG? Recent work on the distribution of AChR using high resolution autoradiography (Porter and Barnard, 1974; Fertuck and Salpeter, 1974) suggests that the receptors are almost entirely restricted to the tops of the folds as illustrated in Fig. 7. In normal mammalian muscle the receptor containing membrane accounts for about 30% of the total but there have been no measurements of this part of the membrane in MG. Moreover, Santa *et al.* (1972) did not take account of the increase in endplate length which may be associated with an increase in the number of terminal expansions. This could compensate for the reduction in membrane area per single nerve terminal, so that the total area of AChR containing membrane per endplate may not be reduced. To resolve this question it will be necessary to either measure the total area of postsynaptic membrane or to find a method for directly localizing AChR under the electron microscope.

Since the amplitude of m.e.p.p. seems to be related to the density, or number per unit area of AChR, rather than the total number per endplate (Albuquerque *et al.*, 1974) the positive correlation between m.e.p.p. amplitude and the number of toxin binding sites that has been found in MG (Ito *et al.*, 1977a) suggests that the reduction in binding could be due to a similar reduction in the density of AChR. This would also account for the reduced ACh sensitivity.

These conclusions are supported by the results of Albuquerque *et al.* (1976b) who have related their physiological data to the ultrastructural appearance of the same endplates. They found that the most marked simplification of the postsynaptic folds and widening of the synaptic cleft was associated with a complete absence of nerve induced depolarization, either spontaneous or evoked, although some ACh sensitivity was still present. On the other hand some endplates looked relatively normal in spite of a reduction to about 30% in the amplitude of m.e.p.p. From these observations they concluded that even though morphological changes must contribute to the defect in transmission, the m.e.p.p. reduction must also reflect a reduction in the density of AChR.

The question remains as to why there should be a reduction in the density of receptors. The most likely explanation relates to the existence of anti-AChR antibodies which are now found in most patients with MG (see below). Whether these antibodies can directly block normal AChR or whether they act by changing their turnover or insertion into the membrane remains to be seen.

Autoimmunity to acetylcholine receptor in myasthenia gravis

The possiblity of an autoimmune basis for myasthenia gravis was suggested by Simpson (1960). This view has since become widely accepted as evidence has accumulated on the role of the thymus in the immune response, and with the demonstration of antibodies which bind to muscle, thyroid and thymus cells in 30% of patients (Feltkamp *et al.*, 1974). However, it is only in the last couple of years that the existence of antibodies which could be directly involved in the aetiology of the neuromuscular defect have been demonstrated.

Cellular immunity to AChR

There have been two reports of cellular reponse to AChR in MG. In both of these thymidine uptake as an indication of lymphocyte transformation in lymphocytes exposed to electric eel AChR has been examined. The stimulation index varied between 1 and 4 in one study (Abramsky *et al.*, 1975a) and a reduction was observed in patients undergoing steroid therapy (Abramsky *et al.*, 1975b). Richman *et al.* (1976) found a stimulation index between 0 and 20 and there was a good correlation between that and the activity of the disease. Moreover in this report there was a correlation between age and the stimulation index, the highest indices being among elderly male patients and those with thymoma. More recently there has been a study of thymidine uptake by lymphocytes from patients with MG exposed to Torpedo membrane fragments rich in AChR (Conti-Tronconi *et al.*, 1977). These authors found a significantly raised uptake only in the presence of autologous serum.

The meaning of these results is not clear. It is somewhat surprising that lymphocytes from patients with MG are sensitized to fish AChR because humoral antibodies to AChR in MG (see below) show very little reaction with fish electroplax AChR (Lindstrom *et al.*, 1976a). It is possible that the sensitized cells are responding to a more conserved region of the receptor. Nevertheless, lymphocyte transformation is not restricted to the cells involved in cell-mediated immunity (antibody producing cells can also be transformed) and it would be a mistake to assume that these results necessarily indicate a cellular attack on the endplate as the cause of the defect in MG.

Anti-AChR antibodies

In rabbits immunized against purified AChR the level of circulating anti-AChR is closely related to the clinical signs of weakness and to the reduction in m.e.p.p. amplitude and α-Bgtx binding which is found in their muscles (Green *et al.*, 1975b; Ito *et al.*, 1978b). The development of experimental autoimmune MG (see Chapters 9 and 16) has stimulated the search for serum factors which might be involved in the human disease.

Several demonstrations of such factors have now been reported. MG sera were able to block α-Bgtx binding to solubilized AChR from denervated, though not from normal, rat leg muscle (Almon *et al.*, 1974; Almon and Appel, 1975). The reduction in toxin binding was limited to about 50% and was also found with IgG prepared from the same sera. A further report shows that there is no correlation between anti-AChR and HLA antigen typing (Appel *et al.*, 1975). Bender *et al.* (1975) showed that MG sera could inhibit immunoperoxidase staining of AChR in cross-sections of normal human muscle, and Ringel *et al.* (1975) found a correlation between this activity and the presence of anti-striated muscle antibodies. Complement fixation in the presence of Torpedo AChR has been found in 80% of sera (Aharanov *et al.*, 1975a) and Mittag *et al.* (1976) have compared various methods for determining anti-AChR activity in MG sera and in thymus extracts.

A survey of 71 patients with MG and 175 controls was made by Lindstrom *et al.* (1976b). They studied IgG binding to solubilized human muscle by precipitation with goat anti-human IgG. The AChR was prelabelled with radioactive α-Bgtx. Anti-receptor activity was present in 87% of MG sera but did not show any particular correlation with age, sex, therapy or duration of symptoms. Most of their sera did not inhibit α-Bgtx binding to the human AChR, a fact which must be considered when evaluating the possible role of these antibodies in producing the reduction in α-Bgtx binding sites at the neuromuscular junction.

We have also measured anti-AChR activity in MG sera using crude Triton X-100 extracts of human muscle (obtained from amputations). The level of AChR in these extracts ranged from 0.5-4.0 picomoles/g tissue. The higher values probably reflect a degree of denervation hypersensitivity which occurs in some pathological conditions. Our results from 50 MG sera are in fair agreement with those of Lindstrom and colleagues and as

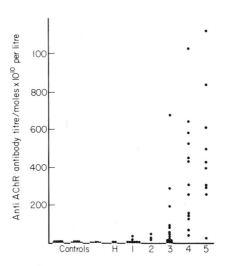

Fig. 8. Anti-AChR antibody levels in 46 controls and 50 MG patients. Human muscle extracted with Triton X-100 was pre-labelled with α-Bgtx. 0.2 picomoles were incubated with 1 μl of serum for 2 hours, followed by addition of excess anti-human IgG (sheep). The precipitate was washed and counted. H, hereditary MG; 1, MG in remission; 2, one muscle group only affected; 3, two groups affected; 4, more than two groups affected plus some reduction in vital capacity; 5, as 4 with marked reduction in vital capacity. Ordinate: anti-AChR antibody titre/moles $\times 10^{10}$ per liter.

can be seen in Fig. 8 there does seem to be some correlation between antibody levels and the severity of the patient's condition as determined by the number of muscle groups involved and the extent of their weakness.

Acetylcholine receptors and the thymus

The role of the thymus in MG is an interesting problem, not simply because of the increasing evidence for its importance in the control of the immune response and its relationship with the development of immunological tolerance. The high incidence of thymic abnormalities in MG, the improvement after thymectomy and in particular the existence of antibodies to striated muscle which cross-react with thymic cells has led to the belief that there may be a specific defect in thymic function which is responsible for the neuromuscular abnormalities (see Osserman, 1969). In 1966 Goldstein and Whittingham reported that some animals immunized against heterologous thymus or muscle developed signs of neuromuscular block. The hypothesis of a circulating factor, thymopoietin (Goldstein and Schlesinger 1975) released from the diseased thymus and responsible for neuromuscular block is attractive, but some groups (e.g. Jones *et al.*, 1971) have failed to reproduce their results, and there is no evidence as to the level of thymopoietin in patients with MG.

The presence of 'myoid' cells in the thymus of birds, reptiles and embryonic mammals has been recognized since first described (Mayer, 1888), and there have been occasional reports of striated cells in the normal human (Feltkamp-Vroom, 1966) and MG thymus (Van de Velde and Friedman, 1970). A cross-reaction between eel AChR and calf thymus has been demonstrated (Aharanov *et al.*, 1975b) and a small number of α-Bgtx binding sites has been shown in rat thymus (Lindstrom *et al.*, 1976a), although there was no apparent localization of α-Bgtx to non-lymphoid cells using autoradiography (Fulpius *et al.*, 1976). It was interesting therefore that Wekerle *et al.* (1975) found striated muscle cells appearing in cultures of rat thymus. Kao and Drachman (1977) have looked more closely at these cultures and find many of the features characteristic of muscle cells – contractility, acetylcholine sensitivity and α-Bgtx binding sites. Although the time course of their appearance in culture suggests that these cells may be derived from 'pluripotential stem cells' rather than any committed precursor (Wekerle *et al.*, 1975) this system offers a new approach to investigating the role of the thymus in MG.

Evidence for a humoral factor in the aetiology of MG:

To what extent could a humoral immune factor be responsible for the neuromuscular defect in MG?

The many unsuccessful attempts to block neuromuscular transmission *in vitro* with MG serum (see Nastuk, 1959 and Namba, 1976) and the failure to demonstrate IgG at the endplate using immunofluorescence (e.g. McFarlin *et al.*, 1966) argue against a humoral blocking factor. Moreover Albuquerque *et al.* (1976a) have investigated the effect of serum on control human and rat muscle with intracellular recordings. They found no effect on the m.e.p.p. amplitude or the acetylcholine sensitivity in relatively short-term experiments (up to 2 hours). Their results confirm our own findings (unpublished) in most instances though we did find one serum which was able to reduce the amplitude of m.e.p.ps to approximately 50% over a period of 5 hours (see Fig. 9). In this experiment m.e.p.p. were recorded from the same endplates before and after application of the serum; there was little change in the resting potential of the fibres, and in the muscle treated with control serum there was no significant change in m.e.p.p. amplitude (see Fig. 9).

In the last few years there have been three reports which do support the relevance of a humoral immune factor in MG. In 1973 Bergström *et al.* showed improvement in patients with MG after thoracic duct drainage. The improvement was not well sustained but its humoral basis was suggested by the marked and rapid deterioration which occurred when the cell-free lymph was reinjected into the patient. In contrast injection of the re-suspended cell fraction produced no effect (Matell *et al.*, 1976). In two

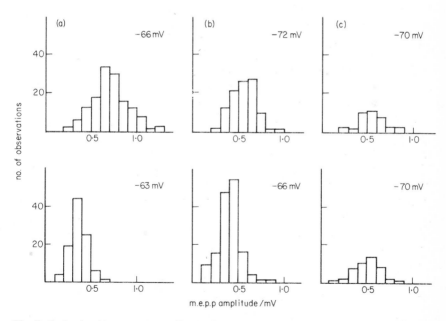

Fig. 9. Reduction in m.e.p.p. amplitude after applying MG serum to normal human inter-costal muscle. (a) and (b) before (top) and after MG serum. (c) before and after control serum. M.e.p.p. were recorded intracellularly in identified fibres. Ordinate: no. of observations; Abscissa: m.e.p.p. amplitude/mV.

papers Toyka *et al.* (1975, 1977) have demonstrated the passive transfer of MG from man to mouse by the daily injection of milligram quantities of IgG concentrated from MG sera. The mice developed weakness, small m.e.p.p. and reduced α-Bgtx binding. In two mice m.e.p.p. were normal but these were both injected with IgG from patients with very low levels of circulating antibodies. In other respects also there was a rough correlation between the level of anti-AChR injected and the severity of the physiological findings. An interesting observation was the reduced effect of passive transfer into mice which had been depleted of the third component of complement (C3). Since absence of the fifth component of complement (C5) did not affect the response these results suggest that binding of the early complement components to antibody-AChR complexes may be an important step in blocking neuromuscular transmission. It will be interesting to see whether morphological changes are found in these animals.

The third factor which supports the relevance of serum antibodies in the pathogenesis of MG is the short term remission which follows plasma exchange in patients with acquired MG (though not in one patient with

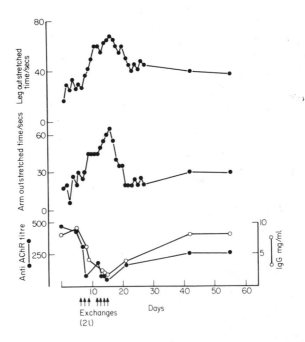

Fig. 10. Anti-AChR antibody levels during and after plasma exchange in a 29 year old woman with an 18 month history of moderately severe MG. She had had a thymectomy 15 months previously. Her clinical state is indicated by the time she could hold her leg or arm outstretched. Ordinates: (a) Leg outstretched time; (b) arm outstretched time; (c) anti-AChR titre; 1gG mg/ml.

congenital MG, c.f. Fig. 8). The clinical results of this procedure are reported elsewhere (Pinching *et al.*, 1976) but Fig. 10 shows the effect of this treatment on anti-AChR antibody levels in one patient, and relates them to the patient's clinical condition. The inverse relationship between antibody and clinical status has now been demonstrated in several patients (Chapter 17) and is consistent with the view that antibody to AChR is playing an important role in the disorder of neuromuscular transmission.

Conclusions

The reduced effect of each quantum of ACh clearly underlies the defect in neuromuscular transmission in MG. Although a reduction in the number of ACh molecules in each quantum cannot be completely ruled out, most of the recent evidence supports the concept of a defect in the postsynaptic membrane. Physiological evidence suggests that there is a marked reduction in the density of functional acetylcholine receptors. Anti-AChR antibody is present in MG sera and in any individual patient appears to show an inverse relationship to their clinical state. The reduction in density of functional receptors may be due therefore to the binding of antibody to the AChR, though this may not directly involve the α-Bgtx binding site. Antibodies binding to other parts of the receptor or to the associated ion channel may be more important. Reduced α-Bgtx binding at MG endplates could be partly attributable to a reduction in the area of postsynaptic membrane.

Since the results of short-term exposure of neuromuscular preparations to MG sera have been largely unconvincing, and there seems to be a time-lag of approximately 12-48 hours before the effect of manipulating antibody levels is seen, one must consider the possibility that the reduction in the amount of functional AChR is the secondary result of antibody-induced changes in the postsynaptic membrane.

Acknowledgements

We are grateful to Mr. M.F. Sturridge, F.R.C.S. for his kind cooperation in obtaining the MG biopsies. This work was supported by the Medical Research Council.

References

Abramsky, O., Aharanov, A., Webb, C. and Fuchs, S. (1975a). *Clin. exp. Immunol.*, **19**, 11-16.
Abramsky, O., Aharanov, A., Teitelbaum, D. and Fuchs, S. (1975b). *Arch. Neurol.*, **32**, 684-687.
Aharanov, A., Abramsky, O., Tarrab-Hazdai, R. and Fuchs, S. (1975a). *Lancet*, **ii**, 340-342.

Aharanov, A., Tarrab-Hazdai, R., Abramsky, O. and Fuchs, S. (1975b). *Proc. Nat. Acad. Sci. USA*, **72**, 1456-1459.

Albuquerque, E.X., Barnard, E.A., Porter, C.W. and Warnick, J.E. (1974). *Proc. Nat. Acad. Sci. USA*, **71**, 2818-2822.

Albuquerque, E.X., Lebeda, F.J., Appel, S.H., Almon, R., Kauffman, F.C., Mayer, R.F., Narahashi, T. and Yeh, J.Z. (1976a). *Ann. N.Y. Acad. Sci.* **274**, 475-492.

Albuquerque, E.X., Rash, J.E., Mayer, R.F. and Satterfield, J.R. (1976b). *Experimental Neurology*, **51**, 536-563.

Almon, R.R., Andrew, C.G. and Appel, S.H. (1974). *Science*, **186**, 55-57.

Almon, R.R. and Appel, S.H. (1975). *Biochem. Biophys. Acta*, **393**, 66-67.

Appel, S.H., Almon, R.R. and Levy, N. (1975). *N. Engl. J. Med.*, **293**, 760-761.

Axelsson, J. and Thesleff, S. (1959). *J. Physiol., Lond.*, **147**, 178-193.

Barnard, E.A., Dolly, J.O., Porter, C.W. and Albuquerque, E.X. (1975). *Experimental Neurology*, **48**, 1-28.

Bender, A.N., Ringel, S.P., Engel, W.K., Daniels, M.P. and Vogel, Z. (1975). *Lancet*, **i**, 607-609.

Bergström, K., Franksson, C., Matell, G. and von Reis, G. (1973). *Eur. Neurol.* **9**, 157-167.

Chang, C.C. and Lee, C.Y. (1963). *Arch. int. Pharmacodyn.*, **144**, 241-257.

Chang, C.C., Chen, T.F. and Chuang, S.-T. (1973). *J. Physiol., Lond.*, **230**, 613-618.

Cöers, C. (1975). *Lancet*, **ii**, 555.

Cöers, C. and Desmedt, J.E. (1959). *Acta Neurol. et Psychiat. Belgica*, **59**, 539-561.

Conti-Tronconi, B.M., Di Padova, F., Morgutti, M., Missiroli, A. and Frattola, L. (1977). *J. Neuropath. and exp. Neurol.*, **36**, 157-168.

Dahlbäck, O., Elmqvist, D., Johns, T.R., Radner, S. and Thesleff, S. (1961). *J. Physiol., Lond.*, **156**, 336-343.

Desmedt, J.E. (1958). *Nature, Lond.*, **182**, 1673-1674.

Elmqvist, D., Hoffmann, W.W., Kugelberg, J. and Quastel, D.M.J. (1964). *J. Physiol., Lond.*, **174**, 417-434.

Elmqvist, D., Johns, T.R. and Thesleff, S. (1960). *J. Physiol., Lond.*, **154**, 602-607.

Elmqvist, D. and Quastel, D.M.J. (1965). *J. Physiol., Lond.*, **177**, 463-482.

Engel, A.G., Lambert, E.H. and Santa, T. (1973). *Neurology (Minneap.)*, **23**, 1273-1281.

Engel, A.G., Tsujihata, M., Lindstrom, J.M. and Lennon, V.A. (1976). *Ann. N.Y. Acad. Sci.*, **274**, 60-79.

Fambrough, D.M., Drachman, D.B. and Satyamurti, S. (1973). *Science*, **182**, 293-295.

Feltkamp, T.E.W., Van den Berg-Looven, P.M., Nijenhuis, L.E., Engelfriet, C.P., Van Rossum, A.L., Van Lochem, J.J. and Oosterhuis, H.J.G.H. (1974). *Brit. Med. J.*, **1**, 131-133.

Feltkamp-Vroom, T. (1966). *Lancet*, **i**, 1320-1321.

Fertuck, H.C. and Salpeter, M.M. (1974). *Proc. Nat. Acad. Sci.*, **71**, 1376-1378.

Fulpius, B.W., Zurn, A.D., Granato, A.A. and Leder, R.M. (1976). *Ann. N.Y. Acad. Sci.*, **274**, 116-129.

Goldstein, G. and Whittingham, S. (1966). *Lancet*, **ii**, 315-318.

Goldstein, G. and Schlesinger, D.H. (1975). *Lancet*, **ii**, 256-259.

Green, D.P.L., Miledi, R., Perez de la Mora, M. and Vincent, A. (1975a). *Phil. Trans. R. Soc. Lond. B.*, **270**, 551-559.

Green, D.P.L., Miledi, R. and Vincent, A. (1975b). *Proc. R. Soc. Lond. B.*,

189, 57-68.

Grob, D., Johns, R.J. and Harvey, A.M. (1956). *Bull. Johns Hopkins Hosp.* **99,** 136-181.

Ito, Y., Miledi, R., Molenaar, P.C., Vincent, A., Polak, R.L., van Gelder, M. and Newsom Davis, J. (1976). *Proc. R. Soc. Lond. B.*, **192,** 475-480.

Ito, Y., Miledi, R., Newsom Davis, J. and Vincent, A. (1978a) (manuscript in preparation).

Ito, Y., Miledi, R. and Vincent, A. (1978b) (manuscript in preparation).

Jenden, D.J., Roch, M. and Booth, R.A. (1973). *Anal. Biochem.*, **55,** 438-448.

Johns, R.J., Grob, D. and Harvey, A.M. (1956). *Bull. Johns Hopkins Hosp.*, **99,** 125-135.

Jones, S.F., Brennan, J.C. and McLeod, J.G. (1971). *J. Neurol. Neurosurg. Psychiat.*, **34,** 399-403.

Kao, I. and Drachman, D.B. (1977). *Science,* **195,** 74-75.

Karlin, A. (1974). *Life Sciences,* **14,** 1385-1415.

Katz, B. (1969). 'The Release of Neural Transmitter Substances' Liverpool University Press.

Katz, B. and Miledi, R. (1976). In 'Motor Innervation of Muscle' (S. Thesleff ed.), pp.31-50. Academic Press, New York and London.

Katz, R. and Miledi, R. (1977). *Proc. R. Soc. Lond. B.*, **196,** 59-72.

Krnjević, K. and Mitchell, J.F. (1961). *J. Physiol. Lond.*, **155,** 246-262.

Lindstrom, J.M., Lennon, V.A., Seybold, M.E. and Whittingham, S. (1976a) *Ann. N.Y. Acad. Sci.*, **274,** 254-274.

Lindstrom, J.M., Seybold, M.E., Lennon, V.A., Whittingham, S. and Duane, D.D. (1976b). *Neurology (Minneap.),* **26,** 1054-1059.

Matell, G., Bergström, K., Franksson, C., Hammarström, L., Lefvert, A.K., Möller, E., von Reis, G. and Smith, E. (1976). *Ann. N.Y. Acad. Sci.,* **274,** 659-676.

Mayer, S. (1888). *Anat. Anz.,* **3,** 97-103.

Mcfarlin, D.E., Engel, W.K. and Strauss, A.J.L. (1966). *Ann. N.Y. Acad. Sci.,* **135,** 656-663.

Miledi, R. (1960). *J. Physiol., Lond.,* **151,** 1-23.

Miledi, R., Molenaar, P.C. and Polak, R.L. (1977). *Proc. R. Soc. Lond. B.,* **197,** 285-297.

Miledi, R. and Potter, L.T. (1971). *Nature, Lond.,* **233,** 599-603.

Mittag, T., Kornfeld, P., Tormay, A. and Woo, C. (1976). *N. Engl. J. Med.,* **294,** 691-694.

Namba, T., Nakata, Y. and Grob, D. (1976). *Ann. N.Y. Acad. Sci.,* **274,** 493-515.

Nastuk, W.L. Strauss, A.J.L. and Osserman, K.E. (1959). *Am. J. Med.,* **26,** 394-409.

Osserman, K.E. (1969). In 'Textbook of Immunopathology' (P.A. Miescher and Müller-Eberhard, eds) vol. 2. pp.607-623. Grune and Stratton, New York.

Pinching, A.J., Peters, D.K. and Newsom Davis, J. (1976). *Lancet,* **ii,** 1373-1376.

Polak, R.L. and Molenaar, P.C. (1974). *J. Neurochem.,* **23,** 1295-1297.

Porter, C.W. and Barnard, E.A. (1974). *J. Memb. Biol.,* **20,** 31-49.

Ringel, S.P., Bender, A.N., Engel, W.K. and Smith, H.J. (1975). *Lancet,* **i,** 1338.

Roberts, D.V. and Thesleff, S. (1969). *Europ. J. Pharmacol.,* **6,** 281-285.

Richman, D.P., Patrick, J., Arnason, B.G.W. (1976). *N. Engl. J. Med.,* **294,** 694-698.

Santa, S., Engel, A.G. and Lambert, E.H. (1972). *Neurology (Minneap.),* **22,** 71-82.

Simpson, J.A. (1960). *Scot. Med. J.*, **5**, 419-436.
Simpson, J.A. (1966). In 'The Biological Basis of Medicine' (E.E. Bittar and N. Bittar, eds) vol. 3. pp.345-390.
Toyka, K.V. Drachman, D.B. Pestronk, A. and Kao, I. (1975). *Science*, **190**, 397-399.
Toyka, K.V., Drachman, D.B., Griffin, D.E., Pestronk, A., Winkelstein, J.A., Fischbeck, K.H. and Kao., I. (1977). *N. Engl. J. Med.*, **296**, 125-131.
Van de Velde, R.L. and Friedman, N.B. (1970). *Amer. J. of Path.*, **59**, 349-368.
Walker, M.B. (1934). *Lancet*, **i**, 1200-1201.
Wekerle, H., Paterson, B., Ketelsen, U.-P., and Feldman, M. (1975). *Nature, Lond.*, **256**, 493-494.

6 Molecular organization of cholinergic receptor in post-synaptic membrane of electric organ of torpedo marmorata

B.CONTI-TRONCONI · C.GOTTI · F.CLEMENTI

*Department of Pharmacology and CNR Center of
Cytopharmacology, University of Milan, Italy.*

The postsynaptic membrane of electric organs of *Torpedo Marmorata* has been increasingly used as a source of nicotinic cholinergic receptor because of its high content of this molecule. Several studies by electron microscope autoradiography (Bourgeois *et al.*, 1973; Fertuck and Salpeter, 1974) and by histochemical detection of α-bungarotoxin (Bender *et al.*, 1976), have clearly localized the maximal concentration of cholinergic receptors on the peaks of the postsynaptic folds and have also indicated that the average number of molecules is about $10,000/\mu m^2$. The morphological structure of postsynaptic membranes, both *in situ* and after isolation by sucrose density gradient, have been examined by freeze-fracture and negative staining by several authors (Heilbronn, 1975; Clementi *et al.*, 1975; Cartaud *et al.*, 1973; Orci *et al.*, 1974; Nickel and Potter, 1973). The structures that have been correlated with the receptor molecule are firstly a regular lattice of small particles, spaced 6 nm, present on the E* face of postsynaptic infoldings, and secondly the rosettes- or doughnut-shaped structures, of 8 nm diameter, seen by negative staining in the isolated postsynaptic membranes. Studies on detergent isolated receptor molecules have also indicated that it is a complex doughnut-shaped structure formed by three to six subunits. However, despite the above mentioned data, there is no clear information about the receptor molecule organization in the subsynaptic membrane and on the number of its subunits. In the present paper we will attempt to illustrate in more detail these points.

The receptor/ionophore complex must be a molecular structure in which the recognition site must project from the external surface of the membrane and the ionophore part lie across the thickness of the membrane. In order to investigate the organization of such a structure, we have analysed the postsynaptic membrane with two different techniques: (1) freeze-fracture of the tissue, thus providing evidence of internal organization of the mem-

---

*In the description of the freeze-fracture images we follow the convention that freeze-fracture exposes two internal faces of the plasmamembrane: the P face, which is left frozen to the cytoplasm, and the E face, which is left frozen to the extracellular fluid (Branton *et al.* 1975).

branes; (2) negative-staining of the isolated membranes, showing their external structures.

For the freeze-fracture examination, pieces of the fresh electric organ of *Torpedo Marmorata* (kindly provided by the Stazione Zoologica of Naples) were fixed in 2·5% glutaraldehyde buffered with 0·14 M phosphate buffer pH 7.3, infiltrated with increasingly concentrated solutions of glycerol, frozen in Freon 22, cooled with liquid nitrogen and freeze-fractured in a Balzer 301 apparatus provided with an electron gun. Negative staining was performed on glutaraldehyde fixed fractions with uranyl acetate or potassium phosphotungstate. Optical diffraction of E.M. negatives was carried out with a Polaron diffractometer using the technique of Horne and Markham (1972). α-Bungarotoxin was isolated from venom of Bungarus multicinctus according to Ong *et al.* (1974) and iodinated with the lactoperoxidase technique (David, 1972).

The freeze-fracture shows very clearly P and E faces of postsynaptic infoldings (Fig. 1). On the E face it is possible to see a regular arrangement of linear arrays of small particles spaced about 6 nm. The distance between the particles (center to center) is 7 nm (Fig. 2). The arrays are localized most frequently on the crests of the postsynaptic folds, but were sometimes present also in the deeper parts. The distances and the type of organization

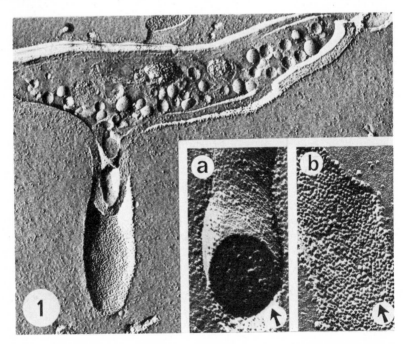

Fig. 1. Freeze-fracture of the electroplax of Torpedo. A nerve ending with a subsynaptic infolding is shown. In the inset the typical aspect of face E (a) and P (b) of the infoldings is illustrated. ×38,000 A× 120,000 B× 130,000.

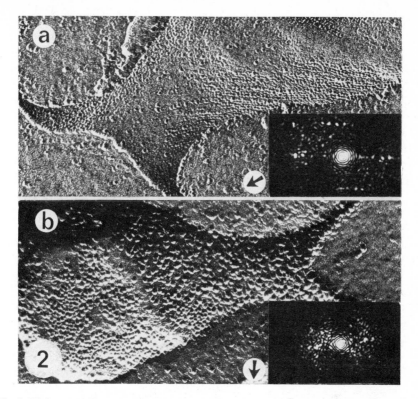

Fig. 2. Higher magnification of the lattice of particles present on both E face (a) and P face (b) of the plasma membrane cleaved at the level of synaptic cleft. The optical diffraction pattern of both images is also shown. ×140,000.

of the particles have been confirmed by optical diffraction (Inset Fig. 2). The P face of the postsynaptic folds was covered by numerous 8 nm spaced particles without any peculiar organization (Fig. 1). This is rather surprising, as it would be expected that a structural organization similar to that of E face would be seen at least in some particular areas such as the crests of the postsynaptic folds. However we found that it was very difficult to cleave the postsynpatic membrane at the level of the synaptic cleft and thus to reveal the receptor-rich zones of the folds. Such peculiar features of the *Torpedo* electric organ have been deduced also by previous workers (Heilbrown, 1975; Cartaud *et al.*, 1973; Nickel and Potter, 1973). Only when the fracture plane exposes the P face of the postsynaptic membrane at the level of the synaptic cleft is it possible to show a population of small particles arranged in regular arrays spaced 7 nm. The distance between the particles (center to center) was 8 nm (Fig. 2).

This organization and these measurements have been checked by optical diffraction (Insert Fig. 2). From our results it seems that the lattice of particles present on the P face is much more specific for the subsynaptic membrane and thus more difficult to show in addition to the afore-mentioned difficulty in cleaving the postsynaptic membrane in this area. This is perhaps the reason why other authors have overlooked it.

To examine the external surface of postsynaptic membranes we have isolated from the electric organ of *Torpedo* a membrane fraction very rich in cholinergic receptor. A sucrose density gradient technique similar to that of Cohen *et al.* (1972) was used. These membranes were examined in the electron microscope after negative staining. They appear to be covered by numerous doughnut-shaped structures that are densely packed together (Fig. 3). These structures have a diameter of 5 nm, a central pit 1.6 nm large and a wall 1.7 nm thick. The distance between the rosettes is 6 nm. Optical diffraction analysis suggest that each structure is formed by six subunits. We have examined different models made by four, five and six subunits structures and only the six subunits models gave a similar diffraction pattern (Fig. 3).

When the membranes were treated with detergent (Sarkosyl N L; Ciba-Geigy, 4% for 30 min at room temperature) it was found possible to peel them off from the doughnut structures and to recover the latter in the supernatant. In detergent treated membranes when several rosette struc-tures have been peeled off, it is possible to recognize organization in parallel arrays of the receptor complexes. Since in these membranes the receptor concentration is about 25% of the membrane protein, we suggest, in agreement with other authors, that these doughnut-shaped structures represent the morphological aspects of the cholinergic receptors. Combining the data obtained from the freeze-fracture and the negative staining we have postulated that the receptor complex has six subunits arranged in an ordinate lattice at the surface of the membrane, and is connected with similarly arranged particles inside the membrane as it is depicted in the drawing in Fig. 3.

In an attempt to investigate the significance of the organization of sub-units and to identify some other protein components of the postsynpatic membranes, we have studied the effects of the binding of different choliner-gic ligands on the physical properties of the cholinergic receptor. Mem-branes were incubated with α-bungarotoxin (6 ng/mg of membrane protein), *Naja naja siamensis* α-toxin (6 ng/mg of membrane protein) and curare

Fig. 3. (a) Negatively stained preparation of isolated membrane showing the structure and pattern of organization of the receptor complexes. In the inset the optical diffraction patterns of the electron micrograph and the six subunits model with its optical diffractogram is shown. ($\times$350,000).
(b) Isolated postsynaptic membrane treated with detergent. The linear arrays of receptor complexes are evident. ($\times$150,000).
(c) A schematic drawing of the arrangement of the receptor molecules of the postsynaptic membrane as it results from freeze-fracture and negative staining preparations.

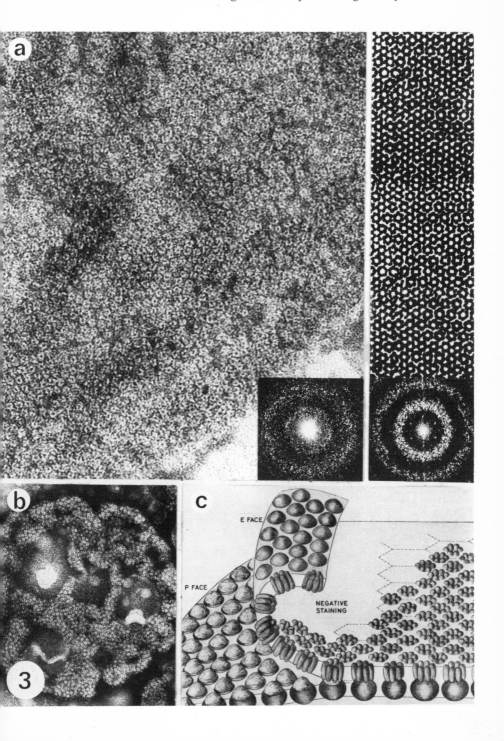

(1 mM) for 30' at room temperature. The membranes were then treated for 20 minutes at room temperature with a solution of Sarkosyl NL 4%. We chose this detergent because it dissolves completely the postsynaptic membranes and interferes only slightly with the α-bungarotoxin binding to cholinergic receptor. The supernatant of the detergent incubated membranes, containing more than 90% of the membrane proteins, was chromatographed on a Sepharose 6B column. The result is shown in Fig. 4.

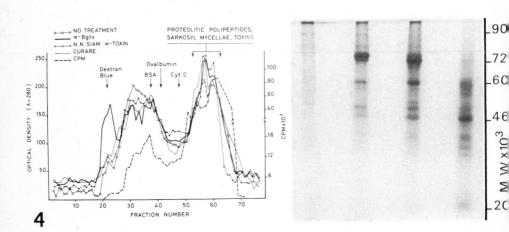

Fig. 4. Elution pattern of purified postsynaptic membranes (after solubilization with Sarkosyl NL) on a Sepharose 6B column. The column (90 cm × 1,5 cm) was previously equilbrated with 0.4% Sarkosyl in 20 mM Tris HCl buffer, pH 7.4 (eventually containing also 1 mM d-tubocurarine). When the membranes are preincubated with bungarotoxin a large peak appears in correspondence with the void volume. The dotted line represents the radioactivity due to ^{125}I when a trace amount of ^{125}I-labelled toxin was added to the cold α-bungarotoxin during the preincubation. The fractions number 22, 31, 37 and 41 were analysed by SDS polyacrylamide gel electrophoresis. The first three fractions able to bind the toxin (22, 31, 37) have a similar protein band composition and different from the last fraction that is unable to bind the toxin.

The solubilized membranes, without any previous drug incubation, were resolved in a large peak, the first part of which had a considerable binding capacity for the toxin. It is difficult to know the molecular weight of the toxin binding peak since the Sarkosyl binds to proteins in micelles of different size. While the treatment of the membranes with reversible binding cholinergic ligands did not modify the chromatographic pattern, a pretreatment with α-bungarotoxin induced the formation of a large peak of high molecular weight in the void volume. The SDS polyacrylamide gel electrophoresis analysis of the this large peak and of the two fractions, that bind the toxin, revealed extensive overlapping with respect to the bands present. A quite different band composition was present in the last fraction of the main peak that did not bind the toxin.

We suggest that toxin can bind to two adjacent subunits of the same or of contiguous doughnut structures. The receptor complex can be stabilized by the bound toxin and becomes more resistant to the action of detergent. This interpretation is supported by previously reported observations that the toxin may have more than one binding site (Fewtrell, 1976) and that each receptor subunit has two binding sites for α-bungarotoxin (Mattson, 1976; Fewtrell, 1976). The similarity of the electrophoretograms from the large peak in the void volume with those from the other two peaks that bind toxin strengthens this interpretation.

References

Bender, A.N., Ringel, S.P. and Engel W.K. (1976). *Ann. N.Y. Ac. Sci.*, **274,** 20-30.

Bourgeois, J.P., Popot, J.L., Ryter, A. and Changeux, J.P. (1973). *Brain. Res.* **62,** 557-563.

Branton, D., Bullivant, S., Gilula, N.B., Karnovsky, M.J., Moor, H., Mühlethaler, K., Northcote, D.H., Packer, L., Satir, B., Satir, P., Speth, V., Staehelin, L.A., Steere, L., and Weinstein, R.S. (1975). *Science,* **190,** 54-56.

Cartaud, J., Benedetti, E.L., Cohen, J.B., Meunier, J.C. and Changeux, J.P. (1973). *FEBS Letters,* **33,** 109-113.

Clementi, F., Conti Tronconi, B., Peluchetti, D. and Morgutti, M. (1975). *Brain Res.,* **90,** 133-138.

Cohen, J.B., Weber, N., Huchet, M. and Changeux, J.P. (1972). *FEBS Letters,* **25,** 43-47.

David, G.S. (1972). *Biochem. Biophys. Res. Comm.,* **48,** 464-471.

Fertuck, N.C. and Salpeter, M.M. (1974). *Proc. Nat. Acad. Sci.,* **71,** 1376-1378.

Fewtrell, C.M.S. (1976). *Neuroscience,* **1,** 249-273.

Heilbronn, H. (1975). In 'Cholinergic mechanisms' P.G. Waser ed. p.343-364, Raven Press, New York.

Horne, R.W. and Markham, R. (1972). In: Practical methods in Electron Microscopy A.M. Glauert, ed. vol.I p.327-434, North Holland, Amsterdam. (1972).

Mattsson, C. (1976). *FOA reports,* **10,** 1-16.

Nickel, E. and Potter, L.T. (1973). *Brain Research,* **57,** 508-517.

Ong, D.E. and Brady, R.N. (1974). *Biochemistry,* **13,** 2822-2827.

Orci, L., Perrelet, A. and Dunant, Y. (1974). *Proc. Nat. Acad. Sci.,* **71,** 307-310.

7 Molecular forms of acetylcholinesterase in electric organ tissue and embryonic skeletal muscle

ISRAEL SILMAN · LILI ANGLISTER · HERBERT GAZIT

*Department of Neurobiology, Weizmann Institute of Science
Rehovot, Israel*

Introduction

The main role of acetylcholinesterase (AChE) is believed to be the termination of impulse transmission by hydrolysis of the neurotransmitter acetylcholine. Subcellular fractionation and cytochemical studies indicate that AChE is associated with the surface membrane of the excitable cell; its precise relationship to the excitable membrane is not, however, clearly understood, and various studies indicate that a significant part of the enzyme is not tightly associated with the plasma membrane. Thus in electric organ tissue much of the AChE is readily solubilized at high ionic strength (Silman and Karlin, 1967), under conditions which do not lead to appreciable solubilization of the acetylcholine receptor (Karlin and Cowburn, 1974; Rosenberg *et al.*, 1977). It is also easily solubilized by limited protease treatment (Massoulié *et al.*, 1970; Dudai and Silman, 1974b; Taylor *et al.*, 1974). In skeletal muscle, too, significant amounts of AChE can be solubilized without detergent (Hall, 1973), and proteases can detach AChE from muscle endplates without affecting the physiological and pharmacological properties of the postsynaptic membrane (Albuquerque *et al.*, 1968; Hall and Kelly, 1971; Betz and Sakmann, 1971). Studies on the molecular structure of AChE are thus important not only for elucidating its mechanism of action, but also for clarifying its mode of association with the excitable membrane, a necessary condition for understanding how AChE fulfils its biological role *in situ*.

Acetylcholinesterase from the Electric Organ of the Electric Eel

The highly specialized electrogenic tissue of electric fish is a particularly rich source, from which AChE was first purified and characterized, thus enabling detailed studies on the molecular structure of AChE. As originally purified from electrogenic tissue of the electric eel, *Electrophorus electricus*, AChE was found to be a globular 11 S protein (Kremzner and Wilson, 1964). It was subsequently shown that 11 S AChE is a tetramer with four similar active-site-bearing subunits, each of M.W. ~80,000, giving an overall M.W. of 300,000-350,000 (for reviews see Rosenberry, 1975; Silman, 1976). The tetramer is actually composed of ~160,000 dimers in which subunits are linked by disulfides (Froede and Wilson, 1970; Dudai and Silman, 1974a; Rosenberry *et al.*, 1974).

The 11 S form of AChE is not, however, present in fresh electric organ tissue, from which three molecular forms can be extracted, with sedimentation constants of 18 S, 14 S and 9 S (Massoulié and Rieger, 1969). These forms, which aggregate reversibly at low ionic strength (Massoulié and Rieger, 1969; Johnson *et al.*, 1977), are all converted by proteolysis or autolysis to the 11 S form which does not aggregate at low ionic strength (Massoulié *et al.*, 1970; Dudai *et al.*, 1972a). Physicochemical and electron microscope studies on purified AChE preparations revealed that all three forms obtained from fresh tissue are asymmetric structures containing a multi-subunit head connected to an elongated tail (Dudai *et al.*, 1973; Rieger *et al.*, 1973a; Bon *et al.*, 1973, 1976). Thus 18 S AChE has a molecular weight of 1.1×10^6, contains ~12 subunits in its head, and has a tail about 500 A long.

Despite the dramatic change in molecular structure caused by proteolysis, SDS-polyacrylamide gel electrophoresis in the presence of reducing agent showed that the elongated forms of AChE contain the same 80,000 polypeptide observed in 11 S AChE (Dudai *et al.*, 1972b), with small amounts of 60,000 and 20,000 components produced from the 80,000 polypeptide by autolysis (Dudai and Silman, 1974a; Rosenberry *et al.*, 1974). However, in the absence of reducing agent a different pattern was observed. Whereas 11 S AChE, under such conditions, contains primarily the 160,000 dimer (Fig. 2D), electrophoresis of 14 S + 18 S AChE without reduction reveals the presence of heavier components. Thus on 3.1% acrylamide gels two species are observed (Fig. 1.; Fig.2A) with molecular weights of ~360,000 and ~460,000, assuming the validity of M.W. calibration using myosin oligomers prepared by chemical cross-linking (Reisler *et al.*, 1973). Electrophoresis of separated samples of 14 S and 18 S AChE showed that the ~360,000 component is derived exclusively from 14 S AChE (Fig. 2B) and the ~460,000 component from 18 S AChE (Fig. 2C). The scanning pattern in Fig. 2A shows that these heavy components comprise close to half the protein applied to the gel, in agreement with earlier experiments using ^{3}H-DFP-labelled AChE, which showed that they accounted for *ca.* 40% of the catalytic subunits (Silman and Dudai, 1975).

Although no distinct polypeptide which might correspond to the tail seen in the electron microscope was observed on the gels, it seemed likely

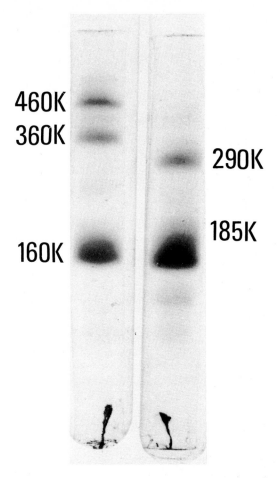

Fig. 1. Effect of collagenase on purified 14 S + 18 S AChE. SDS-acrylamide gel electrophoresis was performed on 3.1% gels and staining was with Coomassie brilliant blue. Left: Before collagenase treatment. Right: After collagenase treatment. Conditions as in legend to Fig. 3.

that the heavy components described above represent head-tail complexes linked by disulfides. Studies mentioned above on the effect of proteases on muscle endplate AChE showed that collagenase released AChE similarly (Hall and Kelly, 1971; Betz and Sakmann, 1971), with concomitant digestion of the basement membrane which contains collagenous polypeptides as major constituents (Kefalides, 1973). It was, therefore, suggested that the tail is collagen-like (Dudai *et al.*, 1973; Dudai and Silman, 1974b; Rieger *et al.*, 1973b), and the experiments described below support this contention.

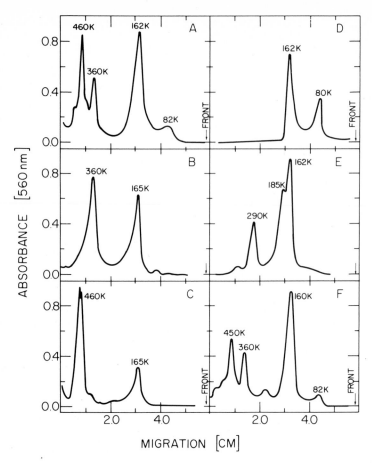

Fig. 2. Densitometer tracings of SDS-polyacrylamide gel electrophoretograms of purified samples of AChE electrophoresed under the conditions described in Fig. 1. (A) 14 S + 18 S AChE. (B) 14 S AChE. (C) 18 S AChE. (D) 11 S AChE. (E) collagenase-treated AChE prepared as described in legend to Fig. 3. (F) AChE incubated with collagenase as in (E) in the presence of 5 mM o-phenanthroline.

If the tail is indeed collagenous, the elongated forms of AChE should contain hydroxyproline and hydroxylysine, amino acids characteristic of this fibrous protein and normally absent from globular proteins. Table 1 shows that 14 S + 18 S AChE contains significant amounts of both hydroxyproline (determined colorimetrically, see Anglister *et al.*, 1976) and hydroxylysine, and that they are essentially absent in 11 S AChE. Furthermore, 14 S + 18 S AChE contains significantly more glycine than 11 S AChE. The amounts of hydroxyproline and hydroxylysine detected in 14 S + 18 S AChE, as well as the increased content of glycine (which may

TABLE 1. AMINO ACID COMPOSITION OF PURIFIED 14S+18S AChE AND 11S
AChE

AMINO ACID	11S AChE	14S+18S AChE
Lys	4.4 ± 0.2	4.4 ± 0.4
His	2.3 ± 0.1	2.5 ± 0.2
Arg	5.3 ± 0.5	5.1 ± 0.3
Asp	12.6 ± 0.7	11.4 ± 0.9
Thr	4.1 ± 0.2	4.3 ± 0.1
Ser	7.9 ± 0.9	7.9 ± 0.3
Glu	10.8 ± 0.8	10.9 ± 0.6
Pro	7.1 ± 0.9	7.1 ± 0.7
Gly	8.4 ± 0.8	11.3 ± 0.6
Ala	6.4 ± 0.5	6.1 ± 0.4
Val	6.5 ± 0.6	6.6 ± 0.7
Met	3.2 ± 1.0	2.6 ± 0.9
ILe	3.7 ± 0.3	3.3 ± 0.2
Leu	9.1 ± 0.6	8.3 ± 0.5
Tyr	3.2 ± 0.8	3.0 ± 0.3
Phe	5.5 ± 0.7	4.8 ± 0.5
Hylys	<0.05	0.60 ± 0.15
HyPro	0.10 ± 0.6	0.83 ± 0.13

Values are expressed as moles per 100 moles of total amino acid recovered ±SEM, averaged
for 9 analyses of 11S AChE and 7 analyses of 14S+18S AChE. Hydroxylysine was analysed
in 5 samples of both 14S+18S AChE and 11S AChE. Hydroxyproline was analysed colorimetrically in 8 samples of 14S+18S AChE and 6 samples of 11S enzyme.

comprise as much as 33% of the amino acid content of collagen), are in
general agreement with the values predicted if the tail were a collagen
triple helix of the length seen in the electron microscope. Similar results
have been reported for elongated AChE from *Torpedo californica*
(Lwebuga-Mukasa *et al.*, 1976). Recently, we have determined the amino
acid composition of separate polypeptides eluted from SDS-acrylamide
gels. Although quantitative data are not yet available, a significant portion
of the hydroxylysine in 14 S + 18 S AChE appears to be associated with
the ~360,000 and ~460,000 polypeptides, providing strong evidence that in
the 'native' enzyme the tail is covalently linked to the catalytic subunit
head.

Since collagenase releases AChE from muscle endplates, it might be
predicted that it would solubilize AChE from electrogenic tissue and also
modify the elongated molecular forms if their tail is indeed collagen-like. It
was shown earlier that collagenase could solubilize electric eel AChE (Dudai
and Silman, 1974b) and convert elongated forms to 11 S AChE with intermediate formation of heavier non-aggregating species (Dudai *et al.*, 1973;

Dudai and Silman, 1974b; Rieger *et al.*, 1973b). However, the action of contaminating non-specific proteases could not be excluded. Lwebuga-Mukasa *et al.* (1976) recently reported conversion of elongated AChE from *Torpedo californica* to the 11 S form by protease-free collagenase. In the following experiments protease-free collagenase from *Clostridium histolyticum* was used which was prepared according to Peterkofsky and Diegelmann (1971).

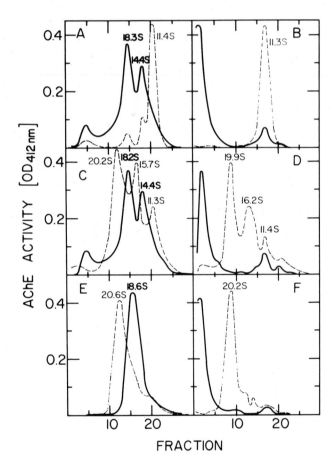

Fig. 3. Action of trypsin and collagenase on purified elongated forms of electric eel acetylcholinesterase. Sucrose gradient centrifugation was performed on 5-20% gradients containing either 1.0 M NaCl − 0.01 M phosphate, pH 7.0 (A,C,E) or 0.1 M NaCl − 0.01 M phosphate, pH 7.0 (B,D,F), before (——) and after (----) digestion with either trypsin or protease-free collagenase. Digestions were performed in 0.2 M NaCl − .05 M Tris, pH 7.0, at 25° for 1 hour. A,B: 14 S + 18 S AChE (1 mg/ml) with trypsin (50 μg/ml). C,D,: 14 S + 18 S AChE (400 μg/ml) with collagenase (20 μg/ml). E,F: 18 S + AChE (100 μg/ml) with collagenase (10 μg/ml).

As can be seen in Fig. 3 the effect of collagenase on purified AChE, assessed by sucrose gradient centrifugation, differs markedly from that of trypsin. Like trypsin, collagenase abolishes the capacity of AChE to aggregate at low ionic strength. However, whereas trypsin converts the elongated forms to the 11 S form (Fig. 3A,B), collagenase converts 18 S and 14 S AChE to non-aggregating species with significantly higher sedimentation coefficients, 20 S and 16 S respectively (Fig. 3C-F). These results are in general agreement with recent observations of Johnson *et al.* (1976), who studied the effect of collagenase on AChE in salt extracts of electric organ tissue.

SDS-acrylamide gel electrophoresis without reduction also showed that collagenase acts differently from trypsin. Whereas trypsin completely converts the heavy components in 14 S + 18 S AChE to the 160,000 dimer found in 11 S AChE, collagenase produces two new components with molecular weights of about 290,000 and 185,000 (Fig. 1, right; Fig. 2E). This process is retarded by the collagenase inhibitor o-phenanthroline (Fig. 2F) as is the change in sedimentation coefficients described above.

The effects of SDS, trypsin and collagenase on elongated forms of AChE can be rationalized by the scheme shown in Fig. 4. The 80,000 M.W. subunits are linked by disulfides to form 160,000 dimers which associate in

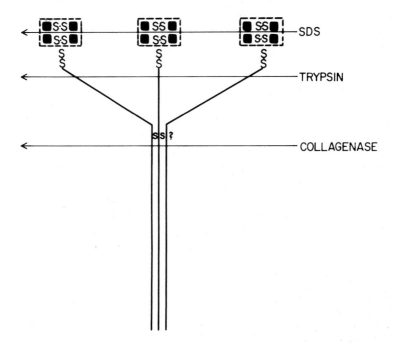

Fig. 4. Scheme showing suggested modes of cleavage of 18 S AChE by sodium dodecyl sulfate, trypsin and collagenase.

pairs to form tetramers. In 18 S AChE each tetramer is attached, presumably by disulfide bonds, to one strand of a collagen triple helix. SDS detaches only those dimers which are not covalently linked to the tail. Trypsin cleaves the tail close to the point of attachment to the catalytic subunits, releasing intact tetramers. Collagenase cleaves at a site within the stem of the tail, removing that part of the tail responsible for aggregation at low ionic strength, but leaving intact a region which holds the tetramers together. The observed increase in sedimentation coefficient may be attributed to the formation, by removal of the tail, of a more symmetric molecular structure, without a significant decrease in molecular weight, since the whole tail probably accounts for less than 10% of the total molecular weight of 18 S AChE. Determination of the Stokes radius and hydroxyproline and hydroxylysine content of the non-aggregating molecular forms produced by collagenase, as well as examination in the electron microscope, should help to determine whether cleavage indeed occurs as proposed in our model.

The data discussed above, from our laboratory and from others, provide strong evidence that the tail of the elongated forms of AChE is indeed collagen-like. The available data suggest that the role of the tail is to anchor the enzyme to the collagenous matrix of the basement membrane. Studies are currently in progress on the purification and chemical characterization of the tail.

Embryonic chick skeletal muscle acetylcholinesterase

AChE increases during development of chick skeletal muscle *in ovo* (Giacobini *et al.*, 1973), and in culture it appears shortly after myoblast fusion, together with the acetylcholine receptor (Prives and Paterson, 1974; Prives *et al.*, 1976). In adult chicken skeletal muscle three forms of AChE are observed, a major 6.5 S form and minor 11 S and 19.5 S components, the latter of which appears to be associated with the endplate (Vigny *et al.*, 1976). Both in cultures of embryonic pectoral muscle and in homogenates of breast muscle from 18-day embryos, we find only one major species of AChE on sucrose gradients, of sedimentation coefficient ~6.5 S (Fig. 5A), whether the enzyme is extracted and centrifuged at low ionic strength (~20% of the total AChE activity), or at high ionic strength in the presence of Triton X-100 (>70% of the total activity). When AChE is similarly extracted from embryonic breast muscle tissue which has been frozen and thawed at least once, very different sedimentation profiles are obtained. A new ~13 S peak is observed, and aggregated material frequently appears (Fig. 5D). It seemed possible that these changes reflect an autolytic process similar to that observed in electric organ tissue. We therefore checked the effects of prolonged autolysis and of tryptic digestion on

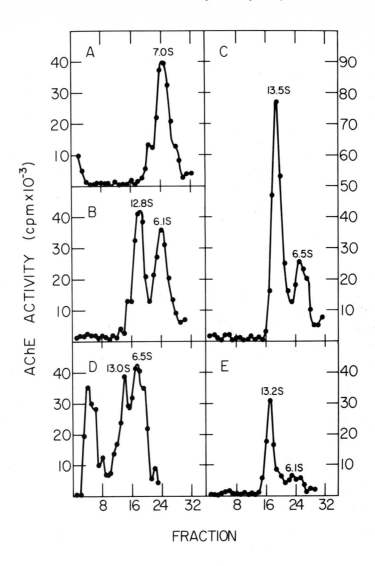

Fig. 5. Sucrose gradient centrifugation profile of acetylcholinesterase activity in homo-genates of embryonic chicken pectoral muscle before and after autolysis or tryptic treatment. Homogenates were prepared by homogenizing 1.3 g muscle tissue from 18-day embryos in 12 ml of 0.05 M Tris chloride, pH 7.5. After the appropriate incubation, homogenates were centrifuged at 100,000 × g for 1 hr at 4°; aliquots of the supernatant were applied to 5–20% sucrose gradients made up in 0.05 M Tris chloride, pH 7.5. Fractions collected were assayed radiometrically. (a) fresh tissue. (b) fresh tissue incubated with trypsin (125 µg/ml) for 15 min at 25°. (c) as in (b) but after 60 min. (d) frozen tissue. (e) fresh tissue after autolysis for 27 hr at 25°. Tryptic digestion was terminated with soybean trypsin inhibitor (125 µg/ml).

embryonic chicken breast muscle homogenates. Both these processes cause increased solubilization of AChE at low ionic strength, with concomitant conversion of the major 6.5 S form to a ~13 S species similar to that observed in frozen tissue. As can be seen in Fig. 5b and 5c, trypsin, under the conditions employed, effects this conversion almost completely in 60 min, subsequent incubation leading to gradual loss of enzymic activity. Autolysis brings about a similar conversion more slowly. After 27 hours, about 50% of the initial AChE activity is retained, and resides almost exclusively in the ~13 S peak (Fig. 5e).

From gel filtration experiments a Stokes radius of about 85 A can be determined for the 6.5 S form of chick muscle AChE and of about 68 A for the 13 S form. From these data one can calculate frictional ratios of ~2.0 for the 6.5 S form, indicating a high degree of asymmetry, and of ~1.4 for the 13 S species, indicating that the latter is a much more 'globular' structure. If it is assumed that the two species migrate on the gradient as proteins with $\bar{v} = 0.73$, molecular weights of about 260,000 and 365,000 can be calculated for the 6.5 S and 12.5 S forms respectively. The molecular parameters of the 6.5 S form of AChE are very similar to those reported by Ott *et al.* (1975) for human erythrocyte AChE, which appears to be a subunit dimer attached to an additional component. In the case of the chick skeletal muscle AChE it may be assumed that the additional component is detached by proteolytic cleavage, and that the free dimers associate in pairs to form a tetramer similar to 11 S electric eel AChE. It is not clear at this stage whether this additional component resembles the collagen-like tail in the elongated forms of electric organ AChE, and how it is involved in attachment of AChE to the surface membrane of the embryonic muscle cell.

Acknowledgements

This research was supported by grants from the Muscular Dystrophy Associations of America and the Israel Committee for Basic Research. We thank Mrs. Esther Roth for expert technical assistance and Mrs. Juliana Conu for performing the amino acid analyses.

References

Albuquerque, E.X., Sokoll, M.D., Sonesson, B. and Thesleff, S. (1968). *Eur. J. Pharm.*, **4**, 40-46.
Anglister, L., Rogozinski, S. and Silman, I. (1976). *FEBS Lett.*, **69**, 129-132.
Betz, W. and Sakmann, B. (1971). *Nature, New Biol.*, **232**, 94-95.
Bon, S., Rieger, F. and Massoulié, J. (1973). *Eur. J. Biochem.*, **35**, 372-379.
Bon, S., Huet, M., Lemonnier, M., Rieger, F. and Massoulié, J. (1976). *Eur. J. Biochem.*, **68**, 523-530.
Dudai, Y. and Silman, I. (1974a). *Biochem. Biophys. Res. Comm.*, **59**, 117-124.

Dudai, Y. and Silman, I. (1974b). *J. Neurochem.*, **23**, 1177-1187.
Dudai, Y., Silman, I., Kalderon, N. and Blumberg, S. (1972a). *Biochim. Biophys. Acta*, **268**, 138-157.
Dudai, Y., Silman, I., Shinitzky, M. and Blumberg, S. (1972b). *Proc. Nat. Acad. Sci.*, **69**, 2400-2403.
Dudai, Y., Herzberg, M. and Silman, I. (1973). *Proc. Nat. Acad. Sci.*, **70**, 2473-2476.
Froede, H.C. and Wilson, I.B. (1970). *Israel J. Med. Sci.*, **6**, 179-184.
Giacobini, G., Filogamo, G., Weber, M., Boquet, P. and Changeux, J.-P. (1973). *Proc. Nat. Acad. Sci.*, **70**, 1708-1712.
Hall, Z.W. (1973). *J. Neurobiol.*, **4**, 343-362.
Hall, Z.W. and Kelly, R.B. (1971). *Nature, New. Biol.*, **232**, 62-63.
Johnson, C.D., Smith, S.P. and Russell, R.L. (1977). *J. Neurochem.*, **28**, 617-624.
Karlin, A. and Cowburn, D. (1973). *Proc. Nat. Acad. Sci.*, **70**, 3636-3640.
Kefalides, N.A. (1973). *Int. Rev. Conn. Tissue Res.*, **6**, 63-104.
Kremzner, L.T. and Wilson, I.B. (1964). *Biochemistry*, **3**, 1902-1905.
Lwebuga-Mukasa, J.S., Lappi, S. and Taylor, P. (1976). *Biochemistry*, **15**, 1425-1434.
Massoulié, J. and Rieger, F. (1969). *Eur. J. Biochem.*, **11**, 441-455.
Massoulié, J., Rieger, F. and Tsuji, S. (1970). *Eur. J. Biochem.*, **14**, 430-439.
Ott, P., Jenny, B. and Brodbeck, U. (1975). *Eur. J. Biochem.*, **57**, 469-480.
Peterkofsky, B. and Diegelmann, R. (1971). *Biochemistry*, **10**, 988-994.
Prives, J.M. and Paterson, B. (1974). *Proc. Nat. Acad. Sci.*, **71**, 3208-3211.
Prives, J.M., Silman, I. and Amsterdam, A. (1976). *Cell*, **7**, 543-550.
Reisler, E.M., Burke, M., Josephs, R. and Harrington, W.F. (1973). *J. Mechanochem. Cell Motility*, **2**, 163-179.
Rieger, F., Bon, S., Massoulié, J. and Cartaud, J. (1973a). *Eur. I. Biochem.*, **34**, 539-547.
Rieger, F., Bon, S. and Massoulié, J. (1973b). *FEBS Lett.*, **36**, 12-16.
Rosenberg, P., Silman, I., Ben-David, E., de Vries, A. and Condrea, E. (1977). *J. Neurochem.*, in press.
Rosenberry, T.L. (1975). *Advances in Enzymol.*, **43**, 103-218.
Rosenberry, T.L., Chen, Y.T. and Bock, E. (1974). *Biochemistry*, **13**, 3068-3079.
Silman, I. (1976). *Trends in Biochemical Sciences*, **1**, 225-227.
Silman, I. and Dudai, Y. (1975). *Croatica Chimica Acta*, **47**, 181-200.
Silman, H.I. and Karlin, A. (1967). *Proc. Nat. Acad. Sci.*, **58**, 1664-1668.
Taylor, P., Jones, J.W. and Jacobs, N.M. (1974). *Mol. Pharmacol.*, **10**, 78-92.
Vigny, M., di Giamberardino, L., Couraud, J.Y., Rieger, F. and Koenig, J. (1976). *FEBS Lett.*, **69**, 277-280.

8 Origin of the acetyl group in acetylcholine at the neuromuscular junction of the rat

PATRICK A. DREYFUS

I.N.S.E.R.M. U 153
Groupe de Biologie et Pathologie Neuromusculaire
Division Risler — La Salpêtrière
47 bd de l'Hôpital, Paris (13è)

Acetylcholine (ACh) at the neuromuscular junction is synthesized in the cytoplasm of axon terminals from choline and acetyl-CoA by the action of choline acetyl-transferase (EC 2.3.1.6.). Studies on the origin of the acetyl radical have given different results according to the material studied: the cortex (Browning and Schulman, 1968) and the neo-striatum (Lefresne *et al.*, 1973) of the rat incorporate pyruvate for the synthesis of the acetyl radical of ACh; acetate is not used. The electric tissue of the Torpedo preferentially incorporates acetate (Israel and Tucek, 1974); as does lobster nerve (Cheng and Nakamura, 1970). Given the anatomical and biochemical similarities of nerve electroplaque junctions and neuromuscular junctions, it is interesting to investigate the origin of the acetyl radical for ACh synthesis in the latter material.

In this work, we have studied the kinetics of the differential incorporation of acetate and pyruvate at the neuromuscular junction. We have used the sternonuclear mastoid muscle of the rat, which has a neural zone visible as a fine striation due to the myelinated axons. The muscles were dissected from male rats (150 to 200 g) anaesthetized with diethyl ether. After ligation of the motor nerve, the muscle, fixed to a support, was submerged in physiological medium which had the following composition: 136-mM $NaC1$; 5.6-mM $KC1$; 1.2-mM NaH_2PO_4, Na_2HPO_4 buffer at pH 7.4; 1.2-mM $MgC1_2$; 16.2-mM $NaHCO_3$; 5.5-mM D-glucose; 2.2-mM $CaC1_2$. This solution was maintained at pH 7.4 by aerating with a mixture of O_2-CO_2 (95%-5%), at a temperature of 38°C. Before incubation 5 μCi/ml (1-^{14}C) acetate (1 mM) with or without 10 mM pyruvate or 5 μCi/ml (2-^{14}C) pyruvate (1 mM) with or without 10 mM acetate, was added. After incubation, the muscle was washed in physiological medium, and rapidly submerged in isopentane cooled by liquid nitrogen. Each muscle was then cut transversely in 1.5 mm thick slices and each slice submerged for about 10 minutes in physiological medium acidified by HCl (pH 3.5 to 4) at 90°C (Israel, 1970). The same results were obtained by acidifying with trichloracetic acid (5% w-v), which in this case was afterwards removed with ether.

Acetylcholine, released into the supernatant, was extracted by tetraphenyl borate dissolved in ethyl butyl ketone (10 mg/ml) (Lefresne *et al.*, 1973). The complex of ACh and tetraphenyl-borate was dissociated by 1.0M HCl. After drying, the extract was solubilized in 20 μl of methanol and analysed by chromatography on a thin layer of cellulose-F, according to the technique described by Marchbanks and Israel (1971). The radioactivity of the acetylcholine spot was measured by scintillation counting. When the extract had been treated with acetylcholinesterase, no acetylcholine spot was found. The value corresponding to the slices of the neural zone is shown as a function of the time of incubation in Figures 1-2.

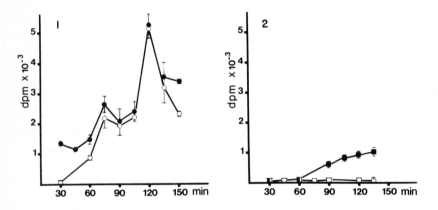

Fig. 1. Radioactivity incorporated into the acetylcholine of the neural zone as a function of time; O–O in the presence of 1mM [¹⁴C] acetate ●—● in the presence of 1mM [¹⁴C] acetate + 10 mM pyruvate.

Fig. 2. Radioactivity incorporated into the acetylcholine of the neural zone as a function of time; ■—■ in the presence of 1mM [¹⁴C] pyruvate □—□ in the presence of 1mM [¹⁴C] pyruvate + 10mM acetate.

In these figures each point represents the mean of three experiments.

The curves show that acetate is incorporated in the ACh of neural zones. Moreover they show that the incorporation of [¹⁴C] acetate is not impaired by a ten-fold excess of pyruvate. [¹⁴C] Pyruvate is also incorporated, but its incorporation is prevented by ten-fold excess of acetate. These results indicate that the acetyl radical of ACh is specifically labelled at the neuromuscular junction, and that acetate is the preferred precursor. The biochemical similarity between the nerve electroplaque junction and the neuromuscular junction is thus apparent. The same mechanism for recycling acetate, as has been proposed for the nerve electroplaque junctions of Torpedo (Dunant *et al.* (1974) seems to occur at the mammalian neuro-muscular junction.

References

Browning, E.T. and Schulman, M.P. (1968). *J. Neurochem.*, **15**, 1391-1405.
Cheng, S.C. and Nakamura, H. (1970). *Biochem. J.*, **118**, 451-455.
Dunant, Y., Gautron, J., Israel, M., Lesbats, B. and Manaranche, R. *J. Neuro-*

Dunant, Y., Gautron, J., Israel, M., Lesbats, B. and Manaranche, R. (1974). *J. Neurochem.*, **23**, 635-643.
Israel, M. (1970). *Arch. Anat. micro. Morphol. exp.*, **59**, 67-98.
Israel, M. and Tucek, S. (1974). *J. Neurochem.*, **22**, 487-491.
Lefresne, P., Guyenet, P. and Glowinski, J. (1973). *J. Neurochem.*, **20**, 1083-1097.
Marchbanks, R.M. and Israel, M. (1971). *J. Neurochem.*, **18**, 439-448.

9 Pathological mechanisms in myasthenia gravis and its animal model, experimental autoimmune myasthenia gravis

JON LINDSTROM

The Salk Institute for Biological Studies
P.O. Box 1809, San Diego,
California, U.S.A. 92112

Introduction

The weakness and fatigability characteristic of skeletal muscles in patients with myasthenia gravis (MG) is now known to result from impaired neuromuscular transmission due to an autoimmune response to skeletal muscle acetylcholine receptors (AChR). Animals immunized against purified AChR develop muscular weakness due to cross reaction between the immune reponse directed at the purified AChR and AChR in their muscles. Animals with experimental autoimmune myasthenia gravis (EAMG) produced in this way have proven excellent models for study of the pathological mechanisms causing impaired neuromuscular transmission in humans with MG. In this chapter studies of EAMG and MG by my collaborators and myself will be reviewed.

Most of our studies have begun with an examination of the animal model, and those features which were defined through studies of EAMG in the rat then tested for in patients with MG. In 1960 John Simpson (Simpson, 1960) proposed that MG might be caused by auto-antibodies which blocked transmission by preventing binding of acetylcholine to its receptor. At that time no biochemical techniques were available for measuring AChR or antibodies to AChR. Lee's demonstration (Lee *et al.*, 1967) that snake neurotoxins bind specifically and with high affinity to the acetylcholine binding site of muscle AChR was a critical advance. Radiolabelled toxins were used to locate and quantitate AChR in muscle (Berg *et al.*, 1972). More importantly, labelled toxin permitted identification of AChR extracted from the membrane (Miledi *et al.*, 1971) and toxin was used on affinity columns to purify AChR from electric organs of eels (Lindstrom and Patrick, 1974). As soon as the first few milligrams of protein were purified by toxin affinity chromatography, it became important to demonstrate that this toxin binding protein was AChR. Jim Patrick and I reasoned

135

that, if antibodies to the purified material could block the response of eel electroplax to carbamylcholine, it would prove that the purified protein was part of the physiological AChR. Although we were aware of the role that Simpson had suggested for antibodies to AChR in impairing neuromuscular transmission in MG, we did not think that the AChR protein from electric eels would be sufficiently similar in structure to the AChR from rat muscle to cross react and we were therefore very surprised to discover that rabbits immunized with the protein purified from electric eels became weak and died. In fact, only a few percent of the antibodies formed against the eel AChR were also able to recognize muscle AChR, but the absolute amount of these antibodies was quite large when compared with the amount of AChR in the muscle of the immunized animal (Lindstrom et al., 1976d, 1977a). Subsequently, in the sera of MG patients we found similar concentrations of antibodies which were directed at AChR from human muscle (Lindstrom et al., 1976e, Lindstrom, 1977). Only a few of these antibodies also recognized AChR from other species (Lindstrom et al., 1976d, Lindstrom, 1977a).

Our results suggest that antibody mediated mechanisms are primarily responsible for impairing neuromuscular transmission in EAMG and MG. Rats given a single injection of purified AChR in Freund's adjuvant and pertussis as additional adjuvant exhibit first an acute and then a chronic form of EAMG (Lennon et al., 1975). If the rats can survive until the immune response has diminished sufficiently, they recover (Lindstrom, 1977c). The course of EAMG in rats is represented diagramatically in Figs. 3-6. Human MG, closely resembles the chronic form of EAMG in the pathological mechanisms impairing neuromuscular transmission, but differs in that in MG there is a continuing immune response specific for human AChR, which is probably stimulated by some endogenous immunogen. In chronic EAMG and MG antibodies impair neuromuscular transmission not only by directly inhibiting AChR activity, but more importantly by causing loss of AChR and morphological alteration of the postsynaptic membrane. Mechanisms by which AChR content is decreased include antibody dependent complement mediated focal lysis of the postsynaptic membrane and antigenic modulation of AChR resulting in an enhanced rate of AChR destruction.

Serum antibodies to AChR in EAMG and MG

Serum antibodies to AChR are usually quantitated using solubilized AChR labelled with ^{125}I-toxin as antigen (Patrick et al., 1973). In this method serum is incubated with aliquots of ^{125}I-toxin labelled AChR and then anti-immunoglobulin is added to precipitate the complexes of antibody-AChR-^{125}I-toxin. Radioactivity of the washed precipitate is measured.

This method in addition to extreme sensitivity, reproducibility, and ease has other virtues in that crude extracts of AChR can be used as well as purified AChR because the specificity of the antigen lies in the specificity of ^{125}I-toxin binding to the AChR. Thus the reaction of antibodies from rats immunized with torpedo AChR or from humans with MG can be quantitated using crude extracts of AChR from rat or human muscle. From a precipitin curve in which increasing amounts of antibody are added to a fixed amount of ^{125}I-toxin labelled AChR two kinds of information are obtained. First, the linear initial slope, under conditions where ^{125}I-toxin-AChR is in great excess, gives a titre for the antiserum in terms of moles of ^{125}I-toxin-AChR which can be bound per litre of serum. Secondly, the plateau, under conditions where antibody is in great excess, provides a measure of AChR concentration. Immunoprecipitation is routinely used to measure the AChR content of extracts of muscle and to measure complexes of antibodies with AChR in these extracts that were found *in vivo* (Lindstrom *et al.*, 1976b, c).

In the sera of animals immunized against AChR purified from electric organs, the concentration of antibodies which recognize only the electric organ AChR is much higher than the concentration of antibodies which also recognize AChR in the animal's muscle (Lindstrom *et al.*, 1976d). However, at late stages in the immune response, the absolute amount of antibody in the serum of an animal with chronic EAMG may be very large with respect to the AChR content of that animal. For example, a rat immunized with torpedo AChR may have a serum titre of 10^{-5} M against torpedo AChR, but only 1×10^{-7} M against rat muscle AChR. Although this means that the serum is highly species specific and cross reacts only 1% with rat muscle AChR, a typical rat having 5 ml of serum would contain 5×10^{-10} moles of antibody, whereas a normal rat contains only about 1/10 this amount, 5×10^{-11} moles, AChR (Lindstrom *et al.*, 1976b,c).

Another important quantitative aspect is that the formation of antibodies provides a great amplification effect. For example, rat muscle AChR is very difficult to purify in large amounts. Immunization of a rat with 2.6×10^{-11} moles of syngeneic rat AChR causes EAMG and thereby the production of an antiserum capable of binding 50×10^{-11} moles of rat AChR (Lindstrom *et al.*, 1976b). The amount of protein used to immunize was too small to study chemically, but the antibodies raised against it provide a useful probe for studying AChR. Electric organ AChR is highly immunogenic. In rats, EAMG has been induced by single immunizations with 1.6 μg of electric eel AChR (Lindstrom *et al.*, 1976d) and 1 μg or less of torpedo AChR (Lindstrom *et al.*, 1977a).

The specificities of antibodies to AChR have been studied by studying the cross reaction between antibodies and AChR extracted from various sources (Lindstrom *et al.*, 1977a). Serum antibodies reacting with AChR extracted from human muscle have been found in 87% of MG patients studied (Lindstrom, 1977a). Antibody concentration averaged 44×10^{-9} M, but ranged from 0-840 $\times$ 10^{-9} M. The antibodies in the sera tested cross-reacted negligeably with AChR extracted from eel electric organ (Lindstrom et al., 1976d) and only slightly more, on the average, with AChR from torpedo (2.5%) or rat (1.9%) (Lindstrom et al., 1977a). Reaction was greater with AChR from squirrel monkey. Although there were these similarities between all MG patients, the degree of cross reaction with various AChR differed between patients, suggesting that they were not all recognizing a single antigenic determinant on AChR (Lindstrom et al., 1977a). Similar cross reaction studies using sera from rats, rabbits, and goats immunized with AChR purified from rats, electric eels, and Torpedo californica have been performed (Lindstrom et al., 1977a). Like the MG patients' sera, sera from the immunized animals were mostly quite species specific. Study of the specificities of these sera suggest that AChR contain a number of antigenic sites, many of which are species specific, but some of which are shared by AChR from other species. All of these sites are not immunogenically equivalent. Specificities of antisera to AChR varied widely depending on the animal immunized, its species, the AChR used as immunogen, and the duration of immunization. Cross reaction between AChR probably involves any of several determinants.

How does antibody effect the function of AChR to which it binds? All the antibodies detected by immunoprecipitation using ^{125}I-toxin-AChR are directed against antigenic determinants other than the acetycholine binding site, which is protected by the ^{125}I-toxin. ^{3}H acetylated eel AChR used as antigen does not have its active site protected, yet precipitin curves using it as antigen are superimposable with those using ^{125}I-toxin-AChR (Patrick et al., 1973). Small amounts of antibodies which were prevented from binding to ^{3}H acetyl-AChR were found in rabbit anti-eel AChR serum (Patrick et al., 1973), but none could be found in goat anti-eel AChR serum (Lindstrom, 1976). Excesses of antibody can prevent binding of ^{125}I-toxin to AChR, but this may result from aggregation or an allosteric effect when many antibody molecules are bound to each AChR (Lindstrom et al., 1976e). Goat anti-eel AChR serum blocks the activity of AChR on eel electric organ cells without substantially reducing ^{125}I-toxin binding (Lindstrom et al., 1977a). Thus, even in membrane bound AChR, binding of antibody need not block the toxin binding site, though large excesses can (Lindstrom, 1976). It is quite possible, however, that although an antibody molecule did not bind at the site where acetylcholine was bound, it could allosterically reduce the binding affinity for acetylcholine. Bound antibodies might also interfere with the regulation or function of the ionophore. AChR extracted from antibody treated electroplax (Lindstrom et al., 1977a) or rats with EAMG (Lindstrom et al., 1976b, c) are crosslinked into aggregates by antibodies. Because sera contain populations of antibodies directed at many determinants on the AChR molecule, and because it is probable that several antibodies can bind simultaneously to an AChR, antibodies probably act simultaneously by several mechanisms to directly impair AChR function in an animal with EAMG. Interestingly,

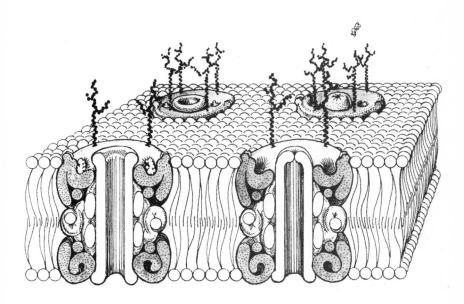

Fig. 1. Hypothetical representation of AChR structure in the postsynaptic membrane. AChR molecules are depicted as integral membrane proteins traversing the membrane and composed of several dissimilar polypeptide chains which contain carbohydrate residues on the extracellular surface. Each receptor is depicted as having two stereospecific binding sites for acetylcholine which allosterically regulate the opening and closing of an ionophore through which cations can traverse the membrane. This diagrammatic representation incorporates some features of AChR structure and function which have recently been reviewed in detail (Karlin *et al.*, 1976; Changeux *et al.*, 1976; Raftery *et al.*, 1976; and Stevens *et al.*, 1976). Although AChR is known to be multimeric, it is not known that it has only two ACh binding sites. And although negatively stained membrane fragments rich in AChR contain doughnut-like structures with negatively staining centers, it is not known whether this corresponds to the ionophore of the AChR macromolecule or whether there is only one ionophore per molecule.

however, studies of acetylcholine noise in the muscles of rats with EAMG have shown that some antibody bound AChR can still pass about 2/3 the normal amount of charge when they are active (Heinemann *et al.*, 1977). A diagramatic representation of the AChR molecule is shown in Fig. 1, and in Fig. 2 antibodies bound to it are depicted.

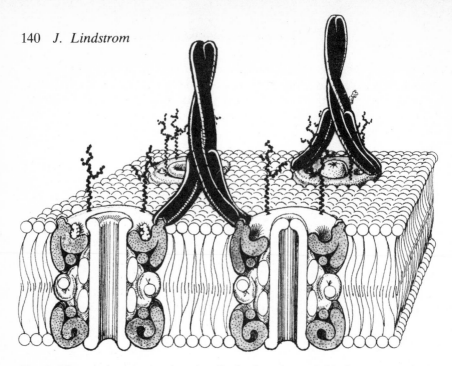

Fig. 2. Diagramatic representation of antibodies bound to acetylcholine receptors in the postsynaptic membrane *in vivo*. Antibodies are depicted as bound to some of the many antigenic determinants on the extracellular surface of the AChR molecule. These antigenic sites are represented as occurring on conformationally important features of the protein, but antibodies to carbohydrate determinants may also exist. *In vivo*, antibodies directed at determinants on the cytoplasmic surface of the AChR molecule cannot bind. Because AChR are multivalent, one antibody is depicted as binding bivalently to a single molecule. Binding of antibody molecules to determinants outside of the acetylcholine binding site may impair AChR activity through allosteric inhibition of acetylcholine binding or through impairing ionophore function. Another antibody is depicted as crosslinking two AChR through symmetrically disposed antigenic determinants. Crosslinking of many closely packed AChR into large aggregates may be a necessary prerequisite for obtaining antigenic modulation, perhaps through endocytosis of these aggregates. Evidence suggests that many of the antibodies bound to AChR are also involved in binding of complement components to the membrane, which causes focal destruction of the membrane.

Pathological mechanisms resulting in impaired neuromuscular transmission in acute and passively transferred EAMG

After rats have been given a single injection of purified AChR in adjuvant, two phases of muscular weakness are seen (Lennon *et al.*, 1975). An acute phase of muscular weakness occurs 8-10 days after injection, followed 28-30 days after the injection by a chonic phase of weakness which persists until the rat dies or until about 100 days when the response to the immunogen diminishes (Lindstrom, 1977c). An obvious phase of acute weakness in rats can be eliminated by immunizing in complete Freund's adjuvant alone without the use of pertussis at other sites as additional adjuvant. Even an obvious chronic phase of weakness can be eliminated by immunization with low doses of AChR. However, rats can lose 60% of their total AChR content and have up to 50% of the remainder bound by antibody and not exhibit clinical weakness (Lindstrom and Lambert, 1977c). This may be because rats have a very large safety factor for neuromuscular transmission resulting from the unusually large amount of quanta in their endplate potentials (Lambert *et al.*, 1976). Responses of animals to immunization with AChR also depend on the immunogen and the species immunized. For example, a goat immunized with eel AChR showed no acute phase, but rapidly developed relatively high concentrations of antibodies cross reacting with muscle AChR and exhibited weakness at 25 days (Lindstrom *et al.*, 1977a). Several goats immunized with equivalent doses of torpedo AChR very quickly developed high titers of highly species specific antibodies to torpedo ($>10^{-6}$ M by 11 days). However, at this time, cross reaction with muscle AChR was extremely low and multiple immunizations were required for at least 60 days until weakness was observed. By this time, the titre against muscle AChR was comparable to that in many rats 30-40 days after a single injection, and the titre against torpedo AChR was $>10^{-5}$ M (Lindstrom *et al.*, 1977a). Unlike rats, rabbits immunized with AChR from eel or torpedo show no acute phase, and many die suddenly at 25 to 30 days after immunization rather than sustain chronic weakness (Patrick and Lindstrom, 1973; and Lindstrom, unpublished).

The remaining discussion of EAMG will be confined to our studies of rats. Figures 3-5 depict a rat neuromuscular junction and show how it is affected by the initial and acute phases of EAMG. All our detailed studies of acute EAMG have used rats given pertussis as additional adjuvant. Since the acute phase can be eliminated by omission of pertussis (Lindstrom and Einarson, unpublished observation), it may be that the phagocytic invasion of the endplate characteristic of acute EAMG is an artifact of this method of immunization. On the other hand, this method may be exaggerating a process which otherwise precedes chronic EAMG in a less concerted fashion.

Binding of antibodies to AChR at the tips of postjunctional folds is the first critical event leading to impaired neuromuscular transmission in EAMG. Focal destruction of the tips of postjunctional folds (Engel *et al.*, 1976a, b), is the first visible evidence of pathology at the junction. Both antibody and the C3 component of complement can be demonstrated in the fragments released into the intersynaptic space during focal destruction (Sahashi *et al.*, 1977). Acute EAMG occurs at a time when concentrations of serum antibody cross reacting with rat muscle are very low (Lindstrom *et al.*, 1976d). By day 10, two-thirds of the serum antibodies are γG and only one-third γM (Lindstrom *et al.*, 1976d). γM is probably not especially important, since γG purified from the serum of rats with chronic EAMG and

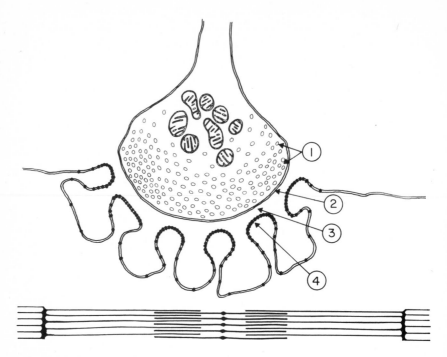

Fig. 3. Diagramatic representation of a normal neuromuscular junction. Numbers on the diagram point out (1) acetylcholine containing vesicles in the nerve ending. (2) The presynaptic membrane of the nerve. (3) The intersynaptic space across which acetylcholine must diffuse after release through specific regions on the presynaptic membrane, and (4) folds in the postsynaptic membrane of the muscle where AChR concentrated at the tips is closely presented to the sites of acetylcholine release.

given intravenously to normal rats causes the same massive phagocytic invasion of the endplate region which characterizes acute EAMG (Lindstrom *et al.*, 1976c). Only a small fraction of muscle AChR is bound by antibodies during passive or acute EAMG (Lindstrom *et al.*, 1976b, c), but the antibody dependent phagocytic invasion which follows destroys a much larger number of AChR. This amplifying effect of the phagocytic invasion accounts for the observation that passive EAMG can be transferred to a rat containing 6×10^{-11} moles of AChR with purified γG sufficient to bind only 1×10^{-11} moles of AChR (Lindstrom *et al.*, 1976c).

The massive phagocytic invasion of the endplate region which characterizes acute EAMG is not observed later in the response (Engel *et al.*, 1976a, b). During the acute phase, mononuclear phagocytic cells and neutrophil leucocytes are observed in the endplate region. The postsynaptic membrane is seen to split away from many fibres, and in some fibres segmental necrosis is observed centered on the endplate region. The same

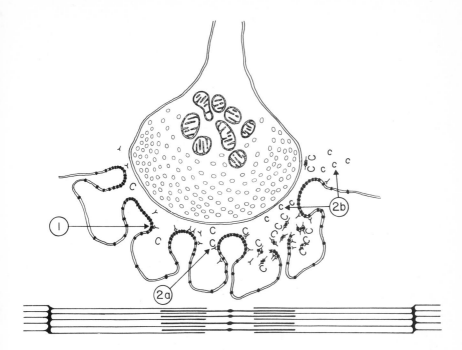

Fig. 4. Diagramatic representation of the initial events in the immune assault on the post-synaptic membrane during EAMG. (1) A small fraction of the AChR in the postsynaptic membrane are bound with antibodies. (2a) Complement is activated by some of the bound antibodies, resulting in focal destruction of the tips of postsynaptic folds where AChR are most concentrated. (2b) Specific proteolytic fragments of complement are released during the complement cascade which induces phagocytic migration to the endplate.

features are observed in normal rats given purified anti-AChR γG from rats with chronic EAMG (Lindstrom *et al.*, 1976c). This suggests that most of the cells seen during the acute phase are dependent on recognition of bound antibody rather than recognition of AChR *per se*. Phagocytic migration into the endplate is probably dependent on chemotactic fragments of complement (e.g. C3A) released during the interaction of antibodies bound to AChR with complement. What terminates the phagocytic invasion is unknown. Because there is so little AChR in a normal rat, it seems unlikely that sufficient amounts of antibody-AChR complexes could be shed to paralyse all peripheral phagocytes. However, this has not been tested in rats, and it may be that AChR turnover in a rat with EAMG is sufficient to generate relatively large amounts of antibody-AChR complexes.

During acute and passively transferred EAMG, AChR content of rat muscle transiently decreases (Lindstrom *et al.*, 1976b, c). This is followed by

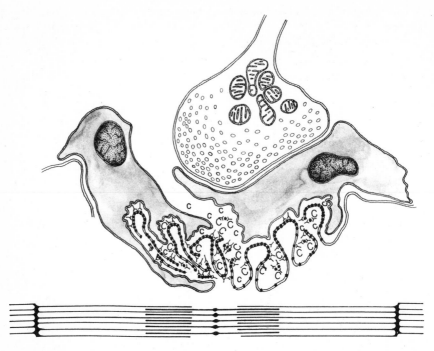

Fig. 5. Diagramatic representation of the acute phase of EAMG and of passively transferred EAMG. These events are seen within 1 day after passively transferring antibodies to AChR to a normal rat or 8-11 days after immunization of a rat with purified AChR. Phagocytes invade the endplate, recognize bound antibody, and strip off large areas of postynaptic membrane. Thus binding of antibodies to a small number of the AChR results in the destruction of large numbers of AChR. Phagocytic processes interposed between nerve ending and postsynaptic membrane may directly impair neuromuscular transmission. When EAMG is passively transferred with antibodies to AChR, all of the phagocytes seen are passively sensitized, and interact with antibody labelled AChR through F_c receptors, but some of the phagocytic cells observed in acute EAMG may be actively immune and have receptors for AChR. If the acute phase is intense, most muscle fibres will be transiently denervated. The acute phase is transient, and after 2-3 days the phagocytic invasion disappears. If pertussis is not used as an additional adjuvant, no clinical signs of an acute phase are seen. It is not known whether the acute phase is an artifact of the use of pertussis or whether it reveals a process that otherwise would occur in a less concerted way in EAMG and perhaps MG.

a transient increase to more than double the normal amount. The decrease is associated with phagocytic destruction of the postsynaptic membrane. The two or three day period following the acute phase when AChR content is abnormally high is probably the result both of repair synthesis as the phagocytic invasion diminshes and of synthesis of AChR at extrajunctional sites due to functional denervation during the acute phase. The final decrease in AChR probably starts as extrajunctional AChR synthesis is terminated by re-innervation, and continues by the mechanisms resulting in chronic EAMG.

Electrophysiological studies of acute and passively transferred EAMG show several features not observed in chronic EAMG or MG. These are (1) decreased electromyogram amplitude (2) absence of evoked potentials in many fibres, and (3) a slight decrease in resting potential (Lambert *et al.*, 1976). The first two of these effects are attributable to complete inhibition of transmission by phagocytes at some junctions and the third effect is attributable to leakages produced during phagocytic destruction of the postsynaptic membrane. As in chronic EAMG and MG, decrementing electromyogram responses to repeated stimulation (Seybold *et al.*, 1976) and reduced mepp amplitude are also observed (Lambert *et al.*, 1976). During passive transfer, the time course of change in these electrophysiological parameters and in clinical signs of muscle weakness all parallel the decrease in AChR content (Lindstrom *et al.*, 1976c).

Pathological mechanisms in chronic EAMG

In rats with chronic EAMG serum antibody titres to rat muscle AChR are usually quite high (10-100 $\times$ 10^{-9} M). A rapid increase in serum antibody titre is noted around the time of onset of clinical weakness (Lindstrom *et al.*, 1976d). Passive transfer experiments demonstrate that these antibodies have ready access to AChR in the postsynaptic membrane (Lindstrom *et al.*, 1976c). The serum antibody content of a rat with a titre of 100×10^{-9} M is sufficient to bind ten times the AChR content of a normal rat.

Receptor content is severely reduced in rats with chronic EAMG (Lindstrom *et al.*, 1976b). Total AChR content of rats with chronic EAMG is not usually reduced below 30-40% of normal (Lindstrom *et al.*, 1977b), but increasing severity of disease is associated with binding of an increasing proportion of the remaining AChR with antibodies (Lindstrom and Lambert, 1977). The content of AChR remaining unbound by antibodies is usually reduced to less than 10% of the normal AChR content before obvious signs of clinical weakness are observed. Nearly moribund rats have virtually all their AChR bound with antibodies. Sucrose gradient sedimentation shows that the antibody-bound AChR are crosslinked into aggregates (Lindstrom *et al.*, 1976b). AChR to which antibodies bound *in vivo* retain their ability to bind toxin, showing that their AChR binding site is not completely obstructed.

Electron microscopic studies of rats with chronic EAMG reveal a greatly simplified postsynaptic membrane structure lacking the normal folds (Engel *et al.*, 1976a, b). The appearance of the endplate suggests a highly dynamic system. Small membrane fragments and larger myelin figures are strewn

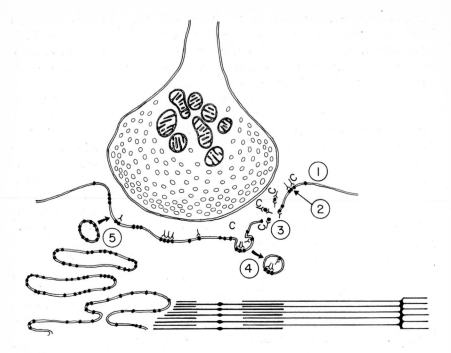

Fig. 6. Diagramatic representation of a neuromuscular junction in chronic EAMG and human MG. Chronic muscular weakness and fatigability characteristic of chronic EAMG appear in rats about 30 days after a single immunization with purified AChR. Serum antibody titre against muscle AChR is nearing a maximum at this time, and if a rat can survive until the response to the immunogen diminishes sufficiently, it will recover. (1) The folded structure of the postsynaptic membrane is greatly simplified and contains a greatly reduced number of AChR. (2) Many of the AChR which remain have antibodies bound. (3) Complement mediated focal destruction of the postsynaptic membrane causes loss of AChR through shedding of complexes and antibody, AChR and complement into the intersynaptic space. (4) Antigenic modulation of AChR causes loss of AChR independent of complement. This may proceed through endocytosis of AChR aggregated by antibodies. In tissue culture, the internalized complexes are degraded to amino acid residues. In any event, antibody enhances the rate of destruction of AChR. (5) Enhanced synthesis of AChR may partially compensate for loss of AChR from the membrane. Newly synthesized AChR may be those not yet labelled by the overwhelming excess of antibodies to AChR in the serum. The simplified structure of the postsynaptic membrane may result from a dynamic balance between AChR destruction and AChR synthesis.

around in the endplate region. Antibodies bound to the postsynaptic membrane can be demonstrated in a patchy distribution by staining with peroxidase conjugated to protein A (Engel *et al.*, 1977a, b and Sahashi *et al.*, 1977). Reduced amounts of AChR distributed in patches along the membrane can be demonstrated by staining with peroxidase conjugated to toxin (Engel *et al.*, 1977a, b and Sahashi *et al.*, 1977). Fragments of membrane which can be stained for both antibody and the C3 component of complement are observed in the intersynaptic space adjacent to areas of focal destruction on the postsynaptic membrane (Engel *et al.*, 1977a, b and Sahashi *et al.*, 1977). This clearly suggests that complement mediated, antibody dependent membrane lysis is responsible for significant amounts of the observed AChR loss in chronic EAMG.

Antigenic modulation of AChR may be another mechanism contributing to AChR loss in chronic EAMG (Lindstrom *et al.*, 1976c). Antibodies from rats with chronic EAMG caused an increase rate of destruction of AChR in the membranes of cultured rat muscle or BC_3H1 cells (Heinemann *et al.*, 1977 and Lindstrom *et al.*, 1977b). Modulation is energy, temperature, and time dependent. Substantial AChR loss occurs in hours. Crosslinking of AChR in the membrane is important for this effect, and it is not observed if monomeric FAb is used instead of divalent antibody (Lindstrom *et al.*, 1977b). AChR in cultured cells are rapidly turned over like those in denervated muscle (Devreotes and Fambrough, 1975), whereas junctional AChR normally turnover very slowly (Berg and Hall, 1974). Antibodies may only increase this ongoing rate of turnover. It is not yet known whether antibodies can cause modulation of intact synaptic AChR at a normal junction. It may be that complement and/or phagocyte mediated destruction of the normal static population of AChR is a necessary prerequisite before antigenic modulation can take place.

The rate of AChR synthesis may be increased in rats with chronic EAMG. No direct evidence for this contention exists. However, since large excesses of antibody are present in serum, and both complement mediated destruction and modulation could be expected to act with a time course of hours, it seems likely that increased AChR synthesis may be an important factor contributing to survival in rats with chronic EAMG. The rapid increase in AChR content in the day or two following the acute phase indicates how rapidly and extensively AChR synthesis can be turned on. Those AChR remaining unbound by antibodies in rats with chronic EAMG may be those most recently synthesized and inserted in the membrane.

The evidence of electrophysiological impairment in rats with chronic EAMG is attributable to both loss of AChR and inhibition of the remaining AChR by bound antibodies. Presynaptic function appears normal, as indicated by a normal number of quanta released per impulse (Lambert *et al.*, 1976). Miniature endplate potentials of decreased amplitude and decrementing electromyograms are observed in chronic EAMG (Lambert *et al.*, 1976). Muscle from rats with EAMG is less sensitive to acetylcholine (Bevan *et al.*, 1976) and more sensitive to curare (Lambert *et al.*, 1976 and Seybold *et al.*, 1976). After the total AChR content in rats with EAMG has decreased to a minimum of approximately 30-40% of normal, increasing weakness is associated with binding of an increasing fraction of AChR by antibodies. This suggests that direct impairment of AChR function by bound antibodies plays an important role in EAMG (Lindstrom and Lambert, 1977). At least some of the AChR to which antibodies are bound retain some function. Study of acetylcholine noise in muscles of rats with chronic EAMG shows that some AChR have a reduced open time (by 15%) and a reduced conductance when open (by 23%) resulting in a net decrease in charge passed of around 33% every time that AChR opens (Heinemann *et al.*, 1977). Partial functioning of antibody-bound AChR in rats having essentially no free AChR remaining could account for the precarious survival of these severely affected rats.

Pathological mechanisms in human MG

Human MG closely resembles the chronic phase of EAMG in rats. These similarities are listed in Table 1. Acute and passive EAMG differ from human MG principally in that they are characterized by a massive phagocytic invasion of the endplates (Engel *et al.*, 1976a, b) and human MG is not (Engel *et al.*, 1971). Chronic EAMG differs from human MG principally in that EAMG results from cross reaction of an immune response to purified AChR and remits when that response diminishes, whereas human MG results from a sustained immune response against muscle AChR triggered and sustained by unknown mechanisms.

Serum antibodies recognizing AChR solubilized from human muscle have been found in 87% of patients tested (Lindstrom, 1977a). These antibodies are highly species specific (Lindstrom *et al.*, 1976d, and Lindstrom *et al.*, 1977a). Like those in rats with EAMG, they are not directed at the acetylcholine binding site of the receptor. Antibody concentration varies from barely detectable levels of 0.7×10^{-9} M to 940×10^{-9} M. The average concentration, 44×10^{-9} M, is comparable to levels of antibody to rat muscle AChR found in rats with chronic EAMG. Antibody concentration does not closely correlate with disease intensity (Lindstrom *et al.*, 1976e). Several factors may help to account for this. First, antibodies to AChR are not acting as simple curare-like antagonists of AChR. Rates of AChR synthesis and destruction and other factors probably influence a patient's ability to withstand the immune assault. Second, antibodies to AChR differing in specificities may differ in their effects on AChR. So total antibody titre may not be so relevant as titre of specific antibody species which can bind *in vivo* and block AChR activity, fix complement, or modulate AChR.

By the same methods used on rats with chronic EAMG, we have shown that AChR content is decreased in muscles of patients with MG to an average value of 36% of normal (Lindstrom and Lambert, 1977). These studies showed that an average of 51% of the AChR which remained were bound with antibodies. These AChR retained the ability to bind toxin. This indicates that the decrease in AChR which could be extracted from these

TABLE 1
Comparison Between Features of Passive, Acute, and Chronic EAMG and MG

	Passive EAMG	Acute EAMG	Chronic EAMG	MG
Clinical				
(1) Weakness	+	+	+	+
(2) Fatigability	+	+	+	+
Electrophysiological				
(1) Decrementing electromyogram	+	+	+	+
(2) Repair of electromyogram with ACh esterase inhibitor	+	+	+	+
(3) Reduced mepp amplitude	+	+	+	+
(4) Increased curare sensitivity	+	+	+	+
(5) Decreased ACh sensitivity	NT	NT	+	+
(6) Reduced muscle action potential amplitude	+	+	−	−
(7) Fibres without end-plate potentials	+	+	−	−
(8) Reduced resting potential	NT	+	−	−
Histological				
(1) Reduced toxin binding at end-plates	NT	NT	+	+
(2) Reduced number of postsynaptic folds	−	−	+	+
(3) Focal destruction of the postsynaptic membrane	+	+	+	+
(4) Antibody-complement complexes in intersynaptic debris	+	+	+	+
(5) Phagocytic invasion of end-plate	+	+	−	−
(6) Segemental necrosis of some fibres	+	+	−	−
Biochemical				
(1) Decreased AChR content	+	+	+	+
(2) Transient increased AChR content	+	+	−	−
Immunological				
(1) 7S antibodies to muscle AChR	+	+	+	+
(2) Average concentration of antibodies to muscle AChR$>10^{-8}$ M	NT	−	+	+
(3) Antibodies highly species specific	+	+	+	+
(4) Antibodies bind to muscle AChR *in vivo*	+	+	+	+
(5) Antibodies not directed at AChR binding site	+	+	+	+
(6) Antibodies block AChR activity *in vitro*	+	NT	+	+
(7) Complement fixation by anti-AChR antibodies *in vitro*	+	NT	+	+
(8) Antibodies cause modulation of AChR on cultured muscle	NT	NT	+	+
(9) Average concentration of antibodies to muscle AChR $<10^{-8}$ M	NT	+	−	−
(10) 19S antibodies to muscle AChR	−	+	−	−
(11) Positive skin test response to AChR	NT	+	−	NT

NT, not tested.

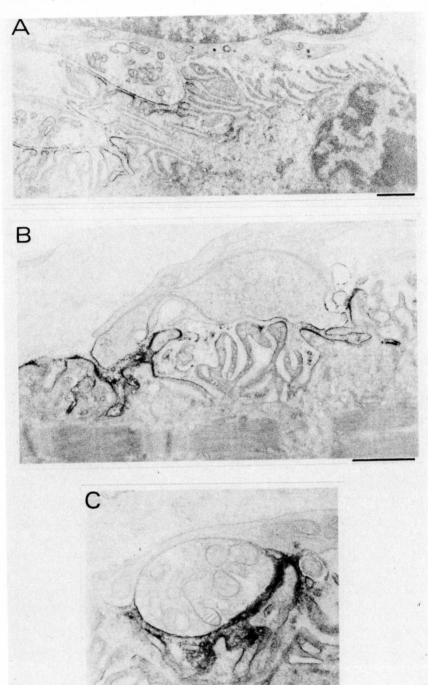

Fig. 7. Localization of AChR, anti-AChR, and bound complement at endplates from myasthenia gravis patients. (a) AChR is localized using α-bungarotoxin conjugated to horseradish peroxidase. The electron dense peroxidase reaction product is present in a patchy distribution along the tips of some postsynaptic membrane folds (from Engel *et al.*, 1977a, by permission). (b) Antibodies bound to AChR are localized using protein A conjugated to horseradish peroxidase (from Engel *et al.*, 1977c, by permission). (c) C3 component of complement bound to the postsynaptic membrane is localized using anti-C3 coupled to horseradish peroxidase. Photograph provided by Dr. Andrew Engel. The bar below each photograph indicates 1μ. Staining for antibody and C3 is most intense in milder cases of MG, where postsynaptic membrane structure is best preserved, because the content of AChR is greatest in these specimens (Engel *et al.*, 1977c). This observation is consistent with the idea (Lindstrom and Lambert, 1977) that AChR loss from these membrane is real rather than apparent due to inhibition of toxin binding to AChR by antibodies.

muscles was real and not due to blockage of toxin binding by antibodies. The content of AChR remaining unbound with antibodies was directly proportional to mepp amplitude in the intercostal muscles studied. These results suggest that loss of functional AChR is the principal factor impairing neuromuscular transmission in MG.

Electron microscopic studies of muscle from patients with MG reveals a simplified postsynaptic membrane structure like that seen in chronic EAMG (Engel *et al.*, 1976a, b and Engel *et al.*, 1977a-c). Total postsynaptic membrane area is reduced and, in particular, the area which can be stained for AChR with peroxidase conjugated to toxin is severely reduced (Engel *et al.*, 1977a). The reduction in AChR staining is directly proportional to the decrease in mepp amplitude in the intercostal muscle biopsy studies (Engel *et al.*, 1977). Thus, both the quantity and distribution of AChR is altered in MG, just as in chronic EAMG. Antibodies and complement bound to the postsynaptic membrane can also be localized (Fig. 7) (Engel *et al.*, 1977c).

Causes of impaired neuromuscular transmission are probably the same in MG and EAMG. These are summarized in Table 2. Although cells sensitized to AChR are present in MG patients (Abramsky *et al.*, 1975), it seems unlikely that the cell mediated destruction of AChR plays a major role. In the first place, massive cellular invasion of the endplates is not

TABLE 2
Causes of Impaired Neuromuscular Transmission in EAMG and MG

(1) *Loss of AChR*
    (a) due to antigenic modulation
    (b) due to complement mediated focal destruction of the postsynaptic membrane
    (c) due to phagocytic invasion — only during acute EAMG
(2) *Inhibition of AChR function*
    (a) antibody bound to an AChR molecule may not completely block activity
(3) *Simplification of postsynaptic membrane structure*
    (a) probably the result of a dynamic balance between AChR loss and AChR synthesis
(4) *Disruption of neuromuscular contact by phagocytes*
    (a) seen only in acute EAMG

seen (Engel *et al.*, 1971). If the morphological changes of the postsynaptic membrane seen in MG and chronic EAMG were the static artifacts of a rare prior invasion by cells, we would have to assume that the neuromuscular junction was quite static and this is unlikely. For example, studies of the time course of EAMG show that AChR content can increase and decrease very quickly (Lindstrom *et al.*, 1976b, c). In the second place, serum antibodies from MG patients can be directly demonstrated to have important pathological roles. γG purified from MG patients can transfer the symptoms of MG to mice (Toyka *et al.*, 1977). The importance of antibodies to the pathology of MG in humans is further indicated by the observation that removal of serum antibodies from patients with MG by plasmaphoresis results in clinical improvement (Pinching *et al.*, 1976). Also, babies with neonatal myasthenia gravis have anti-AChR antibodies in their serum received transplacentally from their myasthenic mothers (Lindstrom *et al.*, 1976d and Keesey *et al.*, 1977). The babies' myasthenia remits as the maternal antibody is cleared from circulation (Keesey *et al.*, 1977). The roles of antibodies in impairing neuromuscular transmission in MG and EAMG are listed in Table 3.

TABLE 3
Pathological Roles of Antibody to AChR in MG and EAMG

(1) *Induce antigenic modulation of AChR*
     (a) crosslinking of AChR by antibody is important
(2) *Induce complement mediated focal destruction of the postsynaptic membrane*
(3) *Directly inhibit AChR function*
(4) *Opsonize the postsynaptic membrane for phagocytic destruction*
     (a) pronounced only in acute EAMG

Cause of human MG

The cause of the autoimmune response to AChR in humans is unknown. It may well involve a genetic predisposition, as indicated by the unusual frequencies of certain HLA types among MG patients (Fritze *et al.*, 1976). An environmental influence may also be important. One possibility is that an antigenic determinant on a bacterium or virus infecting the patient triggers an immune response which cross reacts with the patients' muscle AChR. A second possibility is that a virus causes modification and/or shedding of AChR from some host tissue leading to an immune response. Both mechanisms, or neither, might occur. The second mechanism is considered in Fig. 8.

Studies of the immune response to AChR in rats with EAMG indicate that although syngeneic AChR may be immunogenic, even an antibody dependent cell mediated attack on muscle AChR is not sufficient to trigger a self sustaining autoimmune response. The antibody reponse to muscle AChR in rats with chronic EAMG results from cross reaction with antibodies to purified electric organ AChR used for immunization. Antibodies

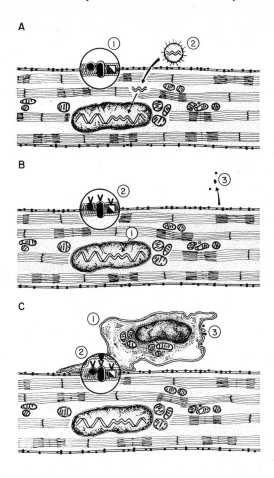

Fig. 8. A possible mechanism for induction of MG in humans. (A) (1) A muscle cell or myoid cell in the thymus contains AChR and other determinants in its surface membrane. (2) A virus specific for this cell type infects the cell. (B) (1) The latent or defective virus produces effects on the cells metabolism, either altering regulation of cellular enzymes or inducing synthesis of some of its own enzymes. These changes may result from attempts to modify the cell surface to prevent infection by other viruses, or may be aborted attempts at budding from the surface by a defective virus. Virus may occasionally interfere with cellular mitotic regulation in AChR containing cells or thymic lymphocytes, causing the thymomas frequently associated with MG. (2) These metabolic alterations may result in changes in post-translational modifications of the AChR and other surface proteins. (3) Alternatively, the virus may cause membrane fragments or proteins to be shed from the cell revealing antigenic determinants to which the immune system is not tolerant. (C) (1) A wandering immuno-competent cell, perhaps of a specificity encountered more frequently with persons of certain genetic backgrounds, encounters material from the infected cell which it recognizes as foreign. The antigens recognized may be in the intact modified membrane (2) and/or shed from the membrane (3). In addition to AChR, or instead of it, other antigens may be recognized. This might account for the observation of myoid antibodies in patients with thymoma and for the increased incidence of other autoimmune diseases in patients with MG.

recognizing rat muscle AChR in a rat immunized with eel AChR are adsorbed by eel electric organ membranes as effectively as the other anti-eel antibodies in the serum (Lindstrom et al., 1976d). The degree of cross reaction increases with time after immunization (Lindstrom, unpublished). EAMG can be induced by immunization of rats with purified syngenic AChR (Lindstrom et al., 1976b). Passive transfer of antibodies to AChR results in phagocytosis of an equivalent amount of AChR in postsynaptic membrane, yet antibody production is not induced (Lindstrom et al., 1976c). Thus the AChR released during the immune response in EAMG is not immunogenic. However, some change associated with removing AChR from the membrane in detergent or purification or emulsification in adjuvant makes rat AChR immunogenic. It is extremely difficult to induce EAMG with heat or SDS denatured electric organ AChR (Lindstrom et al., 1976d). However, multiple immunizations with large amounts over long periods can produce EAMG (Lindstrom, unpublished). Thus comformationally dependent determinants are responsible for the cross reaction between AChR from muscle and electric organ. This suggests that any conformational changes required to render purified rat AChR immunogenic are probably small. Humans, like rats, do not appear to normally mount an immune response to AChR released from damaged muscle, since antibodies to AChR have not been found in the sera of patients suffering from many types of degenerative muscle disease other than MG (Lindstrom et al., 1976e).

Conclusion

Importance of these studies to treatment of human MG

Studies stimulated by the initial description of EAMG (Patrick and Lindstrom, 1973) have led to the understanding that MG is an autoimmune disease directed at the acetylcholine receptor. Realization that the pathology is postsynaptic and autoimmune produces immediate indications for immunosuppressive therapy. Studies of EAMG have revealed much about the pathological mechanisms leading to impaired neuromuscular transmission. These indicate that loss of functional AChR is the principal lesion, and that this results principally from mechanisms mediated by antibodies. Assay of serum anti-AChR antibodies shows promise principally as an additional diagnostic test for MG, and secondarily as a method for monitoring response to immunosuppressive therapy. Direct removal of antibodies through plasmaphoresis coupled with immunosuppressive drugs to inhibit resynthesis is a new therapeutic approach suggested by studies of the pathological mechanisms in EAMG and MG.

Importance of these studies to understanding AChR structure and function

Antibodies to purified AChR and antibodies to AChR from MG patients provide templates which can be used to compare AChR. In particular, it should become possible to prepare antibodies against structurally defined determinants on purified electric organ AChR and use these antibodies to test for the presence of similar or identical determinants on the biochemically less tractable AChR from muscle. Finally, since it is known that antibodies to AChR can inhibit AChR function without simply blocking the acetylcholine binding site (Lindstrom *et al.*, 1977a), antibodies against specific structural determinants on the AChR protein should provide probes for determining the functional role of these structures.

Acknowledgements

Important contributions to the study of pathological mechanisms in EAMG were made by my colleagues Andy Engel, Ed Lambert, Marge Seybold, Steve Heinemann, Vanda Lennon, and Brett Einarson. This research was supported by grants from the National Institutes of Health (NS 11323) and the Muscular Dystrophy Association.

References

Abramsky, O., Aharonov, A., Webb, C. and Fuchs, S. (1975). *Clin. Exp. Immunol.*, **19**, 11-16.

Berg, D. and Hall, Z. (1974). *Science*, **184**, 473-475.

Berg, D.K., Kelly, R.B., Sargent, P.B., Williamson, P. and Hall, Z.W. (1972). *Proc. Natl. Acad. Sci., USA*, **69**, 147-151.

Bevan, S., Heinemann, S., Lennon, V.A. and Lindstrom, J. (1976). *Nature*, **260**, 438-439.

Changeux, J.P., Beneditti, L., Bourgeois, J.P., Brisson, A., Cartaud, J., Devaux, P., Grunhagen, H., Moreau, M., Popot, J.L., Sobel, A. and Weber, M. (1976). *In* 'Cold Spring Harbor Symposia on Quantitative Biology' vol. XL, pp.211-230.

Devreotes, P.N. and Fambrough, D.M. (1975). *J. Cell Biol.*, **65**, 335-358.

Engel, A.G. and Santa, T. (1971). *Ann. N.Y. Acad. Sci.*, **183**, 46-64.

Engel, A., Tsujihata, M., Lambert, E., Lindstrom, J. and Lennon, V. (1976a). *J. Neuropath. Exp. Neurol.*, **35**, 569-587.

Engel, A., Tsujihata, M., Lindstrom, J. and Lennon, V. (1976b). *N.Y. Acad. Sci.*, **274**, 60-79.

Engel, A.G., Lindstrom, J.M., Lambert, E.H. and Lennon, V.A. (1977a). *Neurology*, **27**, 307-315.

Engel, A., Tsujihata, M., Sakakibara, H., Lindstrom, J. and Lambert, E. (1977b). Pathogenesis of human muscular dystrophies, (L.P. Rowland, ed). *Excerpta Medica*, 132-142.

Engel, A., Lambert, E. and Howard, G. (1977c). *Mayo Clinical Proceedings*, **52**, 267-280.

Fritze, D., Herrmann, C., Naeim, F., Smith, G., Zeller, E. and Walford, R. (1976). *N.Y. Acad. Sci.*, **274**, 440-450.

Heinemann, S., Bevan, S., Kullberg, R., Lindstrom, J. and Rise, J. (1977). *Proc. Natl. Acad. Sci.*, **74**, 3090-3094.

Karlin, A., Weill, C.L., McNamee, M.G. and Valderrama, R. (1976). *In* 'Cold Spring Harbor Symposia on Quantitative Biology' vol. XL, pp.203-210.

Keesey, J., Lindstrom, J. and Cokely, A. (1977). *New. Eng. J. Med.*, **296**, 55.

Lambert, E.H. and Elmquist, D. (1971). *Ann. N.Y. Acad. Sci.*, **183**, 183-199.

Lambert, E., Lindstrom, J. and Lennon, V. (1976). *N.Y. Acad. Sci.*, **274**, 300-318.

Lee, C.Y., Tseng, L.F. and Chiu, T.H. (1967). *Nature*, **215**, 1177-1178.

Lennon, V.A., Lindstrom, J.M. and Seybold, M.E. (1975). *J. Exp. Med.*, **141**, 1365-1375.

Lennon, V., Lindstrom, J. and Seybold, M. (1976). *N.Y. Acad. Sci.*, **274**, 283-299.

Lindstrom, J. (1976). *J. Supramol. Struc.*, **4**, 389-403.

Lindstrom, J. (1977a). *J. Clin. Immunol. and Immunopath.*, **7**, 36-43.

Lindstrom, J. (1977b). *In* 'Receptors and Recognition' (P. Cuatrecasas and M.F. Greaves, eds) vol. III, 1-44. Chapman and Hall, London.

Lindstrom, J. (1977c). Pathogenesis of human muscular dystrophies. (L.P. Rowland, ed). *Excerpta Medica,* 121-131.

Lindstrom, J. and Lambert, E. (1977c), *Neurology* in press.

Lindstrom, J. and Patrick, J. (1974). *In* 'Synaptic Transmission and Neuronal Interaction' (M.V.L. Bennett, ed), pp.191-216. Raven Press, New York.

Lindstrom, J., Einarson, B. and Francy, M. (1976a). *Cellular Neurobiology* (Z. Hall, R. Kelly and C.F. Fox, eds) Alan R. Liss Inc., in press.

Lindstrom, J.M., Einarson, B., Lennon, V.A. and Seybold, M.E. (1976b). *J.Exp. Med.*, **144**, 726-738.

Lindstrom, J.M., Engel, A.G., Seybold, M.E., Lennon, V.A. and Lambert, E.H. (1976c). *J. Exp. Med.*, **144**, 739-753.

Lindstrom, J., Lennon, V., Seybold, M. and Whittingham, S. (1976d). *Ann. N.Y. Acad. Sci.*, **274**, 254-274.

Lindstrom, J., Seybold, M., Lennon, V., Whittingham, S. and Duane, D. (1976e). *Neurology*, **26**, 1054-1059.

Lindstrom, J., Campbell, M. and Nave, B. (1977a), in preparation.

Lindstrom, J., Merlie, J. and Heinemann, S. (1977b), in preparation.

Miledi, R., Molinoff, P. and Potter, L.T. (1971). *Nature*, **229**, 554-557.

Patrick, J. and Lindstrom, J. (1973). *Science*, **180**, 871-872.

Patrick, J., Lindstrom, J., Culp, B. and McMillan, J. (1973). *Proc. Natl. Acad. Sci. USA*, **70**, 3334-3338.

Pinching, A.J., Peters, D.K. and Davis, J.N. (1976). *Lancet*, **ii**, 1373-1376.

Raftery, M.A., Vandlen, R.L., Reed, K.L. and Lee, T. (1976). *In* 'Cold Spring Harbor Symposia on Quantitative Biology', vol. XL, pp.193-202.

Sahashi, K., Engel, A.G., Lindstrom, J., Lambert, E.H. and Lennon, V. (1977). *J. Neuropath. and Exp. Neurol.,* in press.

Seybold, M., Lambert, E., Lennon, V. and Lindstrom, J. (1976). *Ann. N.Y. Acad. Sci.*, **274**, 275-282.

Simpson, J. (1960). *Scot. Med. J.*, **5**, 419-436.

Stevens, C.F. (1976). *In* 'Cold Spring Harbor Symposia on Quantitative Biology' vol. XL, pp.169-174.

Toyka, K.V., Drachman, D.B., Griffin, D.E., Pestronk, A., Winkelstein, J.A., Fischbeck, K.H. and Kao, I. (1977). *New Eng. J. Med.*, **296**, 125-131.

10 Role of specific antibodies in the pathogenesis of experimental autoimmune Myasthenia Gravis

ANNE D. ZURN AND BERNARD W. FULPIUS

Department of Biochemistry
University of Geneva
Sciences II
1211 Geneva 4
Switzerland

Recent evidence favours the involvement of the junctional acetylcholine receptors (AChR) in the pathogeny of myasthenia gravis (MG). Fambrough *et al.* (1973) reported a five-fold reduction in the number of AChR molecules at myasthenic neuromuscular junctions as compared with controls. Lindstrom *et al.* (1976b) detected anti-AChR antibodies in more than 90% of myasthenic sera with a radioimmunoassay using human muscle AChR as the antigen. As Fambrough suggested, '... the reduction in the number of AChR in myasthenic junctions, as revealed by the decreased amount of bound ^{125}I-α-Bungarotoxin (α-Bgtx) might reflect an endogenous blockade ... of AChR...'. This supports the hypothesis suggested in 1960 by Simpson according to which '... an antibody to end-plate protein, with the properties of an acetylcholine competitive blocking substance ...' could be involved in the pathogeny of MG.

In the present report, we will review the experimental data favouring a blocking activity of anti-AChR antibodies. Myasthenic serum has been shown to inhibit subsequent binding of ^{125}I-αBgtx on normal human muscle sections (Bender *et al.*, 1975). Immunoglobulins G (IgG) purified from myasthenic sera were reported to inhibit fixation to AChR solubilized from denervated rat muscles (Almon and Appel, 1975) and AChR present on electroplax membrane fragments (Lefvert and Bergström, 1977). In addition, it has been reported that large amounts of these IgG molecules could transfer myasthenic symptoms to mice (Toyka *et al.*, 1975).

Anti-AChR serum has also been obtained from animals immunized with AChR from different sources (for a review, Heilbronn, 1976). These animals develop signs of paralysis similar to those observed in human MG. Their sera were shown subsequently to inhibit toxin binding to AChR solubilized from electroplax membranes (Penn *et al.*, 1976) and AChR

157

present in the membrane of intact electroplax cells (Lindstrom, 1976). The blocking effect of anti-AChR serum was also measured by electrophysiological techniques on isolated electroplax (Patrick and Lindstrom, 1973; Sugiyama *et al.*, 1973; Penn *et al.*, 1976), on nerve-muscle preparations (Berti *et al.*, 1976) and in intact animals (Lindstrom *et al.*, 1976a). These data are summarized in Table 1. They favour a direct blocking effect of anti-AChR antibodies on functional AChR.

TABLE 1

Evidence favouring blocking activity of anti-AChR serum on different AChR preparations.

	AChR preparation	Source of anti-AChR antibodies	Authors
INHIBITION OF TOXIN BINDING	Solubilized AChR	Myasthenic serum	Almon & Appel (1975)
		Anti-eel AChR Serum	Penn *et al.* (1976)
	Electroplax membrane fragments	Myasthenic IgG	Lefvert and Bergstrom (1977)
	Muscle section	Myasthenic serum	Bender *et al.* (1975)
	Cells from the Electroplax	Anti-eel AChR Serum	Lindstrom 1976
ELECTRO-PHYSIOLOGICAL RECORDINGS	electroplax	anti-eel AChR serum	Patrick *et al.* (1973) Sugiyama *et al.* (1973) Penn *et al.* (1976)
	neuro-muscular junction	anti-*Torpedo* AChR serum	Berti *et al.* (1976) Green *et al.* (1975)
	transfer to an animal	myasthenic IgG	Toyka *et al.* (1975)
		anti-eel AChR IgG	Lindstrom & al. (1976)

The following question remains to be answered: is the blocking effect observed due only to a specific subpopulation of anti-AChR antibodies directed against the toxin binding site of AChR or to the overall anti-AChR antibody population? In order to answer this question we developed an assay to measure that particular subpopulation of antibodies (Zurn and Fulpius, 1977), followed it during immunization of a rabbit and compared it with anti-AChR antibodies directed against sites other than the toxin binding site measured by radio-immunoassay. The level of antibodies measured by this latter method is only 1.4 times higher at the onset of paralysis than three weeks before, whereas anti-AChR antibodies directed against the toxin binding site caused at that time a 7-fold higher inhibition of toxin binding than before (Fig. 1).

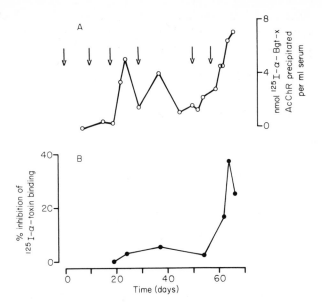

Fig. 1. Measurements of anti-AChR antibodies at different times of the immunization procedure of a rabbit injected with AChR. Days of injection are indicated with arrows. The rabbit was immunized according to the following procedure: the first injection (day 1) was made in complete Freund's adjuvant, the second one (day 10) in incomplete Freund's adjuvant and the two subsequent ones (days 18 and 29) in phosphate buffered saline (PBS). The rabbit was further immunized with complete and incomplete Freund's adjuvant (days 50 and 57) and bled to death at day 66 after severe paralysis had developed. Levels of antibodies directed against other sites than the toxin binding site are shown in A. Amounts of ^{125}I-α-Bgtx-AChR complex precipitated per ml serum were measured by radioimmunoassay. Inhibition of toxin binding due to antibodies directed against the toxin binding site is shown in B. It was expressed in per cent per 0.1 μl serum. These percentages were obtained by measuring the amount of ^{125}I-α-Bgtx bound to soluble *Torpedo* AChR in presence and absence of anti-AChR serum.

These data indicate that there is a direct correlation between the levels of anti-AChR antibodies directed against the toxin binding site and the clinical picture. It should be noticed that the percentage inhibition of toxin binding observed at the onset of the paralysis does not represent the limit above which one has to expect signs of paralysis since, at that time, less pronounced inhibition was observed in other rabbits (unpublished data).

Inhibition of toxin binding was also measured on mouse AChR located within the intact muscle membrane. This preparation reflects in a better way than solubilized AChR what might happen *in vivo*. Portions of mouse diaphragms incubated successively with anti-AChR serum and ^{125}I-α-toxin were sectioned as described by Greene *et al.* (1975) and the radioactivity present in the nerve terminal region was measured. Antiserum taken at the onset of paralysis inhibits toxin binding on AChR *in situ* about ten times more effectively than an antiserum taken three weeks before. This corresponds to the difference found when measured on soluble *Torpedo* AChR and indicates that the effect of the same subpopulation of anti-AChR antibodies is determined with both methods. In conclusion, we propose that only one of the two populations of anti-AChR antibodies studied, the one which inhibits toxin binding, is involved in the appearance of the paralysis observed in this particular case.

References

Almon, R.R. and S.H. Appel (1975). *Biochem. Biophys. Acta.*, **393**, 66-77.

Bender, A.N, W.K. Engel, S.P. Ringel, M.P. Daniels and Z. Vogel (1975). *The Lancet*, **I**, 607-609.

Berti, F.F. Clementi, B. Conti-Tronconi and G.C. Folco (1976). *Br. J. Pharmac.*, **57**, 17-22.

Fambrough, D.M., D.B. Drachman and S. Satyamurti (1973). *Science*, **182**, 293-295.

Green, D.P.L., R. Miledi and A. Vincent (1975). *Proc. R. Soc. London*, **189**, 57-68.

Heilbronn, E. (1976). In: Motor Innervation of Muscle. S. Thesleff ed. Academic Press, p.177-212.

Lefvert, A.K. and K. Bergstrom (1977). *Eur. J. Clin. Invest.*, **7**, 115-119.

Lindstrom, J. (1976). *J. Supramol. Struct.*, **4**, 389-403.

Lindstrom, J., B.L. Einarson, V.A. Lennon and M.E. Seybold (1976a). *J. exp. Med.*, **144**, 726-738 and 739-753.

Lindstrom, J., M.E. Seybold, V.A. Lennon, S. Whittingham and D.D. Duane (1976b). *Neurology*, **26**, 1054-1059.

Patrick, J. and J. Lindstrom (1973). *Science*, **180**, 871-872.

Penn, A.S., H.W. Chang, R.E. Lovelace, W. Niemi and A. Miranda (1976). *Ann. N.Y. Acad. Sci.*, **274**, 354-376.

Simpson, J. (1960). *Scot. Med. J.*, **5**, 419-436.

Sugiyama, H., P. Benda, J.-C. Meunier and J.-P. Changeux (1973). *FEBS Lett.*, **35**, 124-128.

Toyka, K.V., D.B. Drachman, A. Pestronk and I. Kao (1975). *Science*, **190**, 397-399.

Zurn, A.D. and B.W. Fulpius (1977). *Eur. J. Immunol.*, **8**, 529-532.

11 Cellular immune response to acetylcholine receptors in myasthenia gravis

B. CONTI TRONCONI · M. MORGUTTI · F. CORNELIO AND F. CLEMENTI

*Department of Pharmacology and CNR Center of
Cytopharmacology of the University of Milano and
Istituto Neurologico 'Besta', Milano — Italy.*

An experimental disease, similar to human myasthenia gravis can be induced in several mammalian species, from mouse to monkey, by immunization against the nicotinic cholinoceptor (AChR) extracted either from the electric organs of *Torpedo* and electric eel or from mammalian muscles (Patrick and Lindstrom, 1973; Berti *et al.*, 1974, Tarrab-Hazdai *et al.*, 1975; Clementi *et al.*, 1976, Fuchs *et al.*, Chapter 16). The impairment of neuromuscular transmission in the experimental myasthenia is due to an immunological blockade of the muscular cholinoceptor because of common antigenic determinants shared by mammalian and electric organ AChR.

There are clear indications that an immunological blockade of the AChR at the neuromuscular junction is also involved in the pathogenesis of human MG. These include; the presence in the sera of myasthenic patients of antibodies against the cholinoceptor (Ito *et al.* Chapter 5) whose titre is well correlated with the clinical course of the disease (Pinching *et al.*, 1976; Pinching *et al.*, 1977; Lindstrom *et al.*, 1976; Almond and Appel, 1976), the presence of thymic abnormalities in more than 80% of myasthenic patients, the positive response to thymectomy or immunosuppressive therapy, and the significant association with other immune diseases. Moreover, in some newborn children of myasthenic mothers a transient myasthenic syndrome occurs, which is followed by spontaneous remission whose time course is compatible with the clearance of possible neuromuscular blocking antibodies originating from the maternal circulation of the fetal blood stream.

However the thymus involvement, the frequent muscle lymphorrages and the clinical remission obtained with the drainage of lymphocytes from the thoracic duct (Matell *et al.*, 1976) have suggested that a cellular immune reaction may also contribute to the pathogenesis and clinical course of this disease. Recently a positive response of myasthenic lymphocytes against muscle and *Torpedo* AChR has been demonstrated (Abramsky *et al.*,

161

1975b; Conti-Tronconi *et al.*, 1977; Richman *et al.*, 1976). The culture *in vitro* of peripheral blood lymphocytes carried out in the presence of an antigen has been used to demonstrate a previous lymphocytic sensitization to it.

The significance of this test and also its utilization in clinical practice as an aid to diagnosis and prognosis is still a matter of debate, mainly because of the small groups of patients studied up to now and the poor correlations established with their clinical situation. In this study we present results obtained by testing lymphocytes from myasthenic patients, polymyositis patients and healthy subjects, with AChR-rich membranes obtained from *Torpedo Marmorata* electric organ.

Patients and methods

Peripheral blood lymphocytes were obtained from 68 myasthenic patients, 45 females and 22 males, from 9 to 65 years old. The illness dated from 3 months to 7 years. 35 patients were under corticosteroid treatment, 44 patients underwent thymectomy. Control groups were 28 polymyositis patients, ageing from 3 to 62, whose illness dated from 2 months to 5 years, of whom 21 were under steroid treatment and 25 healthy subjects, from 19 to 40 years. Lymphocytes were isolated from venous peripheral blood according to Böyum (1968) and were cultured by the micromethod of Hartzmann *et al.* (1971) with minor modifications.

Lymphocytes were tested both with phytohemoagglutinin (PHA, 10 μl/ml, Wellcome, Beckenham, England) or with our antigen preparation (Ag,50 or 10 μl/ml). The degree of lymphocytic stimulation by antigen was expressed as stimulation index (S.I.), that is the ratio between ^{3}H-thymidine incorporation obtained in the presence of phytohemoagglutinin or antigen and the basal incorporation in the absence of any stimulation. Stimulation indices over 1.5 (the upper value obtained in healthy subjects) were assumed to be positive responses. As antigen, we used a postsynaptic membrane preparation rich in AChR (about 30% w/w of proteins) isolated from *Torpedo Marmorata* electric organs by sucrose density gradient (Clementi *et al.*, 1976). The efficacy of this antigen, in comparison to a mammalian muscle antigen, is low since it does not share all the antigenic determinants of the muscle receptor, but the response is specific (Conti-Tronconi *et al.*, 1977).

Results

Myasthenic lymphocytes were stimulated by AChR in about 55% of cases. The mean stimulation index obtained was 2.06. This sensitization is highly significant ($P < 0.005$) when compared with controls, which had a mean stimulation index of 0.95 (Table 1).

TABLE 1

Means of stimulation indices (± S.E.M.) obtained from lymphocytes stimulated with AChR and phytohemoagglutinin from myasthenics, polymyosytics and controls.

	MYASTHENICS (68 cases)	POLYMYOSITICS (28 cases)	CONTROLS (25 cases)
AChR stimulation index	2.01± 0.19	1.22± 0.13	0.95± 0.06
PHA Stimulation index	62.13± 7.23	60.85± 8.21	83.02± 15

Polymyositis patients had a mean stimulation index of 1.22; the difference between them and normal subjects was not significant. The results obtained with phytohemoagglutinin stimulation showed no difference between the three groups tested.

Table 2 summarizes the results obtained comparing two groups of myasthenic subjects: patients in clinical Stages 2A and 2B (classified according to Ossermann), and patients showing a clinical remission, i.e. in the absence of any pharmacological treatment or with only low doses of anticholinesterase drugs. There is no difference between the mean stimulation index of the two groups. To test the effect of corticosteroid

TABLE 2

Mean stimulation indices from myasthenic patients at different clinical stages.

CLINICAL STAGE	N° OF PATIENTS	MEAN AChR STIMULATION INDEX ± SEM
2A – 2B	21	1.97± 0.34
Remission	12	2.37± 0.56

treatment on lymphocyte response to our antigen, we have compared the results obtained in patients who were under steroid treatment (20-100 mg of prednisone every two days) with those obtained in patients who had never received steroid medications. Again no difference was detectable between the two groups (Table 3).

The last table summarizes the results obtained in the same patients tested before and after thymectomy; this second test was performed from 2 to 6 months after surgery. In this case a significant reduction of lymphocyte reactivity against AChR was observed after surgery in all the five patients tested. The difference between the mean stimulation index before and after thymectomy is significant (P< 0.025).

TABLE 3

Mean stimulation indices obtained after stimulation of lymphocytes from myasthenic subjects with or without corticosteroid treatment.

	N° of patients	Mean AChR stimulation index ± SEM	Mean PHA stimulation index ± SEM
With corticosteroid treatment	18	1.61± 0.41	63.13± 12.51
Without corticosteroid treatment	19	1.98± 0.37	65.99± 12.7

TABLE 4

AChR stimulation indices obtained in the same myasthenic patients before and after thymectomy.

PATIENT (name)	BEFORE	AFTER	%
F.M.	4.44	0.52	−88.29
M.V.	3.16	2.24	−29.12
F.S.	3.44	1.03	−70,06
M.C.B.	2.2	1.77	−19.55
D.M.	1.78	1.13	−36.5
means ± S.E.M.	3.0± 0.47	1.33± 0.3	−48.7

Discussion

From the data reported it appears that the presence and the specificity of lymphocyte sensitization against AChR in myasthenic patients can be accepted as a characteristic feature of myasthenia gravis. The importance of this sensitization in the pathogenesis of the disease is further supported by the fact that in polymyositis, a muscular disorder usually considered of autoimmune origin, the specific sensitization against AChR is only present in a few cases. Moreover, the few above average stimulation indices of polymyositic patients were obtained in subjects with myasthenia-like features. It is surprising that there is no correlation between the degree of lymphocyte response against AChR and the clinical situation of the myasthenic patients. This is at variance with the clear correlation that has been demonstrated between the clinical situation and the level of anti-AChR antibodies in myasthenic sera (Vincent, 1977; Pinching *et al.*, 1976; Pinching *et al.*, 1977; Almond and

Appel, 1976). The lack of correlation may depend upon the fact that blood lymphocytes are a peripheral component of the immune system; moreover the percentage of lymphocytes of the total pool of peripheral blood lymphocytes that are specifically sensitized against AChR is probably rather low, and only one class of cells might be activated by the antigen. It is possible that by testing thymic lymphocytes or lymphocytes present in myasthenic muscles (where they probably act), results could be obtained more closely related to the clinical situation. It is also possible that lymphocyte activation is only one of several immunological disturbances and its significance will be understood only when the overall pattern is known. The steroid treatment did not substantially affect lymphocyte responses either to AChR or to phytohemoagglutinin. A similar observation has been reported by Richman *et al.* (1976) and is in contrast with the results reported from a smaller number of cases by Abramsky *et al.* (1975a).

The effect of thymectomy on lymphocyte response to the antigen is clearcut, but it does not impair their response to PHA; this again suggests the importance of lymphocytic sensitization against AChR in myasthenia gravis since it is known that thymectomy can induce a long lasting improvement. The result reported could be due to the fact that after thymectomy a large pool of lymphocytes is removed. However, in view of a recent hypothesis that suggests that the myoid cells of the thymus, bearing AChR on their surface, are the first target of the autoimmune response in myasthenia (Wekerle and Ketelsen, 1977), it could be that thymectomy causes selective depletion of anti-AChR activated lymphocytes present in thymus and a block in the sensitization of new lymphocytes. Our post-thymectomy tests were carried out not more than 6 months after surgery; it would be interesting to know if the reduction of lymphocytic reactivity towards the AChR antigen remains for a longer time, or reverts to pre-thymectomy values.

In conclusion, it seems that lymphocyte stimulation is of diagnostic value in myasthenia gravis. However because patients showing clinical remission maintain the response, it is not helpful from a prognostic point of view and cannot be of use to the neurologist for the day to day management of myasthenic patients.

References

Abramsky, O., Aharonov, A., Teitelbaum, D. and Fuchs, S. (1975a). *Arch. Neurol.*, **32,** 684-687.
Abramsky, O., Aharonov, A., Webb, C. and Fuchs, S. (1975b). *Clin. Exp. Immunol.*, **19,** 11-16.
Almond, R.R. and Appel, S.H. (1976). *Ann. N.Y. Acad. Sc.*, **274,** 235-243.
Berti, F., Clementi, F., Conti-Tronconi, B. and Omini, C. (1974). *Brit. J. Pharmacol.*, **52,** 468.
Böyum, A. (1968). *Scand. J. Clin. Lab. Invest.*, **21,** suppl. 97.

166   *B. Conti Tronconi, M. Morgutti, F. Cornelio and F. Clementi*

Clementi, F., Conti-Tronconi, B., Berti, F. and Folco, G. (1976). *J. Neuropath. Exp. Neurol.*, **35,** 665-678.
Conti-Tronconi, B.M., Di Padova, F., Morgutti, M., Missiroli, A. and Frattola, L. (1977). *J. Neuropath. Exp. Neurol.*, **36,** 157-162.
Hartzman, R.J., Segall, N., Bach, M.L. and Bach, F.H. (1971). *Transplantation,* **11,** 268-273.
Lindstrom, J.M., Lennon, V.A., Seybold, M.E. and Whittingham, S. (1976). *Ann. N.Y. Acad. Sc.*, **274,** 254-274.
Matell, G., Bergstrom, K., Franksonn, C., Hammarstrom, L., Lefvert, A.K., Möller, E., v. Reis, G. and Smith, E. (1976). *Ann. N.Y. Acad. Sc.*, **274,** 659-676.
Patrick, J. and Lindstrom, J. (1973). *Science,* **180,** 871-872.
Pinching, A.J., Peters, D.K. and Davis, J.N. (1976). *Lancet,* **ii,** 1373-1376.
Pinching, A.J., Peters, D.K. and Davis, J.N. (1977). *Lancet,* **I,** 190-191.
Richman, D.P., Patrick, J. and Arnason, G.W. (1976). *New England J. Med.,* **294,** 694-698.
Tarrab-Hazdai, R., Aharonov, A., Silman, I., Fuchs, S. (1975). *Nature,* **256,** 128-130.
Wekerle, H. and Ketelsen, V.P. (1977). *Lancet,* **i,** 678-680.

12 Inhibition of receptor function in cultured chick myotubes by antiserum to purified acetylcholine receptor (from *Torpedo marmorata*) and myasthenic sera

A.L. HARVEY

Department of Physiology and Pharmology, University of Strathclyde

T. BARKAS · R. HARRISON · G.G. LUNT
Department of Biochemistry, University of Bath

Introduction

A high proportion of sera from patients with myasthenia gravis contains antibodies directed against the acetylcholine receptor of skeletal muscle. This has been demonstrated both by inhibition of binding of α-bungarotoxin (Almon *et al.*, 1974; Mittag *et al.*, 1976), and by immuno-precipitation of labelled receptor (Appel *et al.*, 1975; Mittag *et al.*, 1976). Similarly, the sera of rabbits injected with purified *Electrophorus* or *Torpedo* acetylcholine receptor can partially block the response of the eel electroplax (Sugiyama *et al.*, 1973) or the rat diaphragm (Penn *et al.*, 1976) to bath-applied carbachol. The experiments reported here were performed to test if muscle cells in culture are suitable for investigating the effects of anti-receptor antibodies on the pharmacological properties of the receptor and the possible role of the antibodies in the destruction observed at the neuro-muscular junction in myasthenia.

Monolayer cultures have several advantages over intact tissues in such work:–
1. rapid application and removal of test agents with very little delay due to diffusion into the tissue,
2. long contact periods are possible,
3. the cells are readily observed throughout the experimental period.

Cultured chick myotubes were used, as the presence of 'hot spots' of acetycholine receptors, having about the same receptor density as the neuromuscular junction, has been reported (Vogel *et al.*, 1972; Sytkowski *et al.*, 1973). Agents potentially responsible for the damage observed at the junction can therefore be studied for their effects on the antibody-coated myotubes.

Methods

Tissue culture. Cultures of embryonic chick leg muscle were prepared as described by Harvey and Dryden (1974), except that the initial cell density was 5.10^5 cell/ml. Myotube formation occurred at 2-3 days, and cultures were 7-10 days old when used.

Electrophysiology. Cultures were mounted on an inverted phase contrast microscope and maintained at 37°C with a heated stage. Membrane potentials were measured with an intracellular glass microelectrode filled with 3 M potassium chloride (electrode resistance 10-20 megohms). Responses were obtained to iontophoretic application of acetylcholine. Microelectrodes for iontophoresis were filled with 0.5 M acetylcholine chloride (Sigma Chemical Co.) and connected to a stimulator through one channel of a WPI 750 electrometer. The average resistance of the acetylcholine electrode was 100 Mohm. Care was taken to select electrodes that did not leak drug spontaneously. The dose of acetylcholine is expressed as nanoCoulombs (nC) of charge passed through the electrode. Responses are calculated as depolarization as a percentage of the resting potential. All recordings were made in Eagles' minimal essential medium which was maintained at pH 7.4 by bubbling with CO_2.

The resting membrane potentials of the cells ranged from 25-80 mV (inside negative). However, cells with potential greater than about 50 mV contracted in response to acetylcholine. For this reason, cells with lower potentials were usually chosen for testing drug sensitivity. After exposure to anti-receptor antisera, the cells were quiescent and fibres with higher potentials could be studied.

Sera used. *Torpedo* acetylcholine receptor was purified by affinity chromatography on α-toxin from **Naja** naja siamensis, as described by Cooper and Reich (1972), immobilized on preactivated Sepharose 4B (Pharmacia). Elution was carried out batchwise with 1 M carbachol at room temperature for 3 hours. Antisera to the purified receptor and to receptor-enriched membrane fractions of *Torpedo* were raised in rabbits by intramuscular and subcutaneous injection of antigen in complete Freund's adjuvant at 3 week intervals. Sera from myasthenic patients were provided by Drs. M.J. Campbell and R. Teague, Bristol Royal Infirmary. Patients were treated with anti-cholinesterases or thymectomy; some also had further treatment with steroids. Control sera were obtained from laboratory personnel.

All sera were heat-inactivated at 56°C for 30 minutes prior to use. However, to prevent myolysis, further heat-inactivation (56°C for 60 mins) was required.

Treatment of cells. Cell cultures were incubated with 1 ml of myasthenic or normal serum and 1 ml of medium, or small volumes of anti-*Torpedo* receptor antiserum in a final volume of 2 ml for 2 hr at 37°C. The cells were then washed and tested for drug responsiveness. Treated cells were frozen in ethanol-dry ice and stored at −20°C until assayed for binding of α-bungarotoxin.

Binding of α-bungarotoxin. α-Bungarotoxin was iodinated by the chloramine T method of Hunter (1967) as modified by Urbaniak *et al.* (1973) to a specific activity of 1200 Ci/mmol. Cell cultures were treated with 2 ml of 10 mM phosphate buffer containing 1% Triton and 0.1% BSA, pH 7.4, at 30°C for 2 hrs with continual agitation. The supernatant was removed and assayed for binding of α-bungarotoxin by a modification of the method of Schmidt and Raftery (1973).

Effects of complement or normal lymphocytes. Cells treated with 5 or 10 µl of anti-*Torpedo* receptor antiserum were incubated for up to 6 hrs with 2 ml of a twenty-fold dilution of fresh guinea-pig complement or with 1.10⁶ normal rat (Liverpool Hooded) spleen lymphoid cells prepared as described by Barkas *et al.* (1976), except that all media contained 1% BSA instead of 10% foetal calf serum.

Absorption of lytic sera. 2 ml of four-fold diluted sera were incubated with 0.5 ml of minced chick embryo viscera at 4°C for 90 mins. The supernatant was removed and tested for lytic activity in the presence of guinea-pig complement diluted twenty-fold.

Results

Effect of anti-Torpedo acetylcholine receptor antiserum. The effect of applied antiserum to *Torpedo* receptor on the response of the cells to iontophoretically-applied acetylcholine and on the binding of α-bungarotoxin was investigated. As shown in Figure 1, the depolarization produced by acetylcholine was completely blocked by the addition of 100 µl of anti-*Torpedo* receptor antiserum and considerably decreased by as little as 5 µl of antiserum. In contrast, as much as 1 ml of antiserum to purified receptor-enriched membranes from *Torpedo* produced no effect. Inhibition of α-bungarotoxin binding was estimated to be approximately 80%, using 5 µl of anti-*Torpedo* receptor (Table 1), while 1 ml of anti-*Torpedo* membrane antiserum had no effect.

Effect of myasthenic sera. The effect of 1 ml of myasthenic sera on the cells was studied. Of six sera tested, one showed marked inhibitory activity of the response to acetylcholine, while a further one showed a slight block (Figure 2-4).

No effect on α-bungarotoxin binding was observed with any myasthenic sera (Table 2).

Effect of complement or normal lymphocytes on antibody-coated myotubes. Cells treated with 5 or 10 µl of anti-*Torpedo* receptor antiserum were

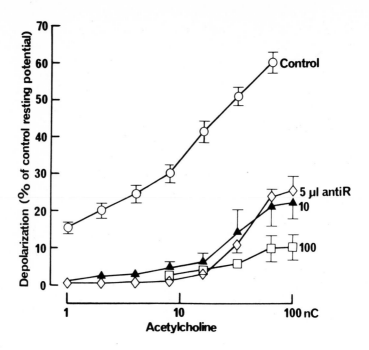

Fig. 1. Effects of anti-*Torpedo* acetylcholine receptor antiserum on the depolization response to acetylcholine. Results are the mean and standard error of 5-7 determinations.

TABLE 1
Effect on anti-*Torpedo* acetylcholine receptor antiserum
on binding of $I^{125}\alpha$-bungarotoxin to chick myotubes

Experiment 1		
SAMPLE	Cpm BOUND	% INHIBITION
Blank – no extract	977± 78 (2)	
Control plate extract	2,479± 197 (2)	
Plate treated with:–		
5μl Antiserum	1,316± 375 (2)	78
10μl	1,296± 189 (2)	79
Experiment 2		
Blank – no extract	1,421± 91 (2)	
Control plate	1,806± 84 (6)	
Treated with 5 μl		
Antiserum	1,503± 33 (2)	79

incubated at 37°C with either guinea-pig complement for periods of up to 6 hr or normal rat spleen lymphocytes overnight. No gross morphological changes were observed in the treated cells.

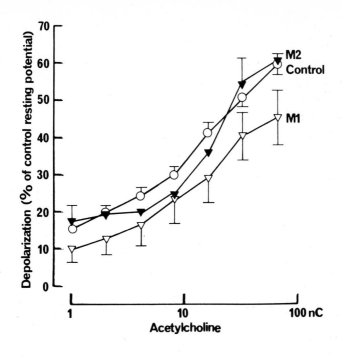

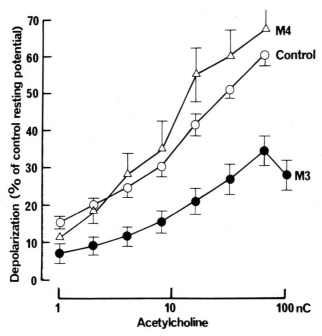

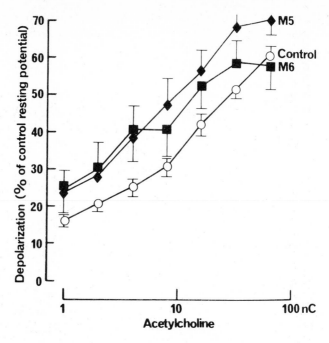

Fig. 2, 3 and 4. Effects of myasthenic sera on the depolarization response to acetylcholine. Results are the mean and standard error of 51 determinations for controls, 9 for M1, 10 for M2, 21 for M3, 10 for M4, 7 for M5, and 6 for M6.

TABLE 2

Effect of myasthenic sera on binding of $I^{125}\alpha$-bungarotoxin to chick myotubes

Experiment 1

SAMPLE	Cpm BOUND
Blank	824± 196 (2)
Control	1728
M5	1978

Experiment 2

Blank	824± 196 (2)
Control	2951± 47 (3)
M1	2564
M3	3425
M4	3165
M6	2813

Natural antibodies to chick cells in sera. In the majority of cases, exposure to heat-inactivated (56°C for 30 min.) sera produced complete lysis of the cells. This effect is shown in Figures 5 and 6, and occurred with both normal and myasthenic human sera, with control rabbit sera and with sera from rabbits injected with *Torpedo* receptor. Lysis was evident after only 5 min. incubation.

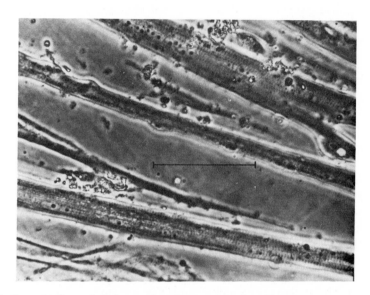

Fig. 5. Control culture of chick myotubes. Bar corresponds to 50 μm.

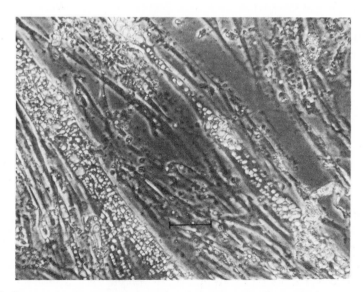

Fig. 6. Culture treated with 1 ml of heat-inactivated serum for 2 hr at 37°C.

The myolytic activity was lost at dilutions of normal sera of sixteen-fold or greater, and could be removed by absorption of the sera with minced chick embryo viscera. The lytic activity was also destroyed by further heat-inactivation (56°C for 60 min.), and could be restored by the addition of fresh diluted guinea-pig serum, which was non-lytic alone.

These results suggest the widespread occurrence of natural anti-chick antibodies.

Discussion and conclusions

Chick embryo muscle in culture provides a useful preparation for the study of the effects of anti-acetylcholine receptor antibodies on both the response to cholinergic drugs and the binding of α-bungarotoxin. Cross-reaction of *Torpedo* and chick receptor was observed. Cross-reaction of *Electrophorus* and chick receptor has been previously reported (Sugiyama *et al.*, 1973). Anti-*Torpedo* receptor antiserum effectively blocked both the response to acetylcholine and the binding of α-bungarotoxin. This may result either from direct blockade, or loss of the receptor from the cell surface, as reported by Lindstrom (Chapter 9).

Some myasthenic sera also block the response to acetylcholine, but not the binding of α-bungarotoxin. This possibly indicates that antibodies may block the depolarization response at a site other than the toxin-binding site, and also suggest cross-reaction of chick and human receptor. The proportion of myasthenic sera with the ability to block the acetylcholine response is low compared with the 70-90% of sera reported to contain anti-receptor antibody as assessed by immuno-precipitation (Appel *et al.*, 1975; Lindstrom *et al.*, 1976; Mittag *et al.*, 1976). This could reflect either relative degrees of sensitivity of the assay systems used, or the presence of anti-receptor antibodies in many myasthenic sera that do not inhibit either the response to cholinergic agonists or α-bungarotoxin binding. Such antibodies may be involved in the pathological changes. However, it is relevant to note that M3, the only myasthenic serum to dramatically inhibit the acetylcholine response, is the only established myasthenic not to have undergone thymectomy or steroid treatment. Inhibition of the response to *Torpedo* acetylcholine receptor of lymphocytes from myasthenics by corticosteroid treatment has been reported (Abramsky *et al.*, 1975), while steroid treatment also decreases the production of anti-receptor antibodies in experimental animals (Chapter 16).

No gross morphological change was observed by light-microscopy after treating the antibody-coated cells with either complement or normal lymphocytes. However, these preliminary results do not preclude the possibility of localized damage to the membrane. The presence of anti-chick antibodies in a high proportion of sera was demonstrated. Whether these antibodies are IgM or IgG in character is not known, but the possibility of the effects of anti-species antibodies should be borne in mind in the design of experiments involving cross-species transfer of serum or serum fractions.

Achnowledgements

We are indebted to the Muscular Dystrophy Assoc. Inc. (A.L.H.) and to the Medical Research Council (T.B., R.H., G.G.L.) for financial support.

References

Abramsky, O., Aharonov, A., Teitelbaum, D. and Fuchs, S. (1975). *Arch. Neurol.*, **32**, 684-687.

Almon, R.R., Andrew, C.G. and Appel, S.H. (1974). *Science*, **186**, 55-57.

Appel, S.H., Almon, R.R. and Levy, N. (1975). *New. Eng. J. Med.*, **293**, 760-761.

Barkas, T., Al-Khateeb, S.F., Irvine, W.J., Davidson, N.McD. and Rosco, P. (1976). *Clin. Exp. Immunol.*, **25**, 270-279.

Cooper, D. and Reich, E. (1972). *J. Biol. Chem.*, **247**, 3008-3013.

Harvey, A.L. and Dryden, W.F. (1974). *Eur. J. Pharmacol.*, **27**, 5-13.

Hunter, W.M. (1967) in 'Handbook of Experimental Immunology'. Ed. D.M. Weir, p.608 Blackwell Scientific Publications, Oxford.

Lindstrom, J.M., Lennon, V.A., Seybold, M.E. and Whittingham, S. (1976). *Annals. New York Acad. Sci.*, **274**, 254-274.

Mittag, T., Kornfeld, P., Tormay, A. and Woo, C. (1976). *New. Eng. J. Med.*, **294**, 691-694.

Penn, A.S., Chang, H.W., Lovelace, R.E., Niemi, W. and Miranda, A. (1976). *Annals New York Acad. Sci.*, **274**, 354-376.

Schmidt, J. and Raftery, M.A. (1973). *Anal. Biochem.*, **52**, 349-354.

Sugiyama, H., Benda, P., Meunier, J.-C. and Changeux, J.-P. (1973). *FEBS Lett.*, **35**, 124-128.

Sytkowski, A.J., Vogel, Z. and Nirenberg, M.W. (1973). *Proc. Nat. Acad. Sci.*, *USA*, **70**, 270-274.

Urbaniak, S.J., Penhale, W.J. and Irvine, W.J. (1973). *Clin. Exp. Immunol.*, **15**, 345-354.

Vogel, Z., Sytkowski, A.J. and Nirenberg, M.W. (1972). *Proc. Nat. Acad. Sci. USA*, **69**, 3180-3184.

13 Acetylcholine receptor antibodies in myasthenia gravis

BY K. BERGSTRÖM · A.K. LEFVERT · G. MATELL[1] · R. PIRSKANEN[2]

*Department of clinical chemistry, Karolinska Institutet,
Karolinska sjukhuset, S-10401 Stockholm Sweden.*

Serum, different lymph protein fractions and spinal fluid have been analysed for antibodies against the nicotinic acetylcholine receptor of human muscle or *Torpedo marmorata*. IgG from the lymph of 6 patients was shown to inhibit binding of ^{125}I-α neurotoxin (Naja naja siamensis) to membrane fragments from the electric organ. This effect was localized to the $F(ab')^2$ fragment of IgG 3 (Lefvert and Bergstrom, 1977). Serum samples from 145 patients with myasthenia gravis was analysed for antibodies to a skeletal muscle receptor preparation. The assay used is based on the binding of myasthenic IgG to a complex between ^{125}I-α-neurotoxin and a detergent extracted receptor (Lefvert and Matell, 1977). The receptor antibody was found in 85% of the patients. Only slight correlations were found between the amount of the receptor antibody and various clinical parameters.

A possible involvement of the central nervous system in myasthenia gravis has been proposed. The recently published observations of decreased rapid eye movement (REM) sleep in these patients (Papazian, 1976) is evidence of CNS involvement, since REM sleep is supposed to depend on cholinergic mechanisms. To test this hypothesis, spinal fluid samples as well as serum from 11 patients were analysed for the receptor antibody. The antibody was found both in the spinal fluid and in the serum of 7 patients and only in the spinal fluid of 1 patient. The ratio between the spinal fluid IgG concentration and the serum IgG concentration was normal except in one patient who had a slightly increased spinal IgG concentration. The ratio between the receptor antibody concentration in the spinal fluid and in the serum was, however, 2-10 times higher than the corresponding ratio for IgG. This indicates a possible local synthesis of the receptor antibody in CSF.

To investigate the kinetic properties of the receptor antibody several determinations of receptor antibody, IgG 3 and total IgG were made in three patients during thoracic duct lymph drainage. These values were used

1. *Myasthenic centre, Södersjukhuset, S-10064, Stockholm, Sweden.*
2. *Department of Neurology, University of Helsinki, Finland.*

in a mathematical model to calculate kinetic parameters. The values found for $t^{1/2}$ and fractional rates of synthesis and catabolism for IgG 3 and for total IgG were shown to agree with those found with other techniques (Morell *et al.*, 1970). The receptor antibody belonged to the IgG 3 subclass but there $t^{1/2}$ was shorter (2-3 days) than the $t^{1/2}$ for IgG (7 days. The fractional rates of synthesis and catabolism were also higher. One explanation for these findings could be strong antigenic stimuli and rapid elimination of the antibody from the circulation by the antigen in this case the cholinergic receptor structures.

References

Lefvert, A.K., Bergstrom, K. (1977). *Eur. J. Clin. Invest.*, **7**, 115-119.
Lefvert, A.K., Matell, G. (1977). *Acta. Med. Scand.*, **201**, 181-182.
Morell, A., Terry, W.D., Waldmann, T.A. (1970). *J. Clin. Invest.*, **49**, 673-680.
Papazian, O. (1976). *Neurology*, **26**, 311-316.

14 Increased decremental response in experimental autoimmune myasthenic rabbits following infusion of human myasthenic IgG

E. STAHLBERG[1] · C. MATTSSON · A. UDDGARD · E. HEILBRONN
L. HAMMARSTRÖM[2] ·E. SMITH[2] · A.K. LEFVERT[3] · A. PERSSON[4] · G. MATELL[5]

*Sect. of Biochemistry, National Defence Research Institute,
S-172 04 Sundbyberg, Sweden.*

In an attempt to clarify the role of AChR antibodies in the pathogenesis of myasthenia gravis (MG), rabbits with experimentally induced myasthenia (EAMG) and normal rabbits were injected with lymph or purified IgG from MG patients. IgG with a high concentration of human AChR antibodies induced a marked additional decrement in EAMG rabbits. The decrement was reversed by Tensilon®. Low titre or normal IgG did not show this property.

Rabbits were immunized with purified nicotinic AChR weekly (Heilbronn and Mattson, 1974), until clinical symptoms of muscle weakness were observed. At that time they were tested with respect to a decremental muscle response after repetitive nerve stimulation (Heilbronn *et al.*, 1975). Before lymph or IgG was injected, the reproducibility of the decrement was checked by stimulation of the nerve every second minute for half an hour. Only rabbits with less decremental variance than 20% were used in transfer experiments. After injection of lymph (crude or fractioned), the decrement was recorded every third minute for two to four hours. Lymph was obtained from patients with severe generalized MG, undergoing thoracic duct drainage (Lefvert and Matell, 1977). Purified IgG was prepared as previously reported (Lefvert and Bergstrom, 1977). Normal human IgG was obtained from KABI AB, Stockholm, Sweden.

Immunized rabbits injected with low titre anti-human AChR or normal IgG showed no change in their decremental response to repetitive nerve stimulation, (Fig. 1). The same result was obtained when non-immunized rabbits were injected with myasthenic lymph. Fig. 2 and Fig. 3 shows the 100% increase in decremental response of immunized rabbits which were

[1] *Dept. Clin. Neurophysiology, Academic Hospital, S-750 14 Uppsala, Sweden.*
[2] *Div. Immunology, Wallenberglab., Lilla Frescati, S-104 05 Stockholm, Sweden,*
[3] *Dept. Clinical Chemistry, Karolinska Hospital, S-104 05 Stockholm, Sweden,*
[4] *Dept. Clin. Neurophysiology, Huddinge Hospital, S-141 86 Huddinge, Sweden,*
[5] *Dept. Medicine, South Hospital, S-100 64 Stockholm, Sweden.*

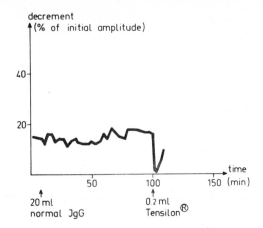

Fig. 1. An immunized rabbit injected with normal IgG. The initial decrement of 15% was not affected by this fraction. The Tensilon® effect is characteristic of *Myasthenia gravis*.

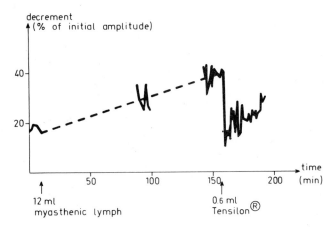

Fig. 2. Effect on receptor immunized rabbit muscle decrement of i.v. injected crude myasthenic lymph.

injected with crude myasthenic lymph and myasthenic IgG respectively. The apparent lack of effect of MG-lymph on normal rabbits may be explained by: (a) a large safety margin of the receptors in the normal neuro-muscular junction, (b) a reduced access of IgG to the receptor at the neuro-muscular endplate in normal rabbits compared to EAMG rabbits. In EAMG rabbits the synaptic cleft is irregular and widened, (Heilbronn *et al.*, 1976), (c) a lack of cross-reactivity between anti-human AChR antibodies and normal rabbit AChR contrary to a supposed cross-reactivity with denervated rabbit AChR. Such differences between junctional and

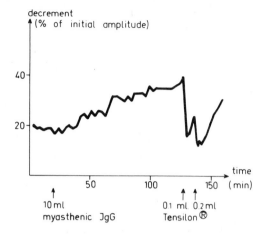

Fig. 3. Effect on the decrement after injection of fractionated myasthenic lymph into immunized rabbit.

extra-junctional receptors have been shown in rats (Almon and Appel, 1975; Almon and Appel, 1976).

We have described an increase in decremental myasthenic muscle response in EAMG rabbits after injection of high titre anti-human AChR lymph or IgG. Neither injections of low titre anti-AChR or normal IgG into EAMG rabbits, nor of high titre lymph to normal rabbits induced any changes in the EMG response. The existence of neonatal myasthenia (Namba *et al.*, 1970) removable by blood transfusion (Dunn, 1976), and the improvement of the clinical status after thoracic duct lymph drainage of myasthenic patients with remission following autologous cellfree lymph or IgG injection (Bergstrom *et al.*, 1973), clearly suggests the presence of a causative agent, possibly an antibody, in sera from such patients.

References

Almon, R.R., Appel, S.H. (1975). *Biochem. Biophys. Acta.*, **393**, 66-77.
Almon, R.R., Appel, S.H. (1976). *Ann. N.Y. Acad. Sci.*, **274**, 235-243.
Bergström, K., Franksson, C., Matell, G., von Reis, G. (1973). *Eur. Neurol.*, **13**, 19-30.
Dunn, J.M. (1976). *Am. J. Obstet, Gynecol.*, **125**, 265-266.
Heilbronn, E., Mattsson, C. (1974). *J. Neurochem.*, **22**, 315-317.
Heilbronn, E., Mattsson, C., Stahlberg, E., Hilton-Brown, P. (1975). *J. Neurol. Sci.*, **24**, 59-74.
Heilbronn, E., Mattsson, C., Thornell, L.E., Sjöström, M., Stahlberg, E., Hilton-Brown, P., Elmqvist, D. (1976). *Ann. N.Y. Acad. Sci.*, **274**, 337-353.
Lefvert, A.K., Matell, G. (1977). *Acta. Med. Scand.*, **201**, 181-182.
Lefvert, A.K., Bergström, K. (1977). *Eur. J. Clin. Invest.* (in press).
Namba, T., Brown, S.B., Grob, D. (1970). *Pediatrics*, **43**, 488-504.

15 Clinical and electroencephalographic changes induced by intracerebral infusion of serum from myasthenia gravis patients and α-bungarotoxin

A. FONTANA · P.J. GROB · R. SAUTER · R. DUBS AND I. MOTHERSILL

Immunology Laboratory, Department of Internal Medicine,
University Hospital, 8091 Zurich, Switzerland and Swiss
Clinic for Epileptics, Zurich, Switzerland

Antibodies have been detected in sera of patients with myasthenia gravis (MG), that inhibit the binding *in vitro* of α-bungarotoxin (α-Bgtx) to motor endplates of skeletal muscle or to acetylcholine receptor (AChR) rich extracts of skeletal muscle or electric tissue (Almon *et al.*, 1974). It has been demonstrated that molecules of the size of antibodies can penetrate the intact neuromuscular junction *in situ* (Zurn and Fulpius, 1976; Fulpius *et al.*, 1976). Furthermore, immunoglobulins have been shown by peroxidase-coupled anti-rat gamma globulin to be present in the endplates of rats with experimental autoimmune myasthenia gravis (EAMG) (Engel *et al.*, 1976). While some authors (Lindstrom *et al.*, 1976; Toyka, 1977) have shown successful passive transfer of EAMG by intravenous or intraperitoneal injection of gamma-globulin fractions from sera of rats with EAMG or of patients with MG, others (Lammers and Van Spijk, 1954; Schwarz, 1952; Namba and Grob, 1969; Namba *et al.*, 1970; Albuquerque *et al.*, 1976) found no alterations of neuromuscular transmission after local or systemic application of MG sera. Preliminary results are presented here that suggest that serum or its IgG-fraction from patients with MG influence central cholinergic transmission.

Methods

Eight cortical and subcortical electrodes and two infusion cannulas were implanted into the caudate nucleus of both hemispheres of rabbits using the LPC-stereotactic apparatus (La Précision Cinématographique, Asnieres/Seine), and taking coordinates from the atlas of Sawyer, Everett and Green (subcortical areas) (1954) and of Rose for cortical areas (1933). Details are given elsewhere (Fontana *et al.*, 1978).

The infusions were performed unilaterally under EEG control using a microinfusion pump (Unita) driven at a constant rate 8.3 μl/min. The usual procedure consisted of 4×7 min. infusion periods interrupted by three intervals of 20 min. 240 μl of the following sera were infused into the caudate nucleus of each of nine rabbits: (1) sera from five MG patients differing in the levels of anti-AChR antibodies as measured by the method described by Monnier and Fulpius (1977). The IgG fraction (28 mg/ml) of one of the MG sera was infused into two rabbits. The MG serum was fractioned by ammonium sulphate precipitation, passed over DEAE-cellulose and eluted with a phosphate gradient (Fahey, 1967). (3) In order to compare the effect of total MG serum or its IgG fraction with α-Bgtx, two rabbits were tested with two different concentrations of α-Bgtx (0.3 mg/ml and 2.3 mg/ml). The crude venom of Bungarus multicinctus was obtained from Miami Serpentarium Laboratories and purified on CM-Sephadex C-50 (Pharmacia) according to the method outlined by Lee et al. (1972) with the modification reported by Zurn and Fulpius (1976). As control 240 μl of the following sera or serum-fractions were infused each into a single rabbit brain: (1) Sera of six healthy individuals and of seven patients with brain damage (post-traumatic epilepsy (five), brain tumor (one), birth injury (one). (2) The IgG-fraction (16 mg/ml) of a healthy individual. (3) The albumin fraction (40 mg/ml) and the gammaglobulin fraction (1.7 mg/ml) eluted from the column at higher phosphate molarities, both fractions originated from MG serum.

Results

Table 1 summarizes the results. Four out of five rabbits showed abnormal discharges in the EEG when infused with MG serum. The electrical discharges were characterized by intermittent single spikes and single sharp waves, by single spike and wave or by sharp and slow wave complexes, these manifestations appearing either generalized or localized to the infused caudate nucleus. Regular auditory click stimulation at a frequency of 1/sec

Table 1. Incidence of EEG-alterations and abnormal clinical symptoms in rabbits infused with different sera/fractions

Infused sera/fraction of:	Number of rabbits tested	Abnormal EEG	Clinical symptom
Patient with MG	5	4	4
Patient with brain damage	7	0	0
Healthy individual	6	0	0
IgG from MG serum	2	2	2
IgG from healthy individual	1	0	0
Albumin from MG serum	1	0	0
Gammaglobulin from MG serum *	1	0	0
α-Bungarotoxin	2	2	0

*Eluted from the column by higher phosphate molarities.

provoked generalized spike discharges at the stimulation rate in one of 5 MG serum injected rabbits tested (Fig. 1). Parallel to the electroencephalographic abnormalities clinical changes occurred. Four of five rabbits manifested general hypotonia with clearly reduced motor activity. They appeared to have little control over their hind legs, walking only with the forepaws and with poor balance.

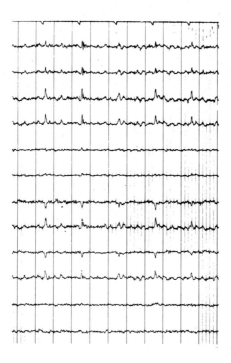

Fig. 1   EEG after intracerebral infusion of MG serum showing click-evoked generalised spike discharges (clicks are indicated by second marker ⌄).

The clinical and EEG responses seemed to correlate with the anti-AChR antibody titres in the infused MG sera. MG serum with 0.125 pmoles/ml anti-AChR antibodies (pmol ^{125}I-α-Bgtx-AChR complex precipitated per ml serum) provoked only rare and focal single spikes and no clinical symptoms in the rabbit mentioned above as non-reactor. In these rabbits receiving MG sera containing 0.7 0.65 and 0.68 pmoles/ml serum AChR antibodies respectively, clinical symptoms and EEG alterations began two to three days after infusion and lasted at least 48 hours. In the rabbit receiving MG serum with the highest amount of antibodies (1.6 pmoles/ml serum) the characteristic changes occurred 24 hours after infusion.

In two of the rabbits showing the above mentioned symptoms injections of 0.005 mg of prostigmine, infused over a period of 12 min. into the same caudate nucleus in which MG serum had been given, resulted in a transitory complete recovery of electroencephalographic and clinical symptoms. The recovery, lasting 20 and 30 min. was followed by generalized repeated bursts of spikes and spike series in the EEG accompanied by contralateral adversive epileptic signs.

In both rabbits, injected with the IgG fraction from serum from patients with MG clinical and electroencephalographic changes occurred, which did not differ from those obtained with the whole MG serum. The infusion of α-Bgtx was followed by only some generalized single spike discharges appearing after 6 hours and lasting 12 hours. During this period no clinical symptoms occurred in the two rabbits tested. At no time after infusion were clinical or electroencephalographic signs of structural or functional damage observed in animals receiving serum from healthy laboratory personnel. In one rabbit 720 μl of such serum had been infused. Also no abnormalities were obtained when similar tests with the sera from patients with brain damage were used.

Discussion

Clinical changes and abnormal bioelectrical discharges in the EEG became visible in rabbits after infusion of MG sera or its IgG fraction into the caudate nucleus. The responses seemed to correlate with the anti-AChR titre in the infused sera. The bioelectrical abnormalities completely disappeared after infusion of prostigmine. We suggest that inhibitory cholinergic neurons were blocked by anti-AChR antibodies. Numerous investigations (Chang, 1953; Feldberg et al., 1957; Rumagai et al., 1952) have shown that D-tubocurarine has a convulsant action when applied topically to the cerebral cortex. The mechanism of its action is still unclear but D-tubocurarine might at least in part antagonize the inhibitory influence of γ-aminobutyric acid (Hill et al., 1972). Other neuromuscular blocking drugs such as gallamine, decamethonium and dihydro-β-erythroidine did not show this convulsive property (Bannerjee et al., 1970). In MG sera immunoglobulins of the IgG class are present which influence the nicotinic cholinergic transmission at the neuromuscular junction. The results presented here imply that this is also true for central nicotinic cholinergic activity. They give further evidence for the assumption that nicotinic cholinergic activity is present in vertebrate brain as has been suggested by others (Krnjevic, 1974). The activity of α-Bgtx binding in rat brain as analysed by radioautography, is highest in synaptosomal preparations, and correlates with regional ACh content. Particularly high α-Bgtx binding is observed in brain stem, thalamic region, caudate nucleus and within the cortex (Salvaterra *et al.*, 1975). The different clinical picture obtained after infusion of MG sera or its IgG fraction compared to the effect of α-Bgtx may be the result of several different binding sites on AChR. Anti-AChR antibodies react with AChR at determinants different from the toxin binding site (Lindstrom, 1976). But also other mechanisms such as a different diffusion rate, different binding affinities have to be taken into consideration. Besides the observations *in vitro* and our data *in vivo*, clinical findings in patients with MG also suggest the possibility that in addition to the well known alterations of neuromuscular transmission central cholinergic functions are also involved in this disorder. Excessive amounts of slow activity and alterations of REM (rapid eye movement) sleep have been observed in the EEG of most MG patients (Hokkanen and Toivakka, 1969; Papazian, 1976).

Summary

Microinfusion of serum of patients with myasthenia gravis (MG) or its IgG fraction into the caudate nucleus of the rabbit brain provokes abnormal bioelectrical discharges, abnormal motor functions and an altered behaviour, transitory phenomena that disappear after application of prostigmine. A correlation between the degree of the abnormal responses and the amount of antibodies against acetylcholine receptors present in the infused MG-sera was noted.

Acknowledgements. We wish to thank Prof. B.W. Fulpius (Dept. of Biochemistry, Science II, University of Geneva) for purification of α-Bgtx and measurement of the antibody titres against human AChR in MG- sera.

References

Albuquerque, E.X., Lebeda, F.J., Appel, S.H., Almon, R., Kaufmann, F.C., Mayer, R.F., Narahashi, T. and Yeh, J.Z. (1976). *Ann. N.Y. Acad. Sci.*, **274**, 475-492.
Almon, R.R., Andrew, C.G., Appel, S.H. (1974). *Science*, **186**, 55-57.
Banerjee, U. Feldberg, W., Georgiev, V.P. (1970). *Br. J. Pharmac.*, **40**, 6-22.
Chang, H. (1953). *J. Neurophysiol.*, **16**, 221-233.
Engel, A.G, Lindstrom, J.M., Lambert, E.H., Lennon, V.A. (1977). *Neurology*, **27**, 307-315.
Fahey, J.L. (1967). *Academic Press, New York/London*, **1**, 321-331.
Feldberg, W., Malcolm, J.L., Darian Smith, I. (1957). *J. Physiol.*, **138**, 178-182.
Fontana, A., Grob, P., Dubs, R., Sauter, R., Mothersill, I. (1978). Neurol.
Fulpius, B.W., Zurn, A.D., Granato, D.A., Leder, R.M. (1976). *Ann. N.Y. Acad. Sci.*, **274**, 116-129.
Hill, R.G., Simmonds, M.A., Straughan, D.W. (1972). *Nature*, **240**, 51-52.
Hokkanen, E., Toivakka, E. (1969). *Acta Neurol. Scand.*, **45**, 556-567.

Krnjevic, K. (1974). *Physiol. Rev.*, **54**, 418-540.
Lammers, W., Van Spijk, D.M. (1954). *Nature*, **173**, 1192-1194.
Lee, C.Y., Chang, S.L., Kan, S.T., Luh, S.H. (1972). *J. Chromatog.*, **72**, 71-82.
Lindstrom, J. (1976). *J. Supramol. Struct.*, **4**, 389-403.
Lindstrom, J.M., Engel, A.G., Seybold, M.E., Lennon, V.A., Lambert, E.H. (1976). *J. exp. Med.*, **144**, 739-753.
Monnier, V.W. Fulpius, B.W. (1977). *Clin. exp. Immunol.* **29**, 16-22.
Namba, T., Grob, D. (1969). *Neurology*, **19**, 173-184.
Namba, T., Brown, S.B., Grob, D. (1970). *Pediatrics*, **45**, 488-504.
Papazian, O. (1976). *Neurology*, **26**, 311-315.
Rose, M., Rose, S. (1933). *J. Psychol. Leipzig.*, **45**, 264-281.
Rumagai, H., Sakai, F., Otsuka, Y. (1962). *J. Neuropharmac.*, **1**, 157-166.
Salvaterra, P.M., Mahler, H.R., Moore, W.J. (1975). *J. biol. chem.*, **250**, 6469-6475.
Sawyer, C.M., Everett, J.W., Green, J.D. (1954). *J. comp. Neurol.*, **101**, 804-844.
Schwarz, H. (1952). *Canad. Med. Assoc. J.*, **67**, 238-241.
Toyka, R.V., Drachmann, D.B., Fischbeck, K.H., Kao, I. (1977). *N. Engl. J. Med.*, **296**, 125-131.
Zurn, A.D., Fulpius, B.W. (1976). *Clin. exp. Immunol.*, **24**, 9-17.

16 Experimental autoimmune myasthenia gravis: a tool for studying the pathogenesis and therapy of myasthenia gravis

SARA FUCHS · REBECA TARRAB-HAZDAI · DANIELA NEVO · DANIEL BARTFELD

Department of Chemical Immunology
The Weizmann Institute of Science
Rehovot, Israel

It was proposed in the early 60's that myasthenia gravis (MG) might be an autoimmune disorder and involve an immunological response towards a protein at the neuromuscular junction (Nastuk *et al.*, 1960; Simpson, 1960). However, in spite of increasing evidence in support of an autoimmune basis for the disease its exact origin was unknown. The reports in 1973 about the decrease in postsynaptic acetylcholine receptors (AChR) in MG (Fambrough *et al.*, 1973) and about the induction in rabbits of symptoms resembling those of MG following injections with purified AChR from electric eel (Patrick and Lindstrom, 1973) shed new light on this issue. Considerable evidence now exists that MG is indeed an autoimmune disease where AChR is a major autoantigen, and that the experimental model disease induced by AChR and designated experimental autoimmune myasthenia gravis (EAMG) is an appropriate model for the human disease. The established similarity between the clinical and experimental diseases, and the involvement of AChR in both of them permits detailed studies on the pathogenesis and therapy of MG. Besides the immediate significance of such a study for MG it is valuable also for the general understanding of autoimmune phenomena in man.

Evidence for an Autoimmune Sensitivity to AChR in Myasthenia Gravis

The possibility that the pathogenesis of MG involves an autoimmune mechanism was based clinically on the association of MG with other autoimmune diseases, the occurrence of thymic abnormalities in a high percentage of myasthenics, and the beneficial effects of thymectomy and steroid therapy. Immunological studies have demonstrated both lympho-cyte-mediated immunological reactions as well as circulating antibodies to muscle and thymic antigens. In view of these studies and of the experimental autoimmune response induced by AChR we tested cellular and humoral sensitivity in myasthenic patients to electric fish AChR.

Peripheral blood lymphocytes from patients with MG were shown to be stimulated when cultured *in vitro* with an electric eel extract enriched with AChR (Abramsky *et al.*, 1975a). These findings suggest that a sensitization *in vivo* of lymphocytes to self AChR is occurring in MG and that cell-mediated autoimmune mechanism may be important in the pathogenesis of the neuromuscular block. Similar results were reported later also by Richman *et al.* (1976) using purified *Torpedo* AChR to stimulate the lymphocytes *in vitro*.

The lymphocyte response to AChR did not seem to correlate with either the clinical condition or the time lapse between onset of the illness and the test. However, there seems to be a correlation between the stimulation indices obtained in the lymphocyte transformation technique *in vitro* and therapy. Higher indices were observed in patients who had undergone neither steroid therapy nor thymectomy whereas lower values were obtained in patients following either of these treatments (Abramsky *et al.*, 1975a). Moreover, as seen in Fig. 1, marked diminution of the cellular response to AChR was shown in patients who displayed clinical improvement after prednisone treatment (Abramsky *et al.*, 1975b).

In addition to cell mediated immunity to AChR, humoral antibodies reacting with AChR were observed in a high percentage of patients with MG (Aharonov *et al.*, 1975a; Bender *et al.*, 1975; Appel *et al.*, 1975; Lindstrom *et al.*, 1976a). The level of circulating antibody estimated depends very much on the assay used and on the cross reactivity between the test antigen and human AChR. Using the microcomplement fixation assay with purified *Torpedo* AChR as the antigen we have observed antibodies to AChR in at least 80% of the patients tested (Aharonov *et al.*, 1975a). Moreover, as seen in Fig. 1, marked diminution of the purified human muscle AChR. Lindstrom *et al.* (1976a) find significant titre of antibodies against human AChR in more than 90% of the patients studies. We observed similar titres in some of our myasthenic patients when testing the sera by the radioimmunoassay with a muscle AChR preparation obtained from denervated rats. However, there seems to be no correlation between the severity of the disease and the antibody titres. There is increasing evidence from several laboratories that circulating antibodies may be actively involved in myasthenia (Matell *et al.*, 1976; Pinching *et al.*, 1976; Toyka *et al.*, 1977), although it is still not fully understood to what extent humoral factors are responsible for the physiological defect in the disease.

Experimental autoimmune myasthenia gravis (EAMG).

EAMG has been induced by several laboratories in various animal species such as rabbits, rats, guinea-pigs, monkeys and mice by injection of purified

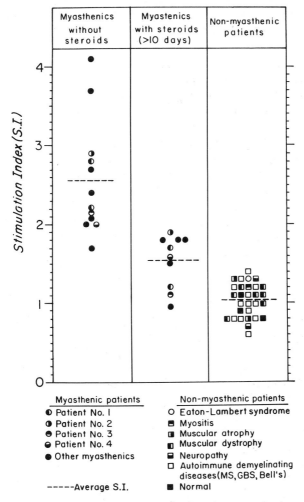

Fig. 1. Lymphocyte response to AChR in myasthenic and nonmyasthenic patients. (From Abramsky *et al.*, 1975b).

AChR from electric organ tissues of *Electrophorus electricus* or from *Torpedo* (Patrick and Lindstrom, 1973; Sugiyama *et al.*, 1973; Tarrab-Hazdai *et al.*, 1975a,b,c; Heilbronn *et al.*, 1975; Green *et al.*, 1975; Lennon *et al.*, 1975; Fuchs *et al.*, 1976). There have been some reports also on the induction of EAMG by purified mammalian AChR (Granato *et al.*, 1976) and by syngeneic preparations of AChR (Lindstrom *et al.*, 1976b; Fulpius, personal communication). Whereas the disease in rabbits, monkeys and occasionally mice seems to be acute and fatal the disease in rats, guinea-pigs and mice is mild and transient.

The AChR-induced myasthenia in monkeys is especially similar to the human disease in its clinical signs (Fig. 2), including difficulties in breathing and swallowing, ptosis, motor weakness, etc., all being reversed temporarily following intramuscular injection of the anticholinesterase prostigmine (Tarrab-Hazdai *et al.*, 1975c).

The clinical, physiological, pharmacological and immunological findings in animals with EAMG closely parallel the observed manifestations of MG. Both humoral and cellular immune responses to the electric organ AChR used as antigen as well as towards self AChR are observed in animals with EAMG. The acquired reactivity towards self AChR, which is lower in extent than the reactivity towards the fish receptor, provides a strong evidence for the autoimmune nature of EAMG.

The mechanism involved in the induction of the experimental disease is not yet fully understood. It appears that both cellular and humoral immune responses may play a role in the pathogenesis of the blockade (Tarrab-Hazdai *et al.*, 1975b; Lindstrom *et al.*, 1976c; Toyka *et al.*, 1977), although cellular factors are probably playing the major role in the initial stages of the attack of the neuromuscular junction. Cytophilic antibodies and macrophages (Engel *et al.*, 1976) also play a role in the pathogenesis of EAMG. We have demonstrated that macrophage cytophilic antibodies with AChR specificity are present in rabbits with EAMG (Martinez *et al.*, 1977). Cytophilic antibodies capable of binding to normal alveolar macrophages are detected in the sera of rabbits 14 days following immunization with AChR, and are maintained through the severe stages of the disease. In addition cytophilic anti-AChR antibodies are bound *in vitro* to macrophages of sick rabbits (Table 1).

The role of cytophilic antibodies in EAMG is not yet established; they may bind first to the AChR in the target tissue and only then bind locally to macrophages via their Fc receptors. Another possibility is that cytophilic antibodies bind first to macrophages with high avidity for the specific antibodies and only then are the antibody coated cells specifically directed to the antigenic target tissue. Since we have observed antibody coated macrophages in the alveolar fluid of sick animals, not associated with the synaptic membrane, and since Engel *et al.* (1976) have reported on the presence of macrophages in the region of the damaged end-plate, we propose that antibody coated macrophages are getting to the target tissue (Martinez *et al.*, 1977).

Fig. 2. Myasthenic monkey one week after fourth injection of purified AChR. The monkey was injected four times at three week intervals intradermally with 100 μg of AChR in complete Freund's adjuvant. The myasthenic monkey was injected intramuscularly with 0.2 mg of Prostigmine. a & b, Before injection of Prostigmine; c, 5 minutes after injection of Prostigmine; d, 10 min after injection of Prostigmine. (From Tarrab-Hazdai, 1975c).

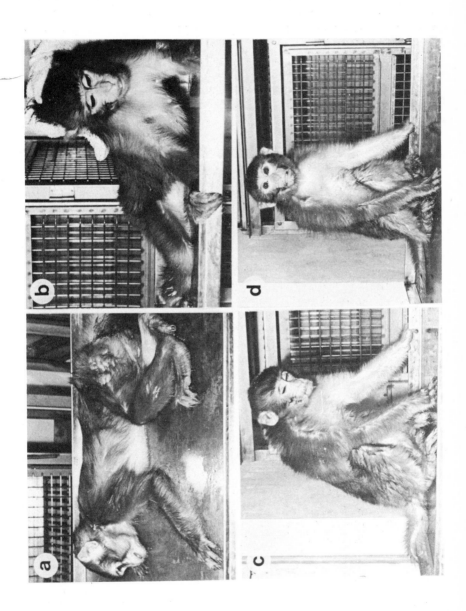

TABLE 1. Binding of ^{125}I-AChR to macrophages of rabbits with EAMG[a]

Injection	^{125}I-AChR bound (pg/2 × 10⁶ macrophages)
AChR (80 µg)[b] in CFA[d]	1260
	1200
	1110
	470
	1200
	760
BSA (150 µg) in CFA[d]	400
	340
CFA[d]	400
	380
Nil[c]	380

[a] The assay was carried out as described by Martinez *et al.* (1977). [b] Macrophages were obtained from rabbits at the severe stage of EAMG. [c] An average of eight rabbits. [d] CFA: Freunds complete adjuvant.

EAMG in mice

An experimental model disease in mice seems of major importance especially for studying genetic aspects of myasthenia gravis and the role of the thymus both as a specific antigenic target in the disease and as a source for immunocompetent helper and suppressor cells. The induction of the disease in mice is more difficult than its induction in other species so far studied. We have succeeded in inducing EAMG in several inbred mouse strains following two immunization with *Torpedo californica* AChR with a nine week interval (Fuchs *et al.*, 1976). EAMG was also induced in BALB/C mice with AChR purified from denervated rat muscle (Granato *et al.*, 1976) and from syngeneic mouse denervated muscle (Fulpius, personal communication).

Our sick mice suffered from weight loss and exhibited signs of fatigue, hypoactivity, ruffled furs and paralysis of the limbs and a motor impairment both of which were accentuated by exercise. Their heads sank and their backs were exaggeratedly humped (Figs. 3 and 4a). Severely sick animals died from the disease whereas in some of the mice the disease seemed to be transient. The clinical symptoms of mice with EAMG were temporarily reversed shortly after intravenous injection of 5 µg edrophonium chloride (Tensilon) (Fig. 4b). In particular there was improvement of such motor performances as gripping and walking.

Cellular and humoral immune responses in the injected mice were determined. The autoimmune response against self AChR in C57BL/6 mice

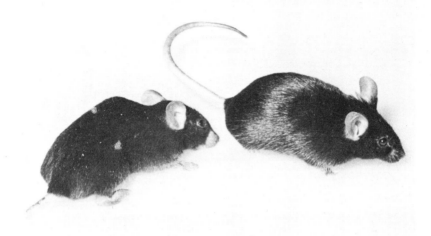

Fig. 3. Posture of a myasthenic C57BL/6 mouse two weeks after second injection of AChR (left) in comparison with a mouse immunized only with complete Freund's adjuvant (right).

injected with AChR was demonstrated by reactivity towards syngeneic muscle extracts. Cellular sensitivity was tested by the *in vitro* lymphocyte transformation technique. Lymphocytes of *Torpedo* AChR-injected mice were stimulated *in vitro* when incubated with the immunogen, as well as with xenogeneic (rabbit) and syngeneic (C57BL/6) muscle extracts (Table 2). Humoral autoimmune response was demonstrated by the ability of

TABLE 2. Incorporation of tritiated thymidine by cultures of lymph node cells from C57BL/6 mice sensitized with AChR.

Antigen added to sensitized lymph node cells (μg/culture)		Stimulation Index[a]	
		day 10	day 42
AChR	(0.50)	9.24	5.16
	(0.25)	10.07	7.14
Mouse (C57BL/6) muscle extract	(5.0)	4.30	Not done
	(2.5)	2.58	Not done
Rabbit muscle extract	(5.0)	6.50	8.66
Lysozyme	(2.0)	1.16	0.88

Micro culture lymphocyte transformation techniques was used. Mice were injected with 10 μg AChR in Freund's complete adjuvant in the foot pads 10 or 42 days prior to the experiments.

[a]Ratio of cpm of experimental to control cultures. Average of 5 experiments.

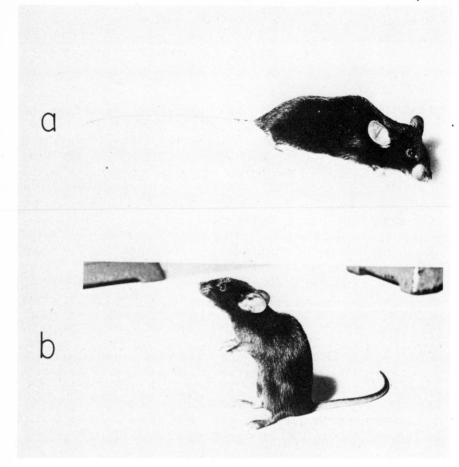

Fig. 4. Myasthenic C57BL/6 mouse two weeks after second injection of AChR. a, Before tensilon test; b, 5 min after intravenous injection of tensilon (5 μg).

mouse anti-AChR sera to bind to syngeneic AChR labelled with ^{125}I-bungarotoxin. However, the humoral cross reactivity with syngeneic AChR should be interpreted with caution and by itself it is not a sufficient criterion for EAMG since similar cross-reactivity was also observed in mice which had high titres of antibodies to *Torpedo* AChR and exhibited no clinical signs of EAMG.

In recent experiments we have injected subcutaneously low doses of cyclophosphamide (20 mg/kg) to C57BL/6 mice 2 days before the administration of *Torpedo* AChR. This low dose of cyclophosphamide was given in order to kill selectively suppressor T-cells (Otterness and Chang, 1976). Indeed, such injected mice exhibited an early phase of EAMG 5-8 days following the AChR injection and a second phase 25-30 days following the receptor injection. It seems that B-cell function was not affected by the cyclophosphamide as the antibody titres of these mice were at least as high as those of AChR-injected mice with no drug treatment.

Genetic aspects

Susceptibility to myasthenia gravis in humans is genetically controlled and associated with the major histocompatibility antigens (HL-A) (Fritze *et al.*, 1976; Pirskanen, 1976; Oosterhuis *et al.*, 1976). EAMG in mice and the availability of many inbred mouse strains provide a valuable tool for studying genetic control of the immune and autoimmune response to AChR. We have demonstrated different susceptibility to EAMG in strains representing different haplotypes of the major histocompatibility complex (H-2) (Fuchs *et al.*, 1976). Mice were injected twice with a nine week interval with 10 μg of purified *Torpedo californica* AChR. Ten days or more after the second injection clinical signs of EAMG were observed in mice of inbred strains with H-2^a, H-2^b, H-2^d and H-2^k haplotypes. The disease was not found in any mice with H-2^q and H-2^s haplotypes (Table 3). It is noteworthy that no correlation between the antibody titres to *Torpedo* AChR and incidence of the disease was found, as mice of all strains tested gave similar high titres. It is possible, however, that there are differences in the specificity of the antibodies. The susceptibility to EAMG

TABLE 3. EAMG incidence and antibody titres against AChR in different strains of mice.

Strain	H-2 Haplotype	Log₂ hemagglutination titre			Animals with clinical signs of EAMG
		Day 21	Day 63	Day 72[a]	
A/J	a	8.2	13.5	20.3	1/5
B10.A	a	7.5	11.2	20.0	2/5
C57BL/6	b	8.0	11.8	18.9	8/12
C3H.SW	b	7.5	11.0	19.3	2/5
CWB	b	7.5	11.5	19.6	2/10
BALB/C	d	7.5	11.2	19.8	2/5
DBA/2	d	8.0	11.0	20.2	2/6
C3H/Hej	k	7.5	12.0	18.5	2/5
CKB	k	7.6	11.3	20.0	2/6
AKR/Cu	k	7.8	11.4	19.0	6/6
DBA/1	q	7.2	11.3	20.2	0/6
SWR	q	8.2	11.4	20.6	0/6
SJL/J	s	8.0	11.8	21.0	0/6
ASW	s	7.3	11.7	20.6	0/6

Mice were injected twice in a nine-week interval with 10 μg of purified *Torpedo* AChR. Antibodies were determined by micro passive hemagglutination technique. Formalinized sheep red blood cells were coated with *Torpedo* AChR (100 μg/ml packed cells) by means of tannic acid. a. 10 days following the booster injection.

may be determined by a genetically controlled ability to respond to a specific determinant or determinants. It has been recently proposed that apart from the possibility that the autoimmune responses to AChR are under genetic control, the capacity of mouse thymic stem cells to differentiate into myogenic cells *in vitro* is inheritable, sex dependent and associated with the major histocompatibility antigens (Wekerle and Ketelsen, 1977).

The role of the thymus

A model involving an autoimmune response to AChR seems to explain adequately many clinical and physiological manifestations of myasthenia gravis. However, any general model for the pathogensis of MG must also take into account the involvement of the thymus in this condition. There is a high incidence of thymic hyperplasia or neoplasia in patients with MG and thymectomy is beneficial in the management of some patients. Immunological studies on myasthenic patients have demonstrated the presence of humoral and cellular immune responses towards thymic tissues. Goldstein (1968) and Kalden *et al.* (1969) have shown that animals immunized with thymic extracts develop an autoimmune thymitis as well as a partial defect in neuromuscular transmission.

The relation between the thymic disorder and the neuromuscular block is not yet understood. An autoimmune response, resulting from antigenic alterations may cause damage to both neuromuscular junctions and to the thymus. They may be both involved together, or one of them may be affected primarily and the other secondarily, due to immunological cross-reaction between them. In view of these possibilities we looked for immunological cross-reaction between AChR and thymus and have shown that electric organ AChR cross-reacts with components of calf thymus, both at the cellular and humoral levels of the immune response (Aharonov *et al.*, 1975b). Such a cross-reaction can provide a molecular basis for the association between neuromuscular block and thymic disorders in MG.

The origin of the cross-reaction between thymus and AChR may stem from 'myoid' cells in the thymus. Cultures of thymus cells from mice, rats and humans were shown recently to yield skeletal muscle colonies possessing demonstrable amounts of AChR on their cell membranes (Wekerle *et al.*, 1975; Kao and Drachman, 1977). It is possible that such cells in the thymus may play a role in the pathogenesis of myasthenia gravis.

We have shown by adoptive transfer experiments (Table 4) that the humoral response against AChR is T-cell dependent. It appears that T -cells are required both for primary and secondary immune responses. Similar results were also obtained by Lennon *et al.* (1976) in rats. It would be interesting to dissociate the need for thymus cells for T-helping or T-suppressing function from the possible specific role of the thymus as a specific antigenic target involved in the pathogenesis of the disease.

TABLE 4. Antibody response to AChR in an adoptive cell transfer experiment in C57BL/6 mice

Group No.	Cells transferred into lethally irradiated mice	AChR injected	$\log^2$ hemagglutination titre[a] Day 7[b]	Day 12	Day 18
1	Normal spleen cells (30×10^6)	$10\,\mu g$ CFA	2.25	5.0	6.37
2	Normal spleen cells treated with ATS[c] (30×10^6) + complement	$10\,\mu g$ in CFA	1.20	1.66	1.75
3	Primed spleen cells[d] (30×10^6)	$10\,\mu g$ in CFA	Not done	13.0	14.75
4	Primed spleen cells treated with ATC (30×10^6) + complement	$10\,\mu g$ in CFA	Not done	1.70	1.88

Cell transfer experiments were performed from normal or primed donors into lethally irradiated mice (800 rad Co^{60} whole body irradiation). [a] Average titre of 10-25 mice [b] Days after injection of AChR [c] Anti-thymocytic serum [d] Cells obtained from mice injected with 10 μg AChR in CFA 3 weeks earlier.

Therapy of EAMG

Aside from the use of EAMG as a tool for studying the pathogeneis of MG it is valuable also for evaluating the mechanism of action and optimal regimens of different drugs used in therapy of MG. Moreover, the availability of an experimental model disease induced by a well characterized antigen (AChR) enables us to attempt the development of specific immunotherapy for MG. We have used the disease in rabbits in order to achieve suppression of EAMG by nonspecific immunosuppressive drugs and by a non-pathogenic derivative of the AChR molecule.

Immunosuppressive drugs

Corticosteroids and the antimetabolite azathioprine were empirically found to be effective in treatment of MG (Jenkins, 1972, Warmotts and Engel, 1972; Seybold and Drachman, 1974; Matell *et al.*, 1976). We have used the same drugs in order to suppress EAMG in rabbits and to follow the mechanism of suppression. Using this model allows us to vary the course of the drug treatments readily and to follow concomitantly several immunological parameters.

Corticosteroids. Rabbits injected with purified *Torpedo californica* AChR were treated with hydrocortisone according to one of two regimens: either early continous administration of high doses hydrocortisone or administration of gradually increasing doses of hydrocortisone. For the early administration course (group A) rabbits injected with AChR on day 0 received hydrocortisone (50 mg) on days 3, 7, 11, 14, 18, 27 and 30. For the gradually increasing course of administration (group B) rabbits injected with AChR on day 0, received 10 mg hydrocortisone on day 0 and the dose was increased by 5 mg daily until a maximum level of 50 mg was reached. From the 9th day, the hydrocortisone administration (50 mg) was given every 3 days for an additional 3 months. In the control group the hydrocortisone treatment was replaced by saline injections.

As can be seen in Table 5 the effect of corticosteroids treatment seems to depend on the regimen. Hydrocortisone administered in gradually increasing doses prevented the appearance of EAMG completely, for at least 4 months after the beginning of the experiment (group B). When hydrocortisone was administered in high doses from the beginning (group A), EAMG appeared earlier and in a more severe form than in the control animals. Nevertheless, this treatment had some suppressive effect, as only four out of the six animals with severe EAMG died before the booster injection. The surviving four animals (two with mild and two with severe signs) lived for an additional 2 to 3 weeks after the second injection of AChR, whereas the animals in the control group died very shortly after the booster injection. The schedule of steroid administration also seems to be of great importance in MG patients particularly in order to minimize side effects; in spite of the overall beneficial effect of steroids in MG, increasing weakness usually occurs early in treatment and can be avoided by a gradually increasing dosage schedule.

The effect of hydrocortisone in suppressing EAMG was paralleled by a diminished cellular sensitization to AChR *in vitro* (Abramsky *et al.*, 1976). This is in agreement with our findings that in human myasthenia decreased cellular sensitization to AChR correlated with clinical improvement during prednisone therapy (Abramsky *et al.*, 1975b).

It appears that the therapeutic action of steroids is by an immunosuppressive mechanism, most probably by suppression of cytolytic effects by sensitized lymphocytes, whereas their early harmful action may be due to an enhancement of immune mechanisms (Stavy *et al.*, 1974). The above experiments describe the successful prevention of the onset of EAMG following appropriate treatment with hydrocortisone. We are now attempting the therapy of EAMG by administration of hydrocortisone to sick animals at various stages of the disease.

Azathioprine. We have shown that azathioprine is effective in suppressing the onset of EAMG in rabbits injected with AChR from *Torpedo californica* and have studied the correlation between clinical effects and several immunological parameters resulting from this immunosuppressive treatment.

Rabbits were injected on day 0 with AChR (80 μg, in complete Freund's adjuvant, intradermally) and with azathioprine (4 mg/kg, intramuscularly). Similar administrations of the drug were given to the rabbits daily for

TABLE 5. Suppression of AChR-induced EAMG by hydrocortisone

Experiment (group)	Treatment	EAMG following 1st immunization				EAMG after booster[a]		
		Onset (days)	Incidence (%)			Surviving after booster (days)	Incidence (%)	
			Mild or moderate	Severe	Death		Clinical signs	Death
Control	Saline	21	50 (4/8)b	50 (4/8)	50 (4/8)c	2 – 7	100 (4/4)	100 (4/4)
A	High dose hydrocortisone	14	25 (2/8)	75 (6/8)	50 (4/8)	14 – 20	100 (4/4)	100 (4/4)
B	Gradually increasing hydrocortisone		0 (0/4)	0 (0/4)	0 (0/4)	>90	0 (0/4)	0 (0/4)

a Second injection was given to all surviving rabbits 35 days after the first immunization. b The numbers in parentheses represent the number of animals. c All rabbits that died exhibited severe signs of the disease beforehand.

15 days and then every 2-3 days for an additional 5 months. In a control group the drug injections were replaced by saline injections.

Azathioprine treatment effectively suppressed the onset of EAMG in rabbits, for at least 12 months, even after discontinuing the drug treatment for 7 months (Table 6). In eight out of ten rabbits there was a complete prevention of EAMG, and these rabbits had a normal electromyographic recording and exhibited no weight loss. Two rabbits in this group died during the experiment but clinical symptoms of EAMG were detected only in one of them. In the control group of AChR-injected rabbits which were not treated with azathioprine, all rabbits exhibited EAMG and showed weight loss and a characteristic decremental electromyographic pattern. It is noteworthy that a second injection of AChR to the azathioprine immunosuppressed rabbits after 12 months, led to the onset of EAMG 6-10 days later, as is the case following a secondary injection of AChR. This behaviour suggests that although EAMG was prevented by azathioprine, immunological memory toward the original AChR injection 12 months earlier was maintained.

TABLE 6. Suppression of AChR-induced EAMG by azathioprine

Treatment[a]	Onset (days)	EAMG Clinical signs (%)	Death (%)	Surviving after 12 months (%)
Saline (control)	21-30	100 (8/8)[b]	100 (8/8)	0
Azathioprine (5 months)	100	10 (1/10)	20 (2/10)[c]	80 (8/10)

[a] All rabbits were injected with 80 μg *Torpedo californica* AChR on day 0. [b] The numbers in parenthesis represent the number of animals. [c] No clinical signs of EAMG were detected in one of these rabbits.

The suppressive effect of azathioprine was accompanied by decreased cellular and humoral immunological reactivity against both the immunizing *Torpedo* AChR and self AChR, with a significantly more pronounced effect on the response to self receptor. The cellular sensitivity towards the *Torpedo* AChR as measured by the lymphocyte transformation technique *in vitro*, was suppressed by about 45% as a result of drug treatment, whereas the reactivity towards self receptor was essentially abolished (Table 7). Azathioprine treatment was shown to be effective also on macrophage bound antibodies and to a lesser extent on lymphocyte bound antibodies (Table 8). Whereas the suppressive effect on the binding of ^{125}I-AChR to lymphocytes amounted to about 40%, the decrease in the binding of ^{125}I-AChR to macrophages was 90%. The specific binding of

^{125}I-AChR to the cells was inhibited by unlabelled AChR and by goat anti-rabbit Ig.

TABLE 7. Lymphocyte transformation with *Torpedo* and self AChR in rabbits treated with azathioprine[a]

Antigen in culture (μg)	AChR with saline	Treatment AChR with azathioprine
	Average Stimulation index.	
Torpedo AChR (1.25)	70	40
(2.25)	91	33
Rabbit muscle AChR (2.5)	9.0	2.00
(5.0)	9.2	2.3
Lysozyme (2.0)	1.5	1.8

a Average of five rabbits in each group. Experiments were done simultaneously on cells of treated and non treated animals 20-30 days after immunization with AChR. Micro culture lymphocyte transformation technique was used.

TABLE 8. Binding of ^{125}I-AChR to lymphocytes and macrophages of rabbits with EAMG and under azathioprine treatment[a]

Treatment[b]	^{125}I-AChR bound (pg per 2 × 10^6 cells)[c]	
	Lymphocytes	Macrophages
Saline	562	725
Azathioprine	312	70

aThe assay of the binding was carried out as described by Martinez *et al.* (1977). b All rabbits were injected with 80 μg *Torpedo* AChR on day 0. c The amount of ^{125}I-AChR bound to lymphocytes or macrophages from animals injected with CFA or other proteins was subtracted. The values represent average of four rabbits in each group. Cells were obtained from rabbits 25-30 days following the injection with AChR.

The effect of the drug on the humoral response towards AChR was measured by analysing total circulating antibodies as well as cytophilic antibodies. The antibody titre against self AChR, representing an auto-immune response, was essentially abolished (Table 9) as was the case also for the cellular sensitivity. However, the titre against the foreign fish receptor was reduced only to a small extent.

The differential effect on the reaction against self and foreign AChR may represent either a change in antibody affinity which may result in a decrease in the cross-reactivity between the two receptors, or a specific effect on a selective antibody population. Our experiments demonstrate that azathioprine is affecting not only the antibody titre but also the antibody class since in the suppressed animals there is a higher proportion of mercaptoethanol-sensitive antibody (IgM). Such a differential effect of thiopurines on 19S and 7S antibody production has been observed also for other immune responses (Borel *et al.*, 1965). Concomitantly with the decrease in total antibody titre there was also a significant decrease in the level of cytophilic antibodies with AChR specificity as measured by their ability to bind to normal rabbit alveolar macrophages (Martinez *et al.*, 1977).

TABLE 9. Anti-receptor antibody concentration in animals with EAMG and animals with azathioprine treatment

Treatment	Antibody titres to *Torpedo* AChR	Antibody titres to rabbit muscle AChR
AChR alone	3×10^{-8} M	1.1×10^{-9} M
AChR with azathioprine	1×10^{-8} M	$< 1.8 \times 10^{-12}$ M

Titres are expressed as moles toxin-binding sites precipitated per litre of serum. The numbers are average of four animals in each group. The tested sera were of bleedings 25-30 days after immunization with 80 μg of pure AChR.

The effect of azathioprine on suppression of EAMG and on the decrease in cellular and humoral immunological reactivity seems to depend on the therapeutic dose. The doses of drug applied in this study (4 mg/kg) appear to be quite optimal since they prevented the onset of the disease beneficially (at least in 8 out of 10 rabbits, Table 6) without causing significant cytotoxic side effects. A higher dose of drug (9 mg/kg) was more effective in preventing onset of the disease, but cytotoxic effects were observed. At this dose, the antibody titre against *Torpedo* AChR was decreased by at least one order of magnitude.

Thiopurines are thought to be particularly active on T-cell delayed hypersensitivity immune responses and much less on humoral antibody responses (Bach, 1975). Since EAMG might be a T-cell mediated disease (Tarrab-Hazdai *et al.*, 1975b; Lennon *et al.*, 1976) one may consider T-cell inactivation as a valid working hypothesis for the immunosuppressive effect of azathioprine on the disease. However, although both cellular and humoral immune responses are present in EAMG, the role and importance of each of them in the pathogenesis of the disease is still a subject of debate. Therefore it cannot yet be concluded whether the immunosuppressive activity of azathioprine on EAMG is due to a decrease in cellular or humoral activity, or in both of them.

The immunosuppressive treatment of EAMG provides a valuable tool for elucidating many aspects of the mechanism of action of non-specific immunosuppressive drugs in the therapy of autoimmune diseases in general, and, in particular, for establishing the optimal conditions for azathioprine therapy of MG.

Specific immunosuppression of EAMG by derivatives of AChR

Although immunosuppressive drugs seem to be useful in the treatment of MG there are disadvantages in using them that stem mostly from their non-specific cytotoxic effects. It is obvious that the treatment of choice, if possible, should be a *specific* one, namely a drug which will affect specifically and selectively the immune reactivity that has led to the neuro-muscular disorder. Having a well defined antigen (AChR) which induces EAMG and which is the autoantigen in MG, one may try by molecular manipulations and immunological analysis to design specific derivatives of the AChR molecule, which will be able to suppress or prevent the disease, and perhaps be of use as specific therapeutic agents.

Immunological characterization of an irreversibly denatured AChR. In attempts to correlate specific structural features of AChR with its unique myasthenic activity, we wanted to cut the AChR molecule into smaller fragments in order to find out where in the molecule the myasthenic function resides and what molecular parameters are governing this function. Since AChR is a multisubunit protein molecule which seems to dissociate only under denaturing conditions, the first step in degrading the molecule was the preparation of an irreversibly denatured AChR derivative obtained by complete reduction and carboxymethylation in 6M guanidine hydro-chloride (Bartfeld and Fuchs, 1977).

The reduced carboxymethylated receptor (RCM-AChR) lost the pharmacological activity of the intact AChR and did not show any detect-able binding of ^{125}I-α-bungarotoxin. RCM-AChR lost also the myasthenic activity of AChR, as rabbits immunized repeatedly with RCM-AChR did not develop any clinical signs of EAMG. However, such rabbits developed high titres of antibodies which cross-react with AChR (Fig. 5). The difference in pathogenicity between RCM-AChR and AChR suggests that there is a difference between their antigenic specificities. Immuno-diffusion experiments (Fig. 6) have demonstrated identity between the reaction of anti-RCM-AChR serum with RCM-AChR and AChR indicating that all the antibodies that are precipitable by the homologous RCM-AChR can be precipitated also by AChR. However, anti-AChR serum shows only a partial cross-reactivity with RCM-AChR suggesting the presence in this antiserum of antibodies against some antigenic deter-minants which do not exist on the denatured receptor.

Similar differences in the antigenic specificities between AChR and RCM-AChR were observed also by inhibition experiments of the binding of the radioactively labelled antigens to the different antisera (Fig. 7). Whereas RCM-AChR and AChR inhibit to the same extent the binding of ^{125}I-AChR to sera of rabbits immunized with RCM-AChR (Fig. 7, top, right), RCM-AChR is a much weaker inhibitor than unmodified AChR

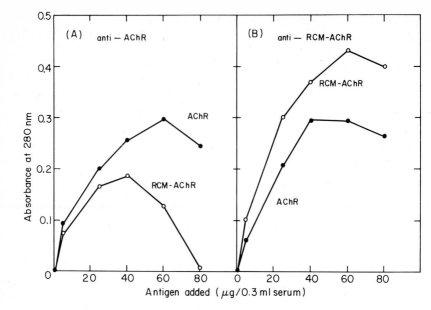

Fig. 5. Precipitin reaction of anti-AChR serum (A) and anti-RCM-AChR serum (B) with AChR (●) and RCM-AChR (o).

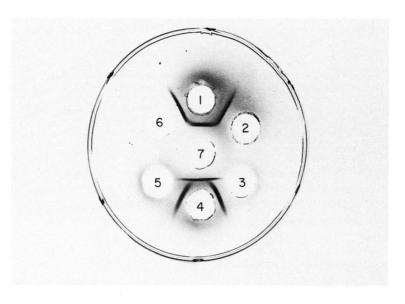

Fig. 6. Immunodiffusion of anti-RCM-AChR serum (well 1) and anti-AChR serum (well 4) with RCM-AChR (wells 2, 3, 5) and AChR (wells 6, 7).

of the binding of ^{125}I-AChR to antisera of rabbits injected with AChR (Fig. 7, top, left). There is no significant difference in the extent of inhibition by RCM-AChR and AChR of the binding of ^{125}I-RCM-AChR to anti-RCM-AChR or anti-AChR sera (Fig. 7, bottom). It thus seems that the major difference between AChR and RCM-AChR leading to their different pathogenicity resides in their different antigenic specificity. The analysis of both systems suggests that some antigenic determinants in the AChR molecule were abolished by the denaturation procedure. However, no additional determinants that were not expressed in the intact molecule became immunopotent after reduction and carboxymethylation.

The difference in antigenic specificity between the two antigens is reflected also by their effects on the binding of bungarotoxin to AChR. Comparison of the effect of antibodies against AChR with that of antibodies against RCM-AChR on the binding of ^{125}I-α-bungarotoxin to AChR

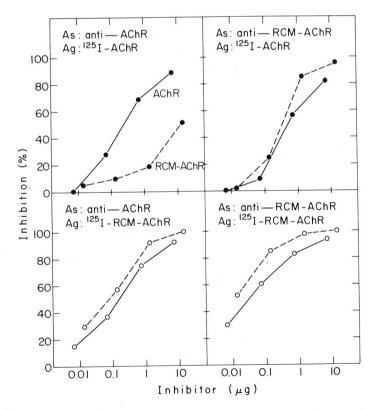

Fig. 7. Inhibition of the binding of ^{125}I-AChR (●) and ^{125}I-RCM-AChR (○) to anti-AChR serum (left) and anti-RCM-AChR serum (right) by AChR (———) and RCM-AChR (----). The assay was carried out as described by Bartfeld and Fuchs (1977).

in vitro shows that whereas anti-AChR antibodies block the binding of ^{125}I-α-bungarotoxin very effectively, anti-RCM-AChR antibodies block this binding only to a very limited extent (Table 10, Fig. 8).

TABLE 10. The effect of specific antibodies on ^{125}I-α-bungarotoxin binding to AChR.

Serum	Serum added to receptor assay	Specific activity α-Bgtx	Inhibition of specific activity by serum (%)
anti-AChR	Before addition of ^{125}I-α-Bgtx	2400	73
	After addition of ^{125}I-α-Bgtx	9300	
anti-RCM-AChR	Before addition of ^{125}I-α-Bgtx	8000	14
	After addition of ^{125}I-α-Bgtx	9300	
Normal rabbit serum	Before addition of ^{125}I-α-Bgtx	9300	0
	After addition of ^{125}I-α-Bgtx	9300	

0.1 ml of a 1/10 dilution of the tested serum was preincubated with AChR for 30 min at 37° before the addition of ^{125}I-α-bungarotoxin, and the receptor assay was continued by measuring the amount of ^{125}I-toxin which coprecipitated with the receptor in 35% saturated ammonium sulphate (Olsen *et al.*, 1972; Aharonov *et al.*, 1977). In the control for this experiment the tested serum was added to the receptor assay after the incubation with ^{125}I-toxin and formation of the AChR-toxin complex.

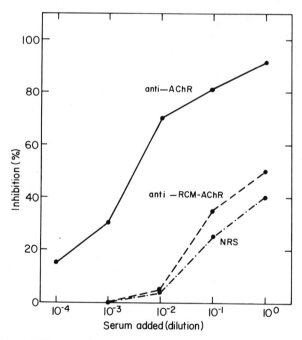

Fig. 8. Inhibition of ^{125}I-α-Bgtx binding to AChR by anti-AChR serum (——), anti-RCM-AChR serum (- - - -) and normal rabbit serum (-·-·-). AChR was incubated with increasing amounts of serum for 30 min at 37° before the addition of ^{125}I-αBgtx and the degree of toxin binding relative to the binding in the absence serum was determined.

The altered antigenic specificity of antibodies to RCM-AChR along with their altered effect in blocking toxin binding to AChR led us to propose that the denaturation of AChR destroyed some antigenic determinant(s) which is (are) important for the induction of EAMG, and which may be located close to the toxin-binding site.

Immunosuppression of EAMG by RCM-AChR. The immunological pharmacological and pathological properties of RCM-AChR make it an appropriate potential candidate for use in immunosuppression of EAMG. Indeed, although RCM-AChR does not induce EAMG, it seems to be effective in being able to prevent the onset of the disease or in curing it in some cases. The immunization schedule and the clinical conditions of several representative rabbits are described schematically in Fig. 9. Rabbits were immunized two or three times with RCM-AChR (100 μg, in complete Freund's adjuvant) and were then injected similarly with the intact AChR. In some cases preimmunization with RCM-AChR had no effect on the onset of the disease which followed the same course as in rabbits which were immunized only with AChR. In about 50% of the rabbits preimmunized with RCM-AChR (a total of 18 rabbits were tested) there was either a delay in the onset of EAMG, i.e. more than two AChR injections had to be given before observing any signs of EAMG, or there was a complete prevention of EAMG for a prolonged period, i.e., rabbits which were injected repeatedly (as many as six times) with AChR following preimmunization with RCM-AChR, displayed no signs of EAMG for at least ten months. In some cases rabbits with EAMG were cured following an injection of RCM-AChR which was given after the disease had developed.

There seems to be a correlation between the therapeutic effect of RCM-AChR as reflected by the clinical conditions of the treated rabbits, and the antigenic specificity of the immune response in those rabbits. Comparison between antisera of protected (rabbit 2) and unprotected (rabbit 1) rabbits at different bleedings show that there are differences both in the titres (Table 11) and antigenic specificity (Fig. 10) between sera of the respective rabbits. In rabbit No. 1 there is a decrease in the binding capacity of ^{125}I-RCM-AChR to serum withdrawn during EAMG, whereas in the protected rabbit (No. 2) the binding capacity of ^{125}I-RCM-AChR to serum withdrawn at the same time is much higher (Table 11). Moreover, the inhibition pattern of the binding of ^{125}I-AChR by RCM-AChR and AChR is different for these two rabbits. In rabbit No. 1, where preimmunization with RCM-AChR did not prevent the onset of EAMG, RCM-AChR is a weaker inhibitor than AChR of the binding of ^{125}I-AChR to the rabbit's serum (Fig. 10, left) as is the case in rabbits injected only with AChR (Fig. 7, top left). In rabbit No. 2 where prevention of EAMG was achieved by preimmunization with RCM-AChR, the difference

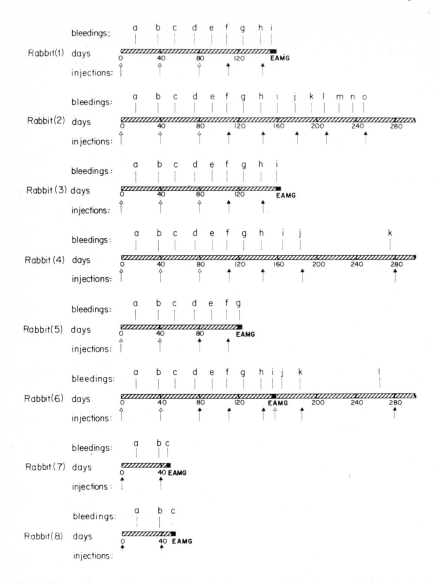

Fig. 9. Schematic description of the immunization schedule, bleedings and development of EAMG in eight representative rabbits. Open arrows represent injection of RCM-AChR (100 μg) and closed arrows represent injection of AChR (100 μg).

between the inhibitory capacity of RCM-AChR and AChR is small after two injections of AChR (Fig. 10, middle) and is completely abolished following three injections with AChR (Fig. 10, right), as is the case in rabbits immunized only with RCM-AChR (Fig. 7, top right).

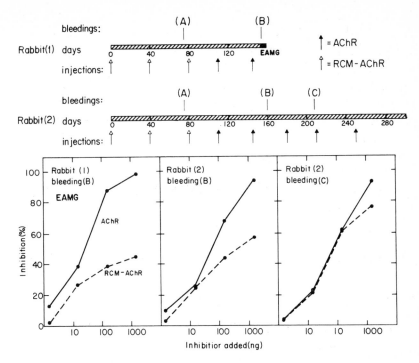

Fig. 10. Inhibition of the binding of ^{125}I-AChR to sera from rabbits No. 1 and No. 2. The immunization course, the bleedings and the development of EAMG are described schematically at the top of the figure.

TABLE 11. Binding of ^{125}I-AChR and ^{125}I-RCM-AChR to antisera of rabbits No. 1 and No. 2 of Fig. 9.

	Rabbit 1		Rabbit 2	
	Binding to ^{125}I-AChR	Binding to ^{125}I-RCM-AChR	Binding to ^{125}I-AChR	Binding to ^{125}I-RCM-AChR
Bleeding				
A	1/800	1/10,640	1/700	1/12,500
B	1/700	1/2,500	1/1,200	1/15,600
C			1/850	1/20,000

Rabbits No. 1 and No. 2 were immunized three times with RCM-AChR and then with AChR (see Fig. 10). At the time of bleeding A none of the rabbits had EAMG. At the time of bleeding B rabbit No. 1 had EAMG whereas in rabbit No. 2 EAMG was prevented (Fig. 10). The radioimmunoassay was performed as described by Bartfeld and Fuchs (1977) and the numbers in the Table represent the serum dilution at 50% binding.

It seems that EAMG can have its onset in rabbits preimmunized with RCM-AChR only if and when the differential specificity of the immune response to AChR as compared to RCM-AChR (as assayed here by the inhibition of the binding of ^{125}I-AChR by AChR and RCM-AChR), is above a certain level. Thus, for instance, in rabbit No. 6 the difference between the inhibition by AChR and RCM-AChR following two injections of AChR is not big enough (Fig. 11b) and EAMG is still prevented. This difference is markedly increased (Fig. 11c) following an additional AChR injection, concomitantly with the onset of EAMG. In line with this pattern, the curative effect of RCM-AChR which was administered to rabbit

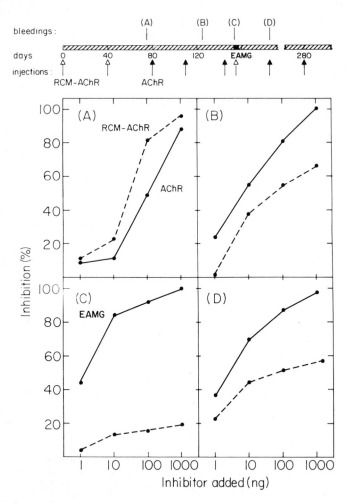

Fig. 11. Correlation between the therapeutic effect of RCM-AChR and the antigenic specificity of the antibodies in rabbit No. 6. Bleedings A and B, before the onset of EAMG; Bleeding C, during clinical signs of EAMG; Bleeding D, after the rabbit was cured following RCM-AChR injection. The immunization course, the bleedings and the development of EAMG are described schematically at the top of the figure.

No. 6 during EAMG is accompanied by a decrease in the differential specificity (Fig. 11d), so that in the cured animal a much smaller difference between the inhibitory capacity of AChR and RCM-AChR is observed.

In addition to the rabbits mentioned above, we have succeeded in curing, by RCM-AChR administration, several myasthenic rabbits in which EAMG was induced by one injection of AChR. Single administration of RCM-AChR to such myasthenic rabbits during the initial stages of clinical development of EAMG led in several cases to complete cure of EAMG, presumably by alteration of the antigenic specificity as described above.

The mechanism of the therapeutic effect of RCM-AChR is not worked out yet and awaits more experimentation. It is possible that the difference in the specificity of the antibodies which accompanies the prevention, appearance or curing of EAMG represents relative levels of two different antibody populations against AChR, one of which is specific to a myasthenic determinant in the AChR molecule and is involved in the disease, whereas the other is directed to other antigenic determinants which are not involved in the disease. AChR can elicit antibodies to both types of determinants and it is the immune response against the myasthenic determinants which is responsible for induction of EAMG. RCM-AChR elicits an immune response to determinants other than the myasthenic determinants and is, therefore, not myasthenic by itself. However, products of this immune response can bind to the native receptor, and probably also to the self receptor and this may be the basis for the preventive and curing effect of RCM-AChR. The curing effect of RCM-AChR may thus be explained by high levels of antibodies to the non-myasthenic determinants which do not block the physiological function of the receptor and compete with antibodies against the myasthenic determinants on the binding to self receptor. Experiments to elucidate the validity of this explanation are now in progress.

Summary

Considerable evidence now exists that myasthenia gravis (MG) is an autoimmune disease in which acetylcholine receptor (AChR) is a major autoantigen. Cellular and humoral immunological sensitivity to AChR are observed in patients with MG. Experimental autoimmune myasthenia gravis (EAMG) induced by the injection of purified AChR has been demonstrated to be an appropriate model for the human disease.

The availability of EAMG allows the elucidation of several aspects of the pathogenesis and therapy of MG. The experimental disease in mice is being used to study genetic aspects of MG and the involvement of the thymus as a specific antigenic target and as a source for immunocompetent cells. A different susceptibility to EAMG is observed in mouse strains representing different haplotypes of the major histocompatibility complex (H-2). Mice of strains with H-2a, H-2b, H-2d and H-2k haplotypes are susceptible to EAMG whereas the disease is not found in any mice with H-2q and H-2s haplotypes.

Non-specific immunosuppressive drugs such as hydrocortisone and azathioprine prevent the onset of EAMG in rabbits injected with AChR from *Torpedo californica*. Although azathioprine has a prolonged suppressive effect, even after the drug has been discontinued immunological memory towards the original AChR challenge is maintained. The suppressive effect of the drug is followed by a decreased cellular and humoral immunological reactivity against the immunizing *Torpedo* AChR and essentially an abolishment of the reactivity against *self* AChR.

Specific immunosuppression of EAMG is being attempted by the use of a non-myasthenic derivative of the receptor. Irreversibly denatured AChR, obtained by complete reduction and carboxymethylation in 6M guanidine, does not induce myasthenia in rabbits, although it elicits antibodies which cross-react with the unmodified AChR. Moreover, this reduced-carboxymethylated AChR (RCM-AChR) has both preventive and therapeutic effects on EAMG. The cross reactivity between AChR and RCM-AChR and the nonpathogenicity of RCM-AChR appears to be crucial in governing the immunosuppressive and therapeutic effects of RCM-AChR on EAMG.

Acknowledgements

Drs. O. Abramsky and A. Aharonov collaborated in the early part of this research. Part of the work described here was supported by grants from the Los Angeles Chapter of the Myasthenia Gravis Foundation and from the United States-Israel Binational Science Foundation (BSF), Jerusalem, Israel. We thank Dr. Israel Silman for helpful discussions and criticism.

References

Abramsky, O., Aharonov, A., Webb, C. and Fuchs, S. (1975a). *Clin. Exp. Imm.*, **19**, 11-16.
Abramsky, O., Aharonov, A., Teitelbaum, D. and Fuchs, S. (1975b). *Arch. Neurol.*, **32**, 684-687.
Abramsky, O., Tarrab-Hazdai, R., Aharonov, A. and Fuchs, S. (1976). *J. Immunol.*, **117**, 225-228.
Aharonov, A., Abramsky, O., Tarrab-Hazdai, R. and Fuchs, S. (1975a). *Lancet*, **ii**, 340-342.
Aharonov, A., Tarrab-Hazdai, R., Abramsky, O. and Fuchs, S. (1975b). *Proc. Nat. Acad. Sci. USA*, **72**, 1456-1459.
Aharonov, A., Tarrab-Hazdai, R., Silman, I. and Fuchs, S. (1977). *Immunochemistry*, **14**, 129-137.

Appel, S.H., Almon, R.R. and Levy, N. (1975). *New. Engl. J. Med.*, **293**, 760-761.

Bach, J.F. (1975). *Frontiers of Biology*, **41**, 93-151.

Bartfeld, D. and Fuchs, S. (1977). *FEBS Lett.*, **77**, 214-218.

Bender, A.N., Ringel, S.P., Engel, W.K., Daniels, M.P. and Vogel, Z. (1975). *Lancet*, **i**, 607-609.

Borel, Y., Fauconnet, M. and Miescher, P.A. (1965). *J. Exp. Med.*, **122**, 263-275.

Engel, A.G., Tsujihata, M., Lindstrom, J.M. and Lennon, V.A. (1976). *Ann. N.Y. Acad. Sci.*, **274**, 60-79.

Fambrough, D.M., Drachman, D.B. and Satyamurti, S. (1973). *Science*, **182**, 293-295.

Fritze, D., Herrmann, C.Jr., Naeim, F., Smith, G.S., Zeller, E. and Walford, R.L. (1976). *Ann. N.Y. Acad. Sci.*, **274**, 440-450.

Fuchs, S., Nevo, D., Tarrab-Hazdai, R. and Yaar, I. (1976). *Nature*, **263**, 329-330.

Goldstein, G. (1968). *Lancet*, **ii**, 119-122.

Granato, D.A., Fulpius, B.W. and Moody, J.F. (1976). *Proc. Nat. Acad. Sci.*, **73**, 2872-2876.

Green, D.P.L., Miledi, R. and Vincent, A. (1975). *Proc. R. Soc. Lond. B.*, **189**, 57-68.

Heilbronn, E., Mattson, C., Stalberg, E. and Hilton-Brown, P. (1975). *J. Neurol. Sci.*, **24**, 59-64.

Jenkins, R.B. (1972). *Lancet*, **i**, 765-767.

Kalden, J.R., Williamson, W.G., Johnson, R.J. and Irvine, W.J. (1969). *Clin. Exp. Imm.*, **5**, 319-340.

Kao, I. and Drachman, D.B. (1977). *Science*, **195**, 74-75.

Lennon, V.A., Lindstrom, J.M. and Seybold, M.E. (1975). *J. Exp. Med.*, **141**, 1365-1375.

Lennon, V.A., Lindstrom, J.M. and Seybold, M.E. (1976). *Ann. N.Y. Acad. Sci.*, **274**, 283-299.

Lindstrom, J.M., Seybold, M.E., Lennon, V.A., Whittingham, S. and Duane, D.D. (1976a). *Neurology*, **26**, 1054-1059.

Lindstrom, J.M., Einarson, B.L., Lennon, V.A. and Seybold, M.E. (1976b). *J. Exp. Med.*, **144**, 726-738.

Lindstrom, J.M., Engel, A.G., Seybold, M.E., Lennon, V.A. and Lambert, E.H. (1976c). *J. Exp. Med.*, **144**, 739-753.

Martinez, R.D., Tarrab-Hazdai, R., Aharonov, A. and Fuchs, S. (1977). *J. Immunol.*, **118**, 17-20.

Matell, G., Bergstrom, K., Franksson, C., Hammarström, L., Lefvert, A.K., Möller, E., von Reis, G. and Smith, E. (1976). *Ann. N.Y. Acad. Sci.*, **274**, 659-676.

Nastuk, W.L., Plescia, O.J. and Osserman, K.E. (1960). *Proc. Soc. Exp. Biol. Med.*, **105**, 177-184.

Olsen, R.W., Meunier, J.C. and Changeux, J.P. (1972). *FEBS Lett.*, **28**, 96-100.

Oosterhuis, H.J.G.H., Feltkamp, T.E.W., can Rossum, A.L., van den Berg-Loonen, P.M. and Nijenhuis, L.E. (1976). *Ann. N.Y. Acad. Sci.*, **274**, 468-474.

Otterness, I.G. and Chang, Y. (1976). *Clin. Exp. Immunol.*, **26**, 346-354.

Patrick, J. and Lindstrom, J. (1973). *Science*, **180**, 871-872.

Pinching, A.J., Peters, D.K. and Newsom Davis, J. (1976). *Lancet*, **ii**, 1373-1376.

Pirskanen, R. (1976). *Ann. N.Y. Acad. Sci.*, **274**, 451-460.

Richman, D.P., Patrick, J. and Arnason, B.G.W. (1976). *New Engl. J. Med.*, **294**, 694-698.

Seybold, M.E. and Drachman, D.B. (1974). *New Engl. J. Med.*, **290**, 81-84.

Simpson, J.A. (1960). *Scot. Med. J.*, **5**, 419-436.
Stavy, L., Cohen, I.R. and Feldman, M. (1974). *Transplantation*, **17**, 173-179.
Sugiyama, H., Benda, P., Meunier, J.C. and Changeux, J.P. (1973). *FEBS Lett.*, **35**, 124-128.
Tarrab-Hazdai, R., Aharonov, A., Abramsky, O., Silman, I. and Fuchs, S. (1975a). *Israel J. Med. Sci.*, **11**, 1390.
Tarrab-Hazdai, R., Aharonov, A., Abramsky, O., Yaar, I. and Fuchs, S. (1975b). *J. Exp. Med.*, **142**, 785-789.
Tarrab-Hazdai, R., Aharonov, A., Silman, I., Fuchs, S. and Abramsky, O. (1975c). *Nature*, **256**, 128-130.
Toyka, K.V., Drachman, D.B., Griffin, D.E., Pestronk, A., Winkelstein, J.A., Fischbeck, K.H. and Kao, I. (1977). *New Engl. J. Med.*, **296**, 125-131.
Warmolts, J.R. and Engel, W.K. (1972). *New Engl. J. Med.*, **286**, 17-20.
Wekerle, H., Paterson, B., Ketelsen, U.P. and Feldman, M. (1975). *Nature*, **265**, 493-494.
Wekerle, J. and Ketelsen, U.P. (1977). *Lancet*, **I**, 678-680.

17 Plasma exchange in myasthenia gravis

A.J. PINCHING. J. NEWSOM DAVIS[1] AND ANGELA VINCENT[2]

Royal Postgraduate Medical School, Hammersmith Hospital

The presence of a postsynaptic defect in myasthenia gravis (MG) is now well established. Morphological changes principally involve the postsynaptic apparatus (Santa *et al.*, 1972), the number of functioning acetylcholine receptors (AChR) is reduced (Fambrough *et al.*, 1973; Vincent *et al.*, this volume), and acetylcholine (ACh) sensitivity is reduced (Albuquerque *et al.*, 1976). The possibility that an immune disorder might underlie the defect in neuromuscular transmission, suggested by Simpson in 1960, is increasingly supported by experimental observation but there is uncertainty about the relative importance of humoral and cell-mediated immune mechanisms.

The occurrence of antibodies to skeletal muscle in virtually all patients with thymoma (Feltkamp *et al.*, 1974) and the coexistence of autoimmune thyroid diseases in some myasthenic patients might suggest a humoral basis for the autoimmunity of MG. On the other hand, the role of the thymus in cell mediated immunity and the fact that the thymus is abnormal in a large proportion of MG patients indicates that cell-mediated mechanisms may also be involved. While the two mechanisms are not mutually exclusive, recent evidence has tended to favour humoral factors.

Serum from MG patients has been found to inhibit the binding *in vitro* of α-bungarotoxin to AChR (Almon, *et al.*, 1974) for which the toxin has a specific affinity, and antibody directed at AChR has been detected in a high proportion of myasthenic patients (Lindstrom *et al.*, 1976; Chapter 5). Toyka *et al.* (1977) have reported that serum from patients with MG can passively transfer a myasthenic illness to mice although other groups have not been successful in similar attempts (Rees *et al.*, 1977).

Thoracic duct drainage is followed by clinical improvement in patients with myasthenia (Bergström *et al.*, 1973), and the active factor is likely

[1]) *National Hospital for Nervous Diseases, Queen Square, London*
[2]) *Department of Biophysics, University College, London*

to be humoral because reinfusion of the cell free lymph caused deterioration. The factor appears to be in the IgG fraction (Lefvert and Bergström, 1976).

We have used plasma exchange to investigate the functional importance of humoral factors in MG. With this technique one can bring about short term changes in serum antibody, and it is known to be clinically valuable in the treatment of autoallergic renal disease, and in particular in the antibody-mediated disease, Goodpasture's syndrome (Lockwood et al., 1976. The clinical response to plasma exchange has been assessed by regular measurements of muscle strength, and this response has been related to the titre of anti-AChR antibody measured by an immunoprecipitation technique.

Up to ten daily exchanges of two litres were undertaken usually over a 10-14 day period. An albumin-rich plasma protein fraction (PPF) replaced the removed plasma. Plasma electrolytes were not materially altered by the procedure. The patients were asked to note any functional changes, such as distance walked, ease of eating, and household tasks. In addition, several indices of muscle function were measured daily at a standard time in relation to medication: vital capacity (maximum expired volume), muscle power graded on a modified MRC scale or tested against a strain gauge, and muscle fatiguability assessed by the time for which arm or leg could be held outstretched against gravity.

All three patients were moderately or severely disabled despite thymectomy, optimal anticholinesterase medication and steroid therapy. Immunosuppression was introduced in Case 1 about one week after the exchange period and in Case 3, one week before the first exchange. Case 2 was studied in more detail with three separate sets of exchange and was immunosuppressed after the second of these. The schedule of immunosuppression in all cases was cyclophosphamide 2-2.5 mg/kg and azathioprine 1 mg/kg for six weeks, followed by the azathioprine alone as maintenance. In Case 2 intolerance caused immunosuppressive drugs to be discontinued after one month.

Case histories of Cases 1 and 2 have already been published (Pinching, Peters and Newsom Davis, 1976); Case 3 was a 55 year old man who had had MG for three years, and who had the serum marker for thymoma (skeletal muscle antibody) but equivocal thymus histology. Control of his disease was strikingly dependent on steroids but he had had a silent perforation of a viscus as a consequence of this therapy. He also suffered from thyrotoxicosis, which was well controlled by carbimazole.

All three patients showed clear improvement following plasma exchange in every index of disease activity, both functional and objective. The pattern of improvement in Cases 1 and 2 was similar, starting 2-3 days after the completion of the set of exchanges, as shown for Case 2 in Fig. 1.

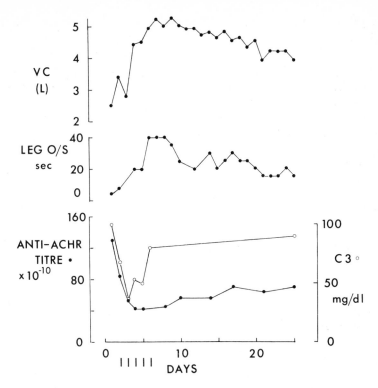

Fig. 1. Effects of plasma exchange (day 2-6, solid bars) on vital capacity (VC), leg outstretched time, anti-AChR antibody titre, and complement C3 in Case 2. Note inverse relationship between clinical indices and antibody titre.

In Case 3, however, although improvement was seen in some muscle groups within a few days, the most striking changes did not occur until about a week after the first exchange, and the peak was delayed for several weeks after the end of the exchange period, as shown by measurements of arm outstretched time in Fig. 2.

The progressive improvement in the objective measurements of muscle power was paralleled by a substantial improvement in the patient's functional abilities. Case 1 had been obliged to eat an almost exclusively liquid diet because chewing and swallowing were very weak but after exchange she was able to eat a normal three course meal without fatigue. Having been unable to fold away clothes, she became able to perform hand washing without difficulty and many other household tasks became possible for the first time for years. She no longer needed to support her head and jaw constantly in the typical myasthenic manner and facial expression was much increased. Case 2 became able to manage a full meal, having found two courses a struggle before, and indeed was able to talk through and after meals. His voice lost its characteristic myasthenic features, illustrated by tape-recordings of his voice before and after exchanges. Whistling to high frequencies became possible. His gait improved, losing the waddling quality caused by proximal weakness, he was able to drive a car and walk considerable distances. Facial expression increased markedly. Case 3 found less fatiguing of his voice, became able to drive a car, mow his lawn and walk over half a mile, activities which had been impossible since the onset of severe disease.

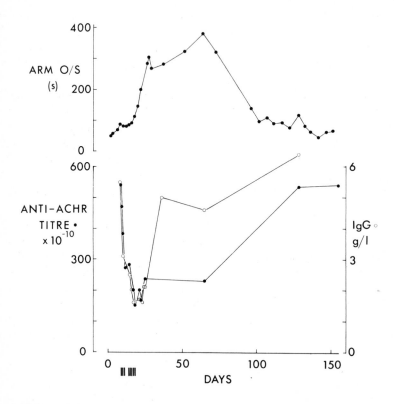

Fig. 2. Effects of plasma exchange on arm outstretched time, anti-AChR antibody and IgG in Case 3. Cyclophosphamide 2 mg/kg given from day 0-42. Note: IgG returns to pre-exchange values before antibody.

While all patients could still be shown to be myasthenic on testing after exchanges, they were nevertheless substantially improved and able to lead more normal lives. In the two cases of relatively short duration, the improvement was sufficient to allow withdrawal of anticholinesterase medication for prolonged periods; in all three cases considerable steroid reduction was possible for the first time without immediate relapse, a fact of major clinical importance because two of them had suffered serious side effects from the high doses required to maintain them at moderate strength.

We have correlated these clinical observations with serial measurements of anti-AChR antibody. Antibody was assayed by precipitation with anti-human IgG of antibody bound to detergent extracted AChR (obtained from amputated human limb muscle) labelled with ^{125}I-α-bungarotoxin (c.f. Lind-strom *et al.*, 1976). The profile of anti-AChR antibody shows a strong inverse association with the patient's clinical state, as illustrated for Case 2 in Fig. 1, in which vital capacity (maximum expired lung volume) was used as the index of muscle strength. This index was paralleled by the times for which the arm and leg could be outstretched against gravity. Plasma exchange brought about a sharp fall in the antibody titre, and this was followed by clinical improvement with a time lag of 48-72 hours. As the antibody titre began to rise again after the series of five exchanges, there was an associated deterioration in the clinical indices of muscle strength.

The profile of the antibody titre was more closely related to the clinical state than the third component of complement (C3) which, after an initial sharp fall, quickly returned close to control values. Serum IgG was reduced in parallel with antibody during the series of exchanges (Fig. 2), but in this subject it had clearly returned to the pre-exchange value before anti-AChR antibody.

If serum anti-AChR antibody was playing no part in the functional block of neuromuscular transmission, or if indeed the antibody was 'protective' (c.f. Aharonov *et al.*, 1975), one would not expect a reduction of serum antibody to be associated with clinical remission. In the event, a remission of symptoms was clearly associated with a reduction of antibody after a time lag of 2-3 days. Conversely, a rise in antibody was associated with clinical deterioration. These preliminary results thus suggest that anti-AChR antibody may be playing an important part in interfering with neuromuscular transmission. This is not to say that other factors will not also be contributing to the defect. Affinity of antibody, the extent of the post-synaptic morphological changes, and the rate of AChR synthesis are all factors that might influence the disorder of transmission.

The apparently close inverse relationship between anti-AChR antibody titre and the patient's clinical state, consistent with a causative role for the antibody, also provides the clinician with an insight into the level of disease activity and an alternative means of monitoring the effects of treatment. It is too early to say whether plasma exchange will have a regular place in the treatment of myasthenia gravis, but our preliminary experience suggests that when undertaken in conjunction with immuno-suppression, plasma exchange may prove to be a useful additional form of therapy in selected cases.

Acknowledgements. We are grateful to the Blood Products Laboratory of the Lister Institute for the supplies of P.P.F. Dr. Angela Vincent is supported by a grant from the Medical Research Council.

References

Aharanov, A., Tarrab-Hazdai, R., Abramsky, O. and Fuchs, S. (1975). *Proc. Nat. Acad. Sci. USA*, **72**, 1456-1459.

Albuquerque, E.X., Lebeda, F.J., Appel, S.H., Almon, R., Kauffman, F.C., Mayer, R.F., Natahashi, T. and Yeh, J.Z. (1976). *Annals of New York Academy of Science*, **274**, 475-492.

Almon, R.R., Andrew, C.G. and Appel, S.N. (1974). *Science*, **186**, 55-57.

Bergström, R., Franksson, C., Matell, G. and von Rees, G. (1973). *European Neurology*, **9**, 157-167.

Fambrough, D.M., Drachman, D.B. and Satyamurti, S. (1973). *Science*, **182**, 293-295.

Feltkamp, T.E.W., van der Berg-Loohen, P.M., Nijenhuis, L.E., Engelfriet, C.P., van Loghen, J.J. and Oosterhuis, H.J.G.H. (1974). *British Medical Journal*, **1**, 131-133.

Lefvert, A.K. and Bergström, K. (1976). *European Society of Clinical Investigation*, **6**, 334.

Lindstrom, J.M., Seybold, M.E., Lennon, V.A., Whittingham, S. and Duane, D.D. (1976). *Neurology (Minneapolis)*, **26**, 1054-1059.

Lockwood, C.M., Rees, A.J., Pearson, T.A., Evans, D.J., Peters, D.K. and Wilson, C.B. (1976). *Lancet*, **i**, 711-715.

Pinching, A.J., Peters, D.K. and Newsom Davis, J. (1976). *Lancet*, ii, 1373-1376.

Rees, D., Behan, P.O., Behan, W.H. and Simpson, J.A. (1977). VII Symposium of Current Research in Muscular Dystrophy, Birmingham, Muscular Dystrophy Group of Great Britain.

Santa, T., Engel, A.G. and Lambert, E.H. (1972). *Neurology (Minneapolis)*, **33**, 71-82.

Simpson, J.A. (1970). *Scottish Medical Journal*, **5**, 419-436.

Toyka, K.V., Drachman, D.B., Griffin, D.E., Pestronk, A., Winkelstein, J.A., Fischbeck, K.H. and Kao, I. (1977). *New England Journal of Medicine*, **296**, 125-131.

Muscular Dystrophy

18 Aspects of the biochemistry of the muscular dystrophies

BY R.J.T. PENNINGTON

Regional Neurological Centre,
Newcastle upon Tyne.

This review will be concerned mainly with some areas of the biochemistry of the muscular dystrophies which have attracted particular attention. Little will be said about the changes in muscle enzyme patterns, since this is dealt with by Dr. Ellis in Chapter 20. Polymyositis, another important muscle disorder, has not received as much attention from biochemists as the muscular dystrophies.

Muscle disorders resulting from a recognized biochemical defect

In spite of much research on muscular dystrophy, which has revealed many changes in muscle chemistry in this group of diseases, there is no known single biochemical abnormality which is sufficiently prominent and specific to be considered the primary genetic defect. There are, however, a number of other muscle disorders which involve a biochemical aberration which appears to represent the primary defect or to be closely related to it; in most cases the abnormality is concerned in the supply of energy to the fibres. Although these conditions are rare, I will discuss them briefly, because of their biochemical interest. The best known is the autosomal recessive disease caused by a deficiency of muscle phosphorylase, first reported by McArdle (1951). It is manifested by fatiguability and by the occurrence upon exercise of painful muscle cramps, a rise in certain serum enzymes and myoglobinuria. In later life a more consistent muscle weakness may be apparent. Biochemically there is increased muscle glycogen (the concentration of which does not exceed 1% in normal muscle) and a failure of blood lactate to increase following ischaemic exercise of the forearm. The latter is a standard test for the blockage of glycolysis from muscle glycogen. Two laboratories have reported immunological evidence that an enzymically inactive phosphorylase protein is present in the muscle in this disease. Recently, however, Feit and Brooke (1976) submitted muscle from three patients (in each of whom muscle phosphorylase could not be detected histochemically) to SDS-electrophoresis. In two, the phosphorylase subunit (M.W. 92000) was absent, but it was present in the third. Roelofs *et al.* (1972) have reported the interesting and puzzling observation that cultures of muscle from a patient with phosphorylase deficiency regained phosphorylase activity.

A patient with clinical symptoms similar to those of muscle phosphorylase deficiency was shown by Tarui *et al.* (1965) to lack another muscle enzyme, phosphofructokinase, and several similar cases have since been reported. Layzer and Rasmussen (1974) have presented evidence that this disease is due to a deficiency of the M-subunit of phosphofructokinase, one of the two types of subunit of this enzyme, which exists as a tetramer. The muscle enzyme is composed wholly of M-subunits and therefore is totally absent. In erythrocytes the enzyme is composed of mixed subunits and displays one-half the normal activity in the patients.

Pompe's disease, characterized by a generalized deficiency of α-1,4-glucosidase, is a rapidly fatal glycogen storage disease of infancy. A milder variant of this deficiency, seen in older children or adults and characterized predominantly by a myopathy, is now well recognized (e.g. Hudgson *et al.*, 1968). Angelini and Engel (1972) showed that whereas in the infantile form of the disease both acid (pH 4.0) and neutral (pH 6.5) α-glucosidase activities are low, only acid α-glucosidase was deficient in their adult cases. The mechanisms by which a deficiency of acid α-glucosidase, a lysosomal enzyme, leads to excess glycogen and to muscle damage is not quite clear. There is a normal rise of blood lactate after ischaemic exercise, indicating that the phosphorylase pathway of glycogenolysis is functioning adequately. A deficiency of amylo-1,6-glucosidase (debranching enzyme) can also affect muscle predominantly, producing a mild myopathy, as well as liver. A case is described in detail by Murase *et al.* (1973).

Recently two disorders of lipid utilization by muscle, associated with specific biochemical changes, have been recognized. Engel and Angelini (1973) and subsequently other groups have described a myopathy in which there is an excess of lipid in the muscles which is accompanied by a low level of muscle carnitine. Carnitine facilities the transport of fatty acids from the cytoplasm into the mitochondria, where they are oxidized. Both Karpati *et al.* (1975) and Angelini *et al.* (1976) have observed clinical improvement of this condition by feeding of carnitine, but in neither case was the muscle carnitine restored to normal levels. A full explanation of the low muscle carnitine cannot yet be given. Carnitine is probably synthesized in the liver, and a defect in the transport of carnitine into muscle or in its retention by the tissue appears to be involved in this condition. However, more than one form of this disease may exist, since the plasma carnitine level was normal in the case described by Angelini *et al.* (1976), but only about 12% of normal in that of Karpati *et al.* (1975);

this suggests that there is a more generalized carnitine deficiency in the latter case. It is of interest that Karpati *et al.*, reported an increased urinary excretion of dicarboxylic acids by their patient, indicating enhanced omega oxidation of fatty acids; this process is not dependent upon carnitine.

Another disease, first identified in two brothers by Bank *et al.* (1975), appears to be due to a deficiency in muscle of carnitine palmityl transferase, the enzyme involved in the transport of long-chain fatty acids into mitochondria via the carnitine cycle. The clinical consequences are very different from and less severe than those of carnitine deficiency, and are characterized by cramps, elevated serum creatine kinase and myoglobinuria, all following exercise and exacerbated by fasting. There is also an elevation of plasma triglycerides, which show a further rise on fasting. Other muscle lipid disorders of unknown etiology have been described (e.g. by Jerusulem *et al.*, 1975). Mention should also be made of the long-recognized polyneuropathy, Refsum's disease. This is an autosomal recessive condition in which there is a block in the oxidative metabolism of phytanic acid (3,7,11,15-tetramethylhexadecanoic acid) which consequently accumulates in the blood and tissues. The defect appears to be in the α-hydroxylation of this compound, which is presumably derived from the diet (Hutton and Steinberg, 1973).

The muscular dystrophies

This discussion will be concerned with Duchenne dystrophy, except where stated otherwise, since the most work has been done on this form of muscular dystrophy. It is a well-defined condition, and is the most serious type of muscular dystrophy.

The biochemical investigation of muscle fibre changes in the muscular dystrophies is complicated by the extensive, and relatively non-specific, morphological changes in the muscles in these diseases. Commonly, there are gross increases in the amounts of fat or connective tissue, invasion by macrophages, and changes in the amounts of nerve and blood vessels relative to the muscle fibres. The presence of muscle fibres in various stages of regeneration must also be taken into account when assessing the possible significance of observed biochemical changes in the whole tissue. Studies on individual fibres by the use of quantitative histochemical techniques, as developed, for example, by Lowry and his collaborators for other tissues, may be of use in overcoming such difficulties, but have not yet been seriously applied in this field. Such problems may also be minimized by studying muscle at early stages of the disease or from female carriers who show slight manifestations of muscle abnormalities.

Any consideration of the nature of the underlying biochemical defect in dystrophic muscle should take into account the nature of the development of the disease as seen under the microscope. It appears that histological abnormalities in muscle are slight or absent at the foetal stage, and thus the earlier stages of development of the muscle fibres seem to be normal. Also fibre regeneration can occur readily in dystrophic muscle, at least in the earlier stages of the disease (Walton and Adams, 1956; Mastaglia and Kakulas, 1969). It would seem therefore that biochemical studies on muscle development in muscular dystrophy are unlikely to help to elucidate the cause of the disease. Structural abnormalities are first seen in fibres which are mature although have not, in most cases at least, attained full adult size. Possibly the earliest observed structural change in the fibre seen under the light microscope is the so-called 'hyalinization' in which the internal structure in a section of the fibre disappears. Bradley *et al.* (1972) have documented the frequency of occurrence of various structural changes at the different stages of the disease, and Cullen and Fulthorpe (1976) have attempted to classify the stages in fibre breakdown as seen under the electron microscope.

Muscle protein metabolism. Normal muscle fibres must clearly maintain a balance between protein synthesis and breakdown, whilst in growing muscle the rate of synthesis exceeds that of breakdown. The manner in which these opposing processes are integrated is unknown. It would be natural to assume that the immediate cause of fibre wasting is either a decrease in protein synthetic activity or an accelerated catabolism of protein, or possibly both. However, Monckton and Nihei (1969) measured the incorporation of [^{14}C]phenylalanine by ribosomes isolated from dystrophic muscle and found that it was actually substantially higher than normal; this was so both in the presence or absence of an artificial messenger-RNA, polyuridylic acid. The rate of amino acid incorporation showed no obvious correlation with the histological changes, and they considered the high rate to be related to a fundamental defect in the muscle. Ionasescu *et al.* (1971) confirmed the higher rate of amino acid incorporation but showed that with ribosomes from dystrophic muscle relatively more of the labelled product was digestible by collagenase, indicating that synthesis of collagen (presumably by ribosomes derived from fibroblasts in the muscle) could account for at least part of the increase. Subsequently these workers also reported an elevated rate of protein synthesis by isolated ribosomes in facioscapulohumeral muscular dystrophy (Ionasescu *et al.*, 1972), in Becker muscular dystrophy (Ionasescu *et al.*, 1973a) and in female carriers of Duchenne muscular dystrophy (Ionasescu *et al.*, 1973b). In each case it was claimed that, in some instances at least, the elevation was not due only to increased collagen synthesis. Recently, Monckton and Marusyk (1976) have studied the incorporation of labelled leucine by small pieces of muscle incubated in a suitable medium. Autoradiography before and after glycerination of the muscle was used to assess the incorporation of isotope into cytoplasm and myo-fibrils respectively. Their results indicated an increased leucine incorporation into cytoplasm and a decrease in its incorporation into myofibrils in the dystrophic muscle. This type of experiment, however, must be interpreted with caution because of possible differences in the rate of transport of the amino acid into the fibres and the further possibility that the interior of the tissue fragments may not be adequately oxygenated. Taken together the preliminary evidence suggests that there is an abnormally high rate of protein synthesis in the cytoplasm of fibres of dystrophic muscle. If confirmed it will explain why anabolic steroids have not proved effective in treating muscular dystrophy. To what extent the high rate of protein synthesis is due to the presence of regenerating fibres is unknown. It is possible that a decline in protein synthesis sets in at some stage in each individual fibre and is largely responsible for the wasting of that fibre. If the proportion of such fibres is small, this could, of course, be masked by an abnormally high rate in the remaining fibres.

If the average rate of protein synthesis is abnormally high in dystrophic muscle, then clearly protein catabolism must be increased to an even greater extent. Unfortunately, little is known about the mechanism of protein catabolism in muscle, or indeed in any tissue. A number of peptide hydrolases have been identified in muscle but their relative importance in the breakdown of protein in normal and pathological states is unknown. It has yet to be established that each of these enzymes is present in the muscle fibres, rather than in other cell types within the tissue. In one case, at least, this does not seem to be so, since a major part of the alkaline proteinase activity in rat muscle homogenates appears to be derived from mast cells (Park *et al.*, 1973). There is an increased proteinase activity over a wide pH range in dystrophic muscle (Pennington and Robinson, 1968; Kar and Pearson, 1972). There is also an increase in cathepsin A (a carboxypeptidase) but not in arylamidase (aminopeptidase) (Kar and Pearson, 1976). The interpretation of such changes is further complicated by the observation (Maskrey *et al.*, 1977) that there is an increase in peptide hydrolase activities (acid proteinase and cathepsin B) in rat diaphragm muscle after denervation, in spite of the fact that denervation causes hypertrophy of the muscle. The existence in muscle of a calcium-activated proteinase (Busch *et al.*, 1972) which can attack myofibril proteins (Dayton *et al.*, 1976) is interesting, in view of the possibility that calcium might enter the fibres from the extracellular space as a result of abnormalities in the sarcolemma. (The concentration of calcium in plasma is about 10^4 times that in resting muscle fibres). Sugita and Toyokura (1976) showed that in Duchenne muscle there is a decrease in troponin-I and troponin-C but less change in troponin-T. In glycerinated muscle fibres the latter was more resistant to treatment with calcium-activated proteinase, and they suggested that this resistance was the reason for its relative preservation in Duchenne muscle.

The urinary excretion of 3-methylhistidine can be used as an index of the rate of catabolism of myosin and actin, most of which are present in the muscles. This amino acid is released by the breakdown of myosin and actin and does not appear to be reutilized (Haverberg *et al.*, 1975). The data of Bank *et al.* (1971) show that in boys with Duchenne dystrophy the mean daily excretion of 3-methylhistidine relative to the excretion of creatinine (taking the latter as a measure of total muscle mass) was approximately doubled, although the two groups overlapped.

More extensive studies on muscle protein synthesis and breakdown have been carried out on mice with hereditary muscular dystrophy. This disease (of which there are two varieties) is commonly used as a model for human muscular dystrophy, as are inherited myopathies in the hamster and chicken (Chapter 26). Such models are important because of the limited availability of human muscle, but it is generally accepted that they are not identical with any of the human dystrophies, although many of the secondary changes in the muscles appear to be similar. In spite of much work, however, the nature of the changes in protein metabolism is still not clear. Several early *in vivo* studies claimed to show an increased rate of muscle protein turnover in the dystrophic mouse. In most cases, however, possible changes in the rate of amino acid uptake into the fibres were not taken into account; there is evidence (Baker, 1964) that this may be increased. Kitchin and Watts (1973) claimed that there was no difference in the incorporation of labelled amino acid, relative to the size of the amino acid pool, into normal and dystrophic muscle proteins. Hayashi *et al.* (1975) concluded that the rate of protein synthesis in dystrophic mouse muscle was normal when related to the amount of muscle DNA. Using autoradiography to measure [³H]leucine incorporation, Monckton and Marusyk (1975) found a decrease in incorporation into myofibrils in dystrophic mouse muscle. Nwagwu (1975) has reported that polyribosomes from dystrophic muscle incorporate amino acids *in vitro* faster than normal, but Petryshyn and Nicholls (1976) have found evidence for a factor in the pH 5 supernatant fraction from dystrophic mouse muscle which inhibits protein synthesis. The inhibitor was a large molecule or was bound to a large molecule, since it was eluted near the void volume when the fraction was submitted to gel filtration on Sephadex G75 columns. It was resistant to heating at 90°C for 5 min, but was sensitive to digestion with pronase, thus indicating that it was a protein.

In the dystrophic mouse, as in human dystrophy, there is an increased activity of both acid proteinase (Weinstock *et al.*, 1958) and alkaline proteinase (Pennington, 1963) in muscle.

A recent study on the dystrophic hamster (Goldspink and Goldspink, 1977) demonstrated that in the diaphragm muscle, an increased rate of protein synthesis and protein breakdown occurred. In this species, however, the increase in synthesis exceeded the increase in breakdown; correspondingly the muscles were larger in the affected animals.

Plasma enzymes. A characteristic feature of the muscular dystrophies is an increase in the level of many enzymes in the blood plasma. From the pattern of the plasma enzyme changes there can be little doubt that they are caused largely or wholly by leakage of enzymes from the muscle fibres. This phenomenon is both an important diagnostic tool and a possibly useful clue in considering the cause of muscular dystrophy. Creatine kinase is the enzyme which is usually measured for diagnostic purposes in muscle disease; it generally shows the largest increase and, being relatively specific to muscle, it is a more specific indicator of muscle damage than most other enzymes.

The early stage of Duchenne or Becker dystrophy is characterized by extremely high levels (several hundred times normal) of this enzyme in the blood. In Duchenne dystrophy an elevation is already present at birth, the level reaches its peak at the age of one or two years, and then gradually declines, as the amount of surviving muscle tissue decreases (e.g. Pearce *et al.*, 1964; Thomson *et al.*, 1974).

It is of great practical importance that many (about two out of three) female carriers of X-linked muscular dystrophy also show a rise in serum creatine kinase. The level of serum creatine kinase in carriers varies over an extremely wide range. This is usually interpreted as a consequence of random inactivation of one of the two X-chromosomes at an early stage of development. The X-chromosome in each nucleus of the carrier's tissue, therefore, will be either normal or will have the abnormal gene. It is considered that the degree of pathological change in the muscle will depend upon the proportion of nuclei which have the abnormal X-chromosome in each fibre. It is puzzling that Roy and Dubowitz (1970) found no consistent relationship between the level of serum creatine kinase and the extent of histopathological changes in the muscle of carriers. There is a slow decline with age in the creatine kinase level in carriers.

In other types of muscular dystrophy the average rise in serum creatine kinase is much less than in Duchenne dystrophy. Active polymyositis may be associated with very high levels. Increases are frequently seen in motor neuron disease, where the primary affliction is in the motor nerve (Williams and Bruford, 1970). In this disease, also, serum enzyme elevations may be more prominent in the earlier stages (Welch and Goldberg, 1972). Increases are found also in the animal dystrophies. Not all muscle wasting conditions lead to an increase in serum enzymes, however. There is no rise in the protein-deficiency disease, kwashiorkor, in myopathy caused by an excess of corticosteroids, or in muscle atrophy resulting from nerve section in rats.

In considering the significance of the serum enzyme changes it may be useful to have some idea of the actual rate at which enzymes leak out of the muscles. This may be done tentatively using the estimate of Bär and Ohlendorf (1970) that the clearance rate of creatine kinase from plasma in humans is about 5% per hour. Taking the creatine kinase concentration in human muscle as about 500 I.U./g (Park and Pennington, 1966), it can be deduced that in a patient with very high serum creatine kinase (10,000 I.U./litre) not more than about 1/150 of the muscle creatine kinase would be lost each day.

There appear to be two general possibilities to account for the leakage. These are a gross disruption of the sarcolemma, which would be expected to allow a relatively indiscriminate efflux of soluble constituents from the underlying region of the muscle fibre, or a membrane change at the molecular level which might be more selective. Mokri and Engel (1975) and Schmalbruch (1975) have recently produced microscopic evidence for holes in the sarcolemma in dystrophic muscle which might support the first possibility, but in order to asses their contribution it is important to know whether these appear at an early stage in the disease, when leakage is high.

There is evidence that leakage of proteins from the diseased muscle is a selective process. Thus in a Duchenne patient with very high serum enzyme levels, the level of creatine kinase may be one-hundred times as high as aldolase, in spite of the fact that the blood clearance rates of the two enzymes are quite similar (Bär and Ohlendorf, 1970) and their activities in muscle are of the same order. There is little or no rise in serum AMP deaminase (Pennington, 1969) whilst phosphofructokinase was undetectable by immunochemical techniques in Duchenne serum (Rowland et al., 1968). The latter workers were also unable to detect myoglobin. It is of interest that the relative levels of different enzymes in serum can vary widely between patients or at different periods in the same patient (Heyck et al., 1966; Harano et al., 1973). The basis of the selectivity appears to bear some relation to the size of the molecule, since both AMP deaminase (320 000) and phosphofructokinase (400 000) are large molecules, and the molecular weight of aldolase (150 000) is greater than that of creatine kinase (81 000). (Very small proteins such as myoglobin may be cleared so rapidly from the blood as to escape detection).

It can therefore be tentatively assumed that there is a membrane change at the molecular level. One qualification must be made, however. A possible factor which may complicate the interpretation of the relative rates of enzyme release is the possibility of the binding of 'soluble' enzymes to intracellular structures (see, for example, Clarke and Masters, 1975). This might lead to a selective release even in the presence of gross damage to the sarcolemma.

To explain adequately the increase in permeability, it is necessary to learn more about the structure of the sarcolemma and the factors which can influence its permeability to protein. One possibility which may be considered, however, is that there is a defect in energy supply to the membrane since there is evidence that interference with energy supply to muscle can lead to increased efflux of enzymes. Hypoxia in dogs was shown to cause an increase in several plasma enzymes (Highman and Altland, 1960). Partial occlusion of the coronary artery in dogs caused transient elevation of plasma aminotransferase without visible damage to the myocardium (LaDue *et al.*, 1955). Mendell *et al.* (1972) found that ligature of the aorta in rats markedly increased many plasma enzymes, although there was little muscle necrosis. Zierler (1958) showed that lack of oxygen or glucose or the presence of the metabolic inhibitors, iodoacetate or cyanide, increased the efflux of aldolase from whole rat muscle incubated *in vitro;* however, this must be interpreted with caution, since the rate of efflux of aldolase *in vitro* appears to be several orders greater than that *in vivo.* The influence of energy supply on membrane permeability to proteins may eventually become clear in the light of modern concepts of the fluidity of membrane structure. The possibility that the enzyme efflux in muscular dystrophy can be explained along these lines is easier to accept than that there is an inherited defect in membrane structure, because of the non-specific nature of the latter phenomenon.

Studies on erythrocytes. The apparent involvement of the sarcolemma in muscular dystrophy has led to speculation that there might be an abnormality in the plasma membranes of other cells. The red blood cell, because of its accessibility, has been the focus of this attention during the past few years, and an impressive list of abnormalities in its membrane has now been reported. The first was by Brown *et al.* (1967) who stated that the ATPase activity of red cell ghosts from patients was stimulated by ouabain, which normally depresses the total ATPase by inhibiting the Na,K-activated component. This has been confirmed by other groups. Acetylcholinesterase has also been reported to display altered kinetics and to respond differently to inhibitors (Watts *et al.*, 1972). The labelling of membrane proteins upon incubation of red cell ghosts with [^{32}P]ATP was found to be higher than normal by Roses *et al.* (1975); the opposite change had previously been observed in myotonic dystrophy by these workers. There is evidence (Roses *et al.* 1976) that the increase in phosphorylation may be particularly marked in one of the components of spectrin. Changes in lipid composition of the red cell membrane have been found (Kunze *et al.*, 1973; Kalofoutis *et al.*, 1977) and an increase in phospholiphase A activity (Iyer *et al.*, 1976). Other reports are of an increase in the rate of potassium efflux (Howland,

1974) and influx (Sha'afi *et al.*, 1975) across the erythrocyte membrane, a high proportion of abnormally shaped cells (Matheson and Howland, 1974), a decrease in deformability (Percy and Miller, 1975) and an increased electrophoretic mobility of the cells (Bosmann *et al.*, 1976). Some of these alterations were found also in red cells from other types of muscular dystrophy and from carriers of Duchenne muscular dystrophy.

It is of interest that some, at least, of these changes could possibly be related to a disturbance in calcium metabolism in the red cell, and this merits further investigation. In view of the ready interchange of lipids between red cells and plasma, it is surprising that more attention has not been given to the possibility that the red cell abnormalities might be due to some change in the chemical composition of the plasma. In this connection, it may be significant that Kohlschütter *et al.* (1976) found no abnormalities in the phospholipids of cultured skin fibroblasts in Duchenne dystrophy, in contrast with the above-mentioned observation by Kunz *et al.* (1973) on erythrocytes. Peter *et al.* (1969), in a small number of cases, incubated normal red cells with serum from patients and found that this treatment induced the abnormal response to ouabain in ghosts prepared from the cells. We have recently been able to confirm this (Siddiqui and Pennington, 1977) and found that the same result could be achieved by incubating the normal ghosts with the Duchenne serum. In our experiments we have not been able to reproduce the large stimulation of ATPase by ouabain, but have found a significantly lower inhibition than normal with the patients' ghosts or after incubation of the normals with serum or plasma from patients. Clearly it is important to ascertain whether the other changes which have been reported in the erythrocytes can be induced in a similar manner. If so, this would weaken the possibility of any primary genetic abnormality in the red cell membrane. The nature of the influence of the plasma also remains to be determined. It could be an alteration in plasma lipids or even an unknown toxic factor affecting the membranes.

Steroid myopathy

I will mention finally an induced condition of muscle wasting, which presents an interesting biochemical problem. Glucocorticoids are widely used in clinical practice, and one of their major side-effects is to produce a myopathy. The net catabolic effect of glucocorticoids upon muscle is also well-known from animal experiments, white muscle being generally more affected than red muscle. Manchester *et al.* (1959) and subsequent workers have shown that cortisol and related steroids cause a decreased incorporation of amino acids into muscle protein, and studies *in vivo* by Goldberg (1969) have confirmed this decrease in protein synthesis. The studies of

Bullock *et al.* (1972 and earlier papers) on isolated ribosomes are in accord with these findings. On the other hand, we have recently been unable to demonstrate any increase in the rate of muscle protein breakdown by cortisone (Shoji and Pennington, 1977).

The mechanism by which glucocorticoids depress muscle protein synthesis is unknown. These hormones are known to induce synthesis of specific proteins in some tissues, e.g. liver. Munck (1971) has suggested that the protein catabolic effect of glucocorticoids on lymphoid tissues results from their stimulation of the synthesis of a protein which depresses glucose uptake. He recognized, however, that glucose uptake by muscle is relatively unresponsive to glucocorticoids. Moreover, Nordeen and Young (1976) have recently provided evidence against this theory. They found that the effects of cortisol could be demonstrated using adenosine as energy source, and various observations suggested that inhibition of oxidative ATP production was responsible for the cortisol-induced changes. Abraham and Sekeris (1971) demonstrated an inhibition of RNA polymerase activity in thymus nuclei by steroids; this appeared to operate without the necessity of the formation of a steroid-cytosol receptor complex as appears to be usual in the action of steroids. Evidently, much more research is required to elucidate the events underlying steroid myopathy.

References

Abraham, A.D. and Sekeris, C.E. (1971). *Biochem. biophys. Acta*, **247**, 562-569.
Angelini, C. and Engel, A.G. (1972). *Arch. Neurol.*, **26**, 344-349.
Angelini, C., Lucke, S. and Cantarutt, F. (1976). *Neurology*, **26**, 633-637.
Baker, R.D. (1964). *Tex. Rep. Biol. Med.*, **22**, (Suppl.1), 880-885.
Bank, W.J., Rowland, L.P. and Ipsen, J. (1971). *Arch. Neurol.*, **24**, 176-186.
Bank, W.J., DiMauro, S., Bonilla, E., Capuzzi, D. and Rowland, L.P. (1975). *New. Eng. J. Med.*, **292**, 443-449.
Bar, U. and Ohlendorf, S. (1970). *Klin. Wschr.*, **48**, 776-780.
Bosmann, H.B., Gersten, D.M., Griggs, R.C., Howland, J.L., Hudecki, M.S., Katyare, S. and McLaughlin, J. (1976). *Arch. Neurol.*, **33**, 135-138.
Bradley, W.G., Hudgson, P., Larson, P.F., Papapetropoulos, T.A. and Jenkinson, M. (1972). *J. Neurol. Neurosurg. Psychiat.*, **35**, 451-455.
Brown, H.D., Chattopadhyay, S.K. and Patel, A.B. (1967). *Science*, **157**, 1577-1578.
Bullock, G.R., Carter, E.E., Elliott, P., Peters, R.F., Simpson, P. and White, A.M. (1972). *Biochem. J.*, **129**, 881-892.
Busch, W.A., Stromer, M.H., Goll, D.E. and Suzuki, A. (1972). *J. Cell Biol.*, **52**, 367-381.
Clarke, F.M. and Masters, C.J. (1975). *Biochim. biophys. Acta*, **381**, 37-46.
Cullen, M.J. and Fulthorpe, J.J. (1976). *J. neurol. Sci.*, **24**, 179-200.
Dayton, W.R., Reville, W.J., Goll, D.E. and Stromer, M.H. (1976). *Biochemistry*, **15**, 2159-2167.
Engel, A.G. and Angelini, C. (1973). *Science*, **179**, 899-902.

Feit, H. and Brooke, M.H. (1976). *Neurology*, **26**, 963-967.
Goldberg, A.L. (1969). *J. biol. Chem.*, **244**, 3223-3229.
Goldspink, D.F. and Goldspink, G. (1977). *Biochem. J.*, **162**, 191-194.
Harano, Y., Adair, R., Vignos, P.J., Miller, M. and Kowal, J. (1973). *Metabolism*, **22**, 493-501.
Haverberg, L.N., Deckelbaum, L., Bilmazes, C., Munro, H.M. and Young, V.R. (1975). *Biochem. J.*, **152**, 503-510.
Hayashi, Y., Suzuki, H.O. and Totsuka, T. (1975). *J. Biochem.*, **77**, 761-768.
Heyck, H., Laudahn, G. and Carsten, P.M. (1966). *Klin. Wschr.*, **44**, 695-700.
Highman, B. and Altland, P.D. (1960). *Am. J. Physiol.*, **199**, 981-986.
Howland, J.L. (1974). *Nature*, **251**, 724-725.
Hudgson, P., Gardner-Medwin, D., Worsfold, M., Pennington, R.J.T. and Walton, J.N. (1968). *Brain*, **91**, 435-462.
Hutton, D. and Steinberg, D. (1973). *Neurology*, **23**, 1333-1334.
Ionasescu, V., Zellweger, H. and Conway, T.W. (1971). *Arch. Biochem. Biophys*, **144**, 51-58.
Ionasescu, V., Zellweger, H., Shirk, P. and Conway, T.W. (1972). *Neurology*, **22**, 1286-1292.
Ionasescu, V., Zellweger, H., McCormick, W.F. and Conway, T.W. (1973a). *Neurology*, **23**, 245-253.
Ionasescu, V., Zellweger, H., Shirk, P. and Conway, T.W. (1973b). *Neurology*, **23**, 497-502.
Iyer, S.L., Katyare, S.S. and Howland, J.L. (1976). *Neuroscience Letters*, **2**, 103-106.
Jerusalem, F., Spiers, H. and Baumgartner, G. (1975). *J. neurol. Sci.*, **24**, 273-282.
Kalofoutis, A., Jullien, G. and Spanos, V. (1977). *Clin. chim. Acta.*, **74**, 85-87.
Kar, N.C. and Pearson, C.M. (1972). *Enzyme*, **13**, 188-196.
Kar, N.C. and Pearson, C.M. (1976). *Proc. Soc. exp. Biol. Med.*, **151**, 583-586.
Karpati, G., Carpenter, S., Engel, A.G., Watters, G., Allen, J., Rothman, S., Klassen, G. and Mamer, O.A. (1975). *Neurology*, **25**, 16-24.
Kitchin, S.E. and Watts, D.C. (1973). *Biochem. J.*, **136**, 1017-1028.
Kohlschutter, A., Wiesmann, U.N., Herschkowitz, N.N. and Ferber, E. (1976). *Clin. chim. Acta*, **70**, 463-465.
Kunze, D., Reichmann, G., Egger, E., Leuschner, G. and Echardt, H. (1973). *Clin. chim. Acta*, **43**, 333-341.
LaDue, J.S., Nydick, I. and Wroblewski, F. (1955). *Circulation*, **12**, 736.
Layzer, R.B. and Rasmussen, J. (1974). *Arch. Neurol.*, **31**, 411-418.
Manchester, K.L., Randle, P.J. and Young, F.G. (1959). *J. Endocrinol.*, **18**, 395-408.
Maskrey, P., Pluskal, M.G., Harris, J.B. and Pennington, R.J.T. (1977). *J. Neurochem.*, **28**, 403-409.
Mastaglia, F.L. and Kakulas, B.A. (1969). *Brain*, **92**, 809-818.
Matheson, D.W. and Howland, J.L. (1974). *Science*, **184**, 165-166.
McArdle, B. (1951). *Clin. Sci.*, **10**, 13-35.
Mendell, J.R., Engel, W.K. and Derrer, E.C. (1972). *Nature*, **239**, 522-524.
Mokri, B. and Engel, A.G. (1975). *Neurology*, **25**, 1111-1120.
Monckton, G. and Marusyk, H. (1975). *Canad. J. Neurol. Sci.*, **2**, 1-4.
Monckton, G. and Marusyk, H. (1976). *Neurology*, **26**, 234-237.
Monckton, G. and Nihei, T. (1969). *Neurology*, **19**, 415-418.
Munck, A. (1971). *Persp. Biol. Med.*, **14**, 265-289.
Murase, T., Ikeda, H., Muro, T., Nakao, K. and Sugita, H. (1973). *J. neurol. Sci.*, **20**, 287-295.

Nordeen, S.K. and Young, D.A. (1976). *J. biol. Chem.*, **251**, 7295-7303.
Nwawgu, M. (1975). *Eur. J. Biochem.*, **56**, 123-127.
Park, D.C. and Pennington, R.J. (1966). *Clin. chim. Acta*, **13**, 694-700.
Park, D.C., Parsons, M.E. and Pennington, R.J. (1973). *Biochem. Soc. Trans.*, **1**, 730-733.
Pearce, J.M.S., Pennington, R.J. and Walton, J.N. (1964). *J. Neurol. Neurosurg. Psychiat.*, **27**, 96-99.
Pennington, R.J. (1963). *Biochem. J.*, **88**, 64-68.
Pennington, R.J. (1969). *In* 'Disorders of Voluntary Muscle' (J.N. Walton, ed) pp.385-410. J. and A. Churchill Ltd., London.
Pennington, R.J. and Robinson, J.E. (1968). *Enzymol. Biol. Clin.*, **9**, 175-182.
Percy, A.K. and Miller, M.E. (1975). *Nature*, **258**, 147-148.£
Peter, J.B., Worsfold, M. and Pearson, C.M. (1969). *J. Lab. clin. Med.*, **74**, 103-108.
Petryshyn, R. and Nicholls, D.M. (1976). *Biochem. biophys. Acta*, **435**, 391-404.
Roelofs, R.L., Engel, W.K. and Chauvin, P.B. (1972). *Science*, **177**, 795-797.
Roses, A.D., Herbstreith, M.H. and Appel, S.H. (1975). *Nature*, **254**, 350-351.
Roses, A.D., Herbstreith, M., Metcalf, B. and Appel, S.H. (1976). *J. neurol. Sci.*, **30**, 167-178.
Rowland, L.P., Layzer, R.B. and Kagan, K.J. (1968). *Arch. Neurol.*, **18**, 272-276.
Roy, S. and Dubowitz, V. (1970). *J. neurol. Sci.*, **11**, 65-79.
Schmalbruch, H. (1975). *Acta Neuropathologica (Berlin)*, **33**, 129-141.
Sha'afi, R.I., Rodan, S.B., Hintz, R.L., Fernandez, S.M. and Rodan, G.A. (1975). *Nature*, **254**, 525-526.
Shoji, S. and Pennington, R.J.T. (1977). *Molec. cell. Endocrinol.*, **6**, 159-169.
Siddiqui, P.Q.R. and Pennington, R.J.T. (1977). *In* Seventh Symposium on Current Research in Muscular Dystrophy. Abs. No.4. Muscular Dystrophy Group of Great Britain, 35, Macaulay Road, London, SW4 0QP.
Sugita, H. and Toyokura, Y. (1976). *Proc. Jap. Acad.*, **52**, 260-263.
Tarui, S., Okuno, G., Ikura, Y., Tanaka, T., Suda, M. and Nishikawa, M. (1965). *Biochem. biophys. Res. Commun.*, **19**, 517-523.
Thomson, W.H.S., Sweetin, J.C. and Elton, R.A. (1974). *Nature*, **249**, 151-152.
Walton, J.N. and Adams, R.D. (1956). *J. Path. Bact.*, **72**, 273-298.
Watts, D.C., Das, P.K. and Coles, H.M.T. (1972). *In* Sixth Symposium on Current Research in Muscular Dystrophy and Related Diseases. Abs. No. 21. Muscular Dystrophy Group of Great Britain, 35, Macaulay Road, London, SW4 0QP.
Weinstock, I.M., Epstein, S. and Milhorat, A.T. (1958). *Proc. Soc. exp. Biol. Med.*, **99**, 272-276.
Welch, K.M.A. and Goldberg, D.M. (1972). *Neurology*, **22**, 697-701.
Williams, E.R. and Bruford, A. (1970). *Clin. chim. Acta*, **27**, 53-56.
Zierler, K.L. (1958). *Ann. N.Y. Acad. Sci.*, **75**, (Art. 1), 227-234.

19 Carrier detection in Duchenne muscular dystrophy: evidence from the study of obligatory carriers and mothers of isolated cases.

J.R. SIBERT · P.S. HARPER · R.J. THOMPSON

Departments of Child Health, Medicine (Medical Genetics) and Medical Biochemistry, Welsh National School of Medicine, Cardiff

Introduction

Since the initial use (Schapira *et al.*, 1960) of the serum creatine kinase (CPK) level as a method of detecting carriers for Duchenne muscular dystrophy a number of studies have been performed (Wilson *et al.*, 1965; Gardner-Medwin, 1971) confirming its usefulness, but in each case showing an extensive overlap of carrier and normal ranges. Attempts have been made to increase the proportion of carriers detected by the integration of genetic and biochemical information (Emery, 1969; Dennis *et al.*, 1976), but the interpretation of results within the normal range remains difficult. The situation has been further complicated by the suggestion (Roses *et al.*, 1976) that the mothers of many isolated cases previously considered to represent new mutations are in fact carriers, despite normal CPK levels. This study presents data relevant to these questions.

Methods

All families in Wales known to contain one or more members affected with Duchenne muscular dystrophy have been investigated, as part of a more general genetic study of the disorder in Wales in which complete ascertainment has been attempted. Criteria for diagnosis included severe disability before the age of 12 years and extreme elevation of serum CPK in addition to the recognized clinical features of the disease, particular care being taken to differentiate families with the Becker form of X-linked dystrophy. 52 families have so far been studied. Healthy, non-pregnant female volunteers of comparable age range were also studied, all blood samples being taken under conditions of normal activity, with avoidance of heavy exercise during the preceding 24 hours. Obligatory carriers were considered in this study to be women with at least one son and one other male relative affected, or with two or more affected sons. CPK levels were

239

determined on a Unicam SP 1800 recording spectrophotometer by the Boehringer (Mannheim) UV-System 10 assay method. Blood samples were either separated within two hours and assayed directly or stored at +4°C overnight. This made no significant difference to the recorded activity. Care was taken to protect sera from light.

Results

The distribution of serum CPK levels in normal controls (59), obligatory carriers (28) and mothers of isolated cases (26) is shown in Fig. 1, results being grouped in 10 mU/ml intervals. The results represent the mean of usually three, and always at least two separate samples. From these distributions a number of conclusions can be derived.

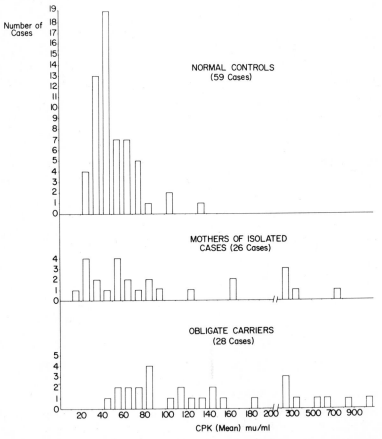

Fig. 1. Mean serum CPK levels in obligatory carriers for Duchenne muscular dystrophy, mothers of isolated cases, and healthy female cotrols. Results are grouped in 10 mU/ml intervals; each result represents the mean of at least two, usually three separate samples.

Approximately 39% of obligatory carriers fall within the 95th percentile of the control series, a value comparable to that found by previous studies and indicating the limitation of the test if values within this range are simply considered as 'normal'. The distributions are not Gaussian, but if logarithmic CPK values are used they approximate to a distribution of this form with the means and standard deviations shown in Table 1.

TABLE 1
Logarithmic CPK levels.

	Geometric Mean CPK (mU/ml)	Mean log CPK	SD log CPK
Controls	48	1.68	0.15
Obligatory carriers	145	2.16	0.37
Mothers of isolated cases	75	1.88	0.42

Odds against an individual being a carrier can be derived for specific values of serum CPK, and are shown in Table 2. These can be combined with prior genetic odds and other information using Bayes theorem, enabling more precise odds to be given for values of CPK within the normal range.

TABLE 2
Odds against being a carrier at various levels of serum CPK. (Determined from mean log. values of control and obligatory carriers CPK levels)

CPK (mU/ml)	Relative odds
30−39.9	6.63
40−	6.12
50−	4.27
60−	2.59
70−	1.46
80−	0.79
90−	0.42
100−	0.22
110−	0.12
120−	0.063
130−	0.034
140−	0.018
150−	0.010

The distribution of CPK values in the mothers of isolated cases is clearly different from both the normal and carrier distributions. Analysis of serum CPK levels from families containing more than one obligatory carrier suggests a correlation of carrier CPK levels within families. The ratio of between-families variance to within-families variance is 8.05 ($p < 0.002$).

Conclusions

Although the use of serum CPK estimations is far from being an ideal method, no more satisfactory alternative has yet been proved to be of value in the detection of carriers for Duchenne muscular dystrophy. The extensive overlap between control and carrier ranges may represent variable X-chromosome inactivation in the hetrozygous females, as well as lack of relationship of the test to the primary biochemical defect in this disease. The derivation of odds for CPK levels within the normal range is shown by our data, as by previous studies of Emery (1969) and Dennis et al. (1976) to contribute considerably to the precision of genetic counselling. Thus a woman with a prior genetic risk of ¼ of being a carrier, and with a mean CPK level of 35 mU/ml, would still have a combined posterior risk of 16.6% of being a carrier if values within the normal range were not distinguished, but a risk of only 4.8% using the data in Table 2.

The distribution of serum CPK levels in isolated cases is comparable with the classical genetic hypothesis of one third of such cases resulting from new mutations in a genetically lethal X-linked recessive disorder (Haldane 1935). The results argue strongly against the hypothesis (Roses et al., 1976) based on the study of phosphorylation of red-cell membrane proteins, that the mothers of almost all such cases are carriers, possibly as a consequence of unequal mutation rate in the sexes. The implications for genetic counselling for families of isolated cases are considerable.

Finally the likelihood raised by our results, that correlation within families exists for levels of CPK in carriers, again has important implications in carrier detection. Thus a relatively low CPK level in a potential carrier where obligatory carriers are also known to have a low CPK level may need to be interpreted with caution. More extensive data on families with multiple obligatory carriers will be required to assess accurately the degree of such a correlation and to allow it to be utilized along with other information.

Acknowledgements

We thank the paediatricians neurologists and other clinicians in Wales who have allowed us to study their patients, the families themselves for their cooperation and Dr Robert Newcombe for statistical advice. We acknowledge gratefully support given to one of us (PSH) by the Muscular Dystrophy Group of Great Britain.

References

Dennis, N.R., Evans, K., Clayton, B. and Carter, C.O. (1976). *Brit. Med. J.*, **2**, 577-579.
Emery, A.E.H. (1969). *J. Neurol. Sci.*, **8**, 579-587.

Gardner-Medwin, D., Pennington, R.J. and Walton, J.N. (1970). *J. Neurol. Sci.*, **13**, 459-474.

Haldane, J.B.S. (1935). *J. of Genetics*, **31**, 317-326.

Roses, A.D., Roses, M.J., Miller, S.E., Hull, K.L. and Appel, S.H. (1976). *New England J. Med.*, **294**, 193-198.

Schapira, F., Dreyfus, J.C., Schapira, G. and Demos, J. (1960). *Rev. Franc. Etud. Clin. Biol.*, **5**, 990-994.

Wilson, K.M., Evans, K.A. and Carter, C.O. (1965). *Brit. Med. J.*, **1**, 750-753.

20 Changes in muscle enzymes in Duchenne dystrophy and their possible relations to functional disturbance

DAVID A. ELLIS

Midland Centre for Neurosurgery and Neurology, Smethwick, U.K.

**Practical and theoretical obstacles to investigation –
Scarcity and variability of material**

Collecting measurements of any sort on dystrophic muscle* takes a time measured in years rather than months; the disease is rare, patients present themselves randomly and not all can be subjected to muscle biopsy. Humans vary; normal muscle for control purposes may be acquired from individuals exercising their muscle in different ways or not at all, and also exercising their free will in dietary matters. 'Normal' variation may mask real changes which may occur in dystrophic muscle. Control tissue is also required from cases of other neuromuscular disease, so that specific changes in dystrophic muscle may be distinguished from more general consequences of muscle disease. Both dystrophic and control muscle may be subject to genetic variation or heterogeneity arising from two causes. In hereditary disease, the same symptoms can arise from mutation affecting each of several different enzymes acting as one of an integrated functional group because in each case the functional group suffers. This has been shown for deficiencies in the ornithine cycle (Harris, 1970; Brock 1972). The second cause is multiple allelism (Harris, 1970) in which *separate* lesions of the *same* structural gene produce a family of diseases which may differ markedly in severity; e.g., the haemoglobinopathies, and Lesch-Nyhan disease (Brock, 1972). Ultimately we may recognize as many forms of Duchenne disease as there are haemoglobinopathies, perhaps with as wide a range of severity; even now classification of clinical symptoms tends to further subdivision of pseudohypertrophic dystrophy (Walton and Gardner-Medwin, 1974).

*For the sake of brevity 'dystrophic muscle' is used instead of 'muscle from patients affected with Duchenne-type muscular dystrophy', unless the context specifies otherwise.

Clinical status of patients

Thomson *et al.* (1975) pointed out the extreme functional variation affecting the muscle of an active four-year old Duchenne boy when compared with a twelve-year old boy in a wheelchair; the first is subjecting his surviving muscle to great stress and training, while in the latter the remaining vestiges of muscle will be atrophying from disease. This adds to difficulties of interpretation.

The object of investigation

Since empirical treatment has failed, rational therapy for dystrophy must await at least a broad understanding of the disease, and preferably a knowledge of which gene group (Katsantoni, 1976) is affected. Absolute deficiencies of enzymes are rare in human genetics; frequently, as in glycogen disease (Ryman, 1974) there is absence of one protein component among several tissue-specific proteins, leading to partial enzyme dificiency. Complete loss of the activity of any of the fundamental enzymes of, for example, glycolysis or energy production would probably be lethal. The gradual insidious change in dystrophy perhaps bespeaks of a *modification* of binding properties of enzymes or proteins which would exert a slow cumulative malignant effect rather than their complete absence which would be immediately fatal.

Putative basic causes have to account for; the possibility of at least four non-allelic forms of pseudohypertrophic disease (Walton and Gardner-Medwin, 1974; Warner Kloepfer and Emery, 1974), the 'wearing-out' of proximal muscles before distal (e.g., Bonsett, 1963) and of white fibres before red (Baloh and Cancilla, 1972; see below) the slow involvement of diaphragm, heart, smooth muscle and liver, and the accumulation of triglyceride (Grundmann and Beckmann, 1962; Bonsett, 1963, 1969; Huvos *et al.*, 1967; Thomson, 1964).

Changes observed in muscular dystrophy

Proteins are the primary gene products, but it is their function as catalysts, contractile elements, membrane components and translocators which is usually studied first; examination of the proteins themselves often follows adduction of evidence for a functional disturbance. In this review results will deal not only with enzyme changes but also with functional change testified to by substrates or products.

Effects of muscle wasting and replacement by other tissue elements

Obviously, as effective muscle mass diminishes, most purely muscle constituents will also diminish. The problem is to decide whether measured diminution is more than that which would be expected at a given stage of muscle degeneration. What follows is a subjective selection of results.

Contractile apparatus. Contraction is the *raison d'être* of muscle and the myofibrillar proteins have received due attention in dystrophy, the most severe affliction of motor function. Hoagland (1946) and Horvath (1958) found a greatly reduced quantity of myosin, but did not observe any abnormality in it. Schapira *et al.* (1954) concluded from streaming bire-fringence of the solution that myosin from dystrophic muscle contained more small particles and fewer large ones, probably the effect of frag-mentation. Samaha and Gergely (1969) Furukawa and Peter (1971, 1972) and Samaha (1972) studied actomyosin and the troponin system which regulates its contraction; although troponin content was reduced, and actomyosin displayed reduced Mg-ATPase activity, it appeared that though reduced in quantity the contractile machinery in dystrophy showed no deficiences.

Energy Provision. The oxygen-carrying protein myoglobin was found to show some abnormality in spectroscopic properties and it was speculated that dystrophy might by a muscular analogy of haemoglobinopathy (reviewed by Macciotta *et al.*, 1963; Whorton *et al.*, 1961; Miyoshi *et al.*, 1963, 1968) but Rowland *et al.* (1968) and Romero-Herrera *et al.* (1973) concluded that, as with myosin and the contractile system and also poly-ribosomes (see below) the observed differences could be attributed to partial fragmentation.

Muscular content of creatine, creatine phosphate and usually ATP are reduced in dystrophy (Debré *et al.*, 1936; Reinhold and Kingsley, 1938; Ronzoni *et al.*, 1958) as is creatine kinase (Vignos and Lefkowitz, 1959; Vignos and Warner, 1963). Depletion of creatine seems to be a conse-quence of reduced muscle mass (Pennington, 1974). Shields *et al.* (1975) showed that by depleting muscle creatine by drug treatment in rats several dystrophy-like symptoms resulted including a reduction in creatine kinase. Vester *et al.* (1968) concluded that surviving muscle fibres probably contain normal levels of creatine kinase. It seems likely that the loss of or failure to absorb creatine by damaged fibres could explain the tissue reductions of creatine phosphate and creatine kinase, and may suggest a general reason for the low levels of some enzymes in dystrophic muscle.

Heyck *et al.* (1963) studied a variety of enzymes in a sizable group of patients which were grouped according to the stage of degeneration of the muscle; this remains a monumental contribution to the subject, and many of its implications are not yet understood. As a general hypothesis explaining why different groups of enzymes should diminish at different stages, they suggested that subcellular membranes became damaged suc-cessively, releasing and losing waves of enzymes as degeneration advanced. Thomson *et al.* (1975) relate membrane health and the release of enzymes into the plasma to ATP levels. Berthillier *et al.* (1967) suggested ATP itself leaked from dystrophic fibres. Enzymes disappearing from muscle are not all found increased in serum (Pennington, 1975), and the loss of substrates or other low-molecular weight material may in turn, as with creatine (Shields *et al.*, 1975), ulimately influence the level of enzymes. Heyck *et al.* (1963) found activity of glutamate dehydrogenase, phosphogluconate dehydrogenase, glucose 6-phosphate dehydrogenase and isocitrate dehydrogenase to be increased in dystrophy, while most other enzymes diminished progressively and others increased at first but then diminished. The effect of substrates and effectors upon gene activity in maintaining enzyme levels may be invoked to explain these findings.

Changes in tissue composition during disease. Increases in NADP-linked dehydrogenases (as mentioned above) were considered by Pennington (1975) to be a possible result of infiltration by macrophages. Other changes may be expected from the unusual tissue composition, involving variable replacement of specific muscle protein by collagenous tissue (Lilienthal *et al.*, 1950, and others) and fat deposits (Reinhold and Kingsley, 1938, and others). Lysosomal enzymes increase probably in response to cell death. Sorbitol dehydrogenase (Kleine and Chloud, 1967) and several phosphatases (Beckett and Bourne, 1957; Bourne and Golarz, 1959; Kar and Pearson, 1972a and b, 1973) are thought to be have increased activities as a result of proliferating connective tissue.

Retention or appearance of primitive features in dystrophic muscle

Mature human muscle is a mixture, a mosaic in cross-section of three types of fibre; types I, II and 'intermediate'. Type I fibres are thinner, slower to contract, red and have more mitochondria which are distributed throughout the fibre. They rely predominantly on oxidative metabolism and their contraction is 'tonic', rather than 'phasic'. Type II fibres are of larger diameter, fast in action, white and have mitochondria only at the fibre periphery. They are capable of rapid, powerful contraction at the expense of anaerobic glycolysis. The third, a red fast-twitch type, has characteristics intermediate between the two extremes. Foetal muscle up to 18 weeks gestation lacks this mosaic structure, and is composed of homogeneous fibres (Dubowitz, 1974). The action of motor-nerves seems to initiate and maintain the mature mosaic of specialized fibres. Exercise may modify considerably the degree of specialization achieved in any individual (Pernow and Saltin, 1971).

Loss of specialization in dystrophy. In most groups of patients, effects of use and disuse will be present in addition to the effects of disease, so there is considerable difficulty of interpretation.

McComas and Thomas (1968) found a slowed contraction time in dystrophic muscles, and Tsukiyama and Ueda (1966) observed a parallel between electrophysiological changes and the reduction in white-fibre patterns of lactate dehydrogenase. Histochemical study brought Baloh and Cancilla (1972) to the view that in dystrophy the confusing picture is best explained as a change from glycolytic to oxidative metabolism. DiMauro *et al.* (1967) showed that several glycolytic enzymes waned as the disease advanced, and the fibre-types became indistiguishable. They suggested that selective loss of the more highly-specialized type II fibres was occurring. Glycogen phosphorylase, present in large amounts only in type II fibres was lost from a very early stage, while glycogen synthetase, an enzyme present equally in types I and II, was lost later. Samaha and Gergely (1969) also attributed to preferential involvement of type II fibres the reduction in sarcoplasmic reticulum calcium-activated ATPase that they reported. The well-known preservation of mitochondrial enzymes until late in the disease (Dreyfus *et al.,* 1956) would also be expected if the type I fibres rich in mitochondria were spared.

These effects would tend to make dystrophic muscle redder, but in fact the red pigment myoglobin diminishes early in the disease (Macciotta *et al.,* 1963), probably as a result of accelerated catabolism.

Resemblances to the foetal condition. In a study of mouse muscle, John (1976) showed the scope and delicacy with which motor innervation controls muscle proteins during maturation. Some, but not all myofibrillar proteins occur in different molecular forms in fast-twitch and slow-twitch muscle, evidently specified by different structural genes and regulated by the activity patterns imposed by the nerve upon each fibre. In foetal mouse muscle further differences occur between structures of these proteins, and in the 'dystrophic' mouse some of these characteristic foetal forms were found. During maturation the synthesis of purely foetal forms is evidently normally repressed, and the type of innervation causes selection of the structural genes activated.

Such complexity of regulation of the protein constitution of mature muscle should lead us to expect disease to alter the functional constituents; such alterations have been observed particularly in those proteins having easily-recognized differences between their molecular variants, the isoenzymes.

Isoenzymes are homologous, but not identical proteins, often dimers or tetramers of more than one polypeptide species, and usually with different tissue specificities. Lactate dehydrogenase is the prime example, it occurs as tetrameric isoenzymes the subunits of which can be combination of 'H' — ('heart') or 'M' — ('muscle') types (Goodfriend and Kaplan, 1964). The H and M subunits are specified by separate genes, one probably X-linked (Ruddle *et al.*, 1970). The H-type is inhibited by pyruvate at lower concentration than is the M-type (Goodfriend and Kaplan, 1964). Thus the M subunit is adapted to the glycolytic situation of muscle, and presumably represents a more specialized form. H is more anodic than M, and electrophoretic patterns differing from normal were observed by Wieme and Lauryssens (1962). Dreyfus *et al.* (1962) observed the similarity between the foetal and dystrophic patterns of lactate dehydrogenase. Different patterns of creatine kinase and aldolase led Schapira *et al.*, 1968 and Schapira, 1968 to the postulate that disease in general conferred a metabolic pattern in which 'mature' forms of enzymes disappeared and 'immature' forms replaced them.

All five lactate dehydrogenase isoenzymes were present in normal muscle, (Emery, 1964; Shepard *et al.*, 1965; Katz and Kalow, 1966; Cao *et al.*, 1966), but in the case of creatine kinase (Takahashi *et al.*, 1972) and aldolase (Tzvetanova, 1972) the abnormal pattern in disease showed the emergence of a 'brain-type' isoenzyme where none existed in normal muscle. Although the change in lactate dehydrogenase isoenzyme pattern was common to all *chronic* disease of muscle Tollersund (1971) showed in lambs made deficient in Vitamin E for 2-3 weeks that although early signs of muscle disease appeared, there was no change in isoenzyme pattern in so short a time. Ito (1972) studied the evolution of isoenzyme patterns with the course of Duchenne disease, and concluded that the M subunit was gradually disappearing. Ito inferred that between 4 and 9 years of age the dystrophic boy suffers the effective loss of all his type II fibres, only red fibres remaining thereafter. Górecka (1974) concluded that the dystrophic pattern of lactate dehydrogenase is more mature than that of foetal muscle, thus implying that dystrophic muscle does not simply fail to mature but rather that its development is overlain by the malignant effects of disease.

Other isoenzymes in which analagous changes have been found in dystrophy include those of iso-citrate dehydrogenase (Katz and Kalow, 1966), malate dehydrogenase (Cao *et al.*, 1966; Ideo *et al.*, 1966), aldolase (Ideo and Cao, 1966; Ito, 1972; Tzvetanova, 1972), adenylate kinase (Schirmer and Thuma, 1972), and enolase (Goldberg *et al.*, 1976). In the case of aldolase, the gradual appearance in muscle of the brain-type C-subunit (Tzvetanova, 1972) shows behaviour opposite to that of lactate dehydrogenase, in which M subunits gradually disappear. Presumably the aldolase C is made by derepressing a structural gene already present in the fibre, while the lactate dehydrogenase M structural gene becomes repressed by the effects of chronic disease.

These changes can probably be summarized as responses of individual fibres to the stimulus of disease, uncovering thereby the potential to make polypeptides of which there is little need during health and implying also that these changes help in a regenerative manner to combat disease. Since isoenzyme changes represent readily investigable examples of moves towards regeneration, there probably occur similar changes in other less readily investigable proteins.

Consideration of the protein changes occurring in disease leads to the expectation that de-specialization of metabolism will follow. This is more difficult to recognize, although the fructose pathway of glucose utilization developed in dystrophic and present in foetal muscle (Ellis *et al.*, 1973) may be one example. End-products of metabolism are more recognizable, and Hughes (1972) drew particular attention to the similarity in phospholipid composition between dystrophic and foetal muscle (in both human and mouse disease) and argued that this reflected de-differentiation.

Regeneration and protein synthesis. The high serum levels of some muscle enzymes in dystrophy has prompted calculation of their synthesis and breakdown rates (Pennington, 1974). Monckton and Nihei (1966) showed, despite the loss of muscle during dystrophy, that the synthesis rate of creatine kinase was maintained fairly well until the late stages of the disease. By contrast the synthetic rate of aldolase was reduced throughout. They found RNA in dystrophic muscle to be adequate in amount, and to function properly, though fewer of the large polyribosomes could be prepared from it than from normal muscle. Ionasescu *et al.* (1971, 1973) showed that dystrophic muscle from early stages of the disease contained fewer polysomes, but that they had increased rates of turnover. 'Soluble fraction' from dystrophic muscle was less capable of supporting the incorporation of amino acids by either normal or dystrophic muscle polysomes, and it was concluded that dystrophic muscle lacked a repressor of collagen synthesis, so that less normal protein, but more collagen was made. The authors pointed out that their findings might in part be explained by fragments, rather than whole polysomes being studied. The turnover of proteins requires breakdown as well as synthesis and as Millward *et al.* (1975) have shown the two processes are coupled. The increase in proteolytic enzymes (Pennington, 1975) in diseased muscle is important for re-cycling of dead material.

There is of yet no unequivocal explanation of the increased activity of cytoplasmic NADP-linked enzymes (Heyck *et al.*, 1963; Kar and Pearson, 1972c) and the variation in enzymes of the glyoxalase system (Kar and Pearson, 1975) that are concerned, respectively, with flow through synthetic pathways (Eggleston and Krebs, 1974) and with the growth regulators promine and retine (Szent-Györgyi, 1967).

Effects of disorganization of muscle structure

Total disintegration of most fibres eventually occurs as the disease progresses. Of interest is evidence for structural faults existing in earlier stages when a larger proportion of intact fibres remain. The release of muscle enzymes into the blood is the most striking of such changes, and gave rise to the hypothesis that the basic lesion in dystrophy is at the surface membranes. However, severe disease of any large organ leads to massive leakage of enzymes to the blood fulfilling diagnostic functions in the case of hepatomas and brain infarcts as well as in myopathy. Kleine (1970) has suggested that generalized release of enzymes into the blood occurs from all tissues in dystrophy, since raised serum levels of enzymes not found in muscle can be detected.

Membrane lipids

Investigation of muscle phospholipids in dystrophy has revealed differences (Kunze and Olthoff, 1970; Hughes, 1972; Kunze et al., 1973, 1975) in that lecithin content was reduced and sphingomyelin increased relatively. Kunze et al. (1975) found a deficiency in the acylation of choline phosphatidic acid, oleate (18:1) being substituted for linoleate (18:2) to give a lecithin deficient in poly-unsaturated acids. Hughes (1972) believed the changed pattern to be a consequence of de-differentiation suggesting that these results probably follow gene activation changes rather than being inborn errors. This does not, of course, reduce their possible impact on membrane stability, and may describe in chemical terms the biological lability some dystrophic membranes display.

Membrane function

The intact membrane is maintained against oxidation and other destructive effects by enzymes and vitamins, notably the fat soluble vitamins (Lucy and Dingle, 1964). Glutathione reductase is one such protective enzyme which Kleine and Chloud (1966) found essentially unaltered in dystrophy. Nor did Folkers et al. (1972) find consistent changes in coenzyme Q metabolism. Vitamin E deficiency has long been a model of muscle disease in animals and it is probable that a primary effect of such deficiency will be to increase membrane permeability (Diplock and Lucy, 1973; Ahkong et al., 1973). There are many potential ways of affecting membrane function, and it is not believed that vitamin E or its deficiency plays any part in Duchenne dystrophy. Thomson et al. (1975) consider reduced availability of ATP to be a common mechanism in muscle disease whereby membrane function may be disturbed.

The sarcolemma. This, the biological membrane limiting each fibre has attached to it several enzyme activities connected with transport phenomena that all appear to depend upon ATP the phosphorolysis of which is harnessed against concentration gradients. Three such enzymes were studied by Dhalla *et al.* (1973) in two Duchenne patients of unspecified age. The sodium-potassium ATPase was diminished, while calcium ATPase and magnesium ATPase were slightly increased. These results were considered to indicate some compensatory changes in already unhealthy membranes.

Adenyl cyclase, important in mediating hormone action at the cell-surface was shown by Susheela *et al.* (1975) and Canal *et al.* (1975) to have reduced activity in dystrophy, although the selective activating effect of fluoride restored normal activity. Mawatari *et al.* (1976) found an increased level in dystrophic muscle cells in culture. Canal *et al.* (1975) found reduced levels of adenyl cyclase in other neuromuscular diseases, but in Duchenne dystrophy there was a reduced level of the specific diesterase responsible for destroying cyclic nucleotides, whereas there was an increase in other muscle diseases.

Mokri and Engel (1975) have found by electron-microscopy evidence of early damage in focal regions of the sarcolemma. However, amongst several control specimens from other muscle diseases they also found similar changes in one patient with dystrophic myotonica. It would appear likely that membrane damage occurs sooner or later in muscle disease generally, and that therefore only a particularly significant and specific alteration in membrane *function* (rather than its structure) could provoke the complete observed range of disturbance in dystrophy.

Sarcoplasmic reticulum. One function associated with this membrane structure is the uptake and release of calcium ions that regulates contraction. A pump requiring ATP is involved and measured by a calcium-activated ATPase. This has been investigated by Samaha and Gergely (1969) who found a reduced quantity, but with normal properties. Takagi *et al.* (1973) confirmed this and also examined the magnesium-activated ATPase which was slightly diminished. Takagi *et al.* also found the protein and lipid composition of the reticulum to differ from the normal in having less lecithin as does dystrophic muscle generally.

Mitochondrial membrane. Studies of respiration and coupled phosphorylation (Ionasescu *et al.*, 1967) and of fatty acid oxidation (Lin *et al.*, 1972) have shown abnormalities of dystrophic muscle mitochondria which may reflect abnormal swelling. Swelling and contraction cycles occur in normal mitochondria in response to changes in metabolic status (Mahler and Cordes, 1966) and appear to relate to osmotic effects mediated through permeability changes (Blondin and Green, 1967). Degenerative changes in dystrophy would, perhaps, be expected to result in such alterations in membrane permeability, as do also exhaustive exercise, hypoxia and ischaemia (Gollnick *et al.*, 1971).

Lipid changes in general

The organization of higher organisms necessary to prevent incompatible processes from interfering with one another is achieved by a complex of membranes, of which lipids form integral parts. The turnover of lipids is obviously important from a structural viewpoint.

Synthesis of lipids is accelerated by muscle dysfunction, but this increase appears to be mainly of fat (Audova, 1923; Reinhold and Kingsley, 1938; Kunze and Olthoff, 1970; West *et al.*, 1977). In dystrophy the appearance of fat in fibres otherwise little affected by degenerative change was observed by Ostenda and Sluga (1971) and was considered to be one of the first noticeable changes occurring when the basal membrane was still intact. Phospholipid content, however, in contrast to neutral lipid, is reduced in dystrophy (Hoagland, 1946) and changes in its composition have been noted above but do not appear to be the result of a specific defect.

The potential effects of altered lipid metabolism on the development of dystrophy were recognized by Dreyfus and Schapira (1960), but the relations of fat accumulation and membrane change to altered intermediary metabolism and lipogenesis are still obscure.

Alterations in use of fuels and energy production

Fatty acids are by far the most important fuel of resting muscle (Greville and Tubbs, 1968), implying aerobic metabolism in which substrate oxidation by mitochondria is paramount. During exercise the glycogen store serves as fuel for glycolysis (Saltin and Karlsson, 1971) and, as exercise continues, an increasing amount of blood glucose is taken up (Wahren *et al.*, 1971). In severe exercise, glycogen stores may become exhausted. The effects of training are; to increase myoglobin content and oxidative capacity (Holloszy *et al.*, 1971) including both the size and number of mitochondria (Morgan *et al.*, 1971; Kiessling *et al.*, 1971), to increase glycogen reserves (Morgan *et al.*, 1971) and to increase the rather low capacity of muscle to use its own fat stores as fuel (Fröberg *et al.*, 1971).

White fibres play little part in resting muscle metabolism, but are increasingly recruited as the demand for power increases. Presumably the intermediate fibres also play a greater role in sustained exercise. In the classic study of Dreyfus *et al.* (1954, 1956) the rate of glycogen breakdown to lactate, and the activities of glycogen phosphorylase, phosphoglumutase and aldolase were found to be drastically reduced in dystrophic muscle, findings confirmed and amplified by Aronson and Volk (1957), Vignos and Lefkowitz (1959), Ronzoni *et al.* (1961), Heyck *et al.* (1963), Di Mauro *et al.* (1970) and Davidenkova *et al.* (1970). However, it has been generally found that many mitochondrial enzyme activities are retained at normal levels until the disease is well advanced (Dreyfus and Schapira, 1960; Heyck *et al.*, 1963), and the respiratory quotient of dystrophic muscle was found to remain normal (Hoagland, 1946). It is now generally agreed that the reduction in glycolysis, like that of fatty acid oxidation (Lin *et al.*, 1972) progresses with the disease (Hooft *et al.*, 1966; DiMauro *et al.*, 1967) and reflects loss of healthy muscle but the story is not quite so simple, hence the next section.

Mitochondrial function

Aconitase, succinate dehydrogenase, succinoxidase, fumarase and cyto-chrome oxidase activities were retained at the same levels in relation to non-collagen protein (Dreyfus and Schapira, 1960), similarly malate dehydro-genase and isocitrate dehydrogenase (Heyck *et al.*, 1963). Duma *et al.* (1967) found reduced oxygen uptake by dystrophic muscle which added substrates were unable to improve. Blood citrate level is low in dystrophy (Ionasescu and Luca, 1965; Niebrój-Dobosz and Hausmanova-Petruszewicz, 1965) but Niebrój-Dobosz (1971) found raised muscle levels of the extra-mito-chondrial enzymes citrate lyase, acetyl coenzyme A synthetase and isocitrate dehydrogenase which would tend to remove any citrate which escaped into the sarcoplasm and might account for its low level in the blood.

Ionasescu *et al.* (1967) and Olson *et al.* (1968) in studies of oxidative phosphorylation in dystrophic muscle showed a decline in oxygen uptake with progress of the disease, and a decline in the control ratio by which coupling of substrate oxidation to phosphate esterification is measured. The efficiency of phosphorylation was, however, maintained throughout suggesting that a state of 'loose coupling' prevails as during the swelling-contraction cycle in normal mitochondria.

Thus, biochemical studies largely support the anatomical observations of Ostenda and Sluga (1971) that mitochondria remain relatively un-damaged until the disease is far advanced in each fibre. The preferential loss of white fibres suggests the same. Stengel-Rutkowski and Barthelmai (1973) have shown early diminution of glycerol phosphate oxidase, a membrane bound mitochondrial enzyme which transports electrons from the glycolysis system to the respiratory chain. Its association with the glycolytic system suggests that its decline may be related to that, rather than to mitochondrial function.

Glycolysis

Enzyme levels. Although phosphorylase activity was reduced, the activation of the *b* form was apparently normal (Dreyfus *et al.*, 1954). Most of the enzymes of the Embden-Meyerhof pathway have been determined, and eventually most show a diminution in terms of non-collagen nitrogen, some more rapidly than others (Heyck *et al.*, 1963; DiMauro *et al.*, 1967). Exceptions were hexokinase (Ronzoni *et al.*, 1961; Heyck *et al.*, 1963; Davidenkova *et al.*, 1970) and glycerol phosphate dehydrogenase (Heyck *et al.*, 1963), which retained normal activities throughout. Functionally-linked enzymes like those of glycolysis form 'constant-proportion' groups (Pette, 1971) and their activities are regulated in concert; hexokinase is clearly not part of the glycolysis group (Pette, 1971; Huston *et al.*, 1975; Bylund *et al.*, 1976).

The pacemaker, or overall rate-controlling activity of glycolysis under most conditions is phosphofructokinase (Krebs, 1972) and DiMauro *et al.* (1967) reported that this declined along with the aldolase, lactate dehydrogenase and glycogen synthetase as the disease advanced. Chibisov and Sitnikov (1973) found two other enzymes of glycogen metabolism, amlyo-1:6-glucosidase and acid maltase to be retained normally.

Substrates. Mösberg (1930) noted fasting blood lactate to be raised in dystrophy, but neither pyruvate nor lactate levels were found by Ionasescu and Luca (1964, 1965) to rise normally during ischaemic exercise; these authors concluded that for the same amount of work done, dystrophic muscle took up the same amount of glucose, but produced less lactate, implying a similar change in glucose metabolism as has been found in diabetes (Beloff-Chain *et al.*, 1971). Changes in muscle levels of intermediates are difficult to interpret, since levels at any time of assay give no clue to flux rates; what is required is 'crossover analysis' (Williamson, 1965), of levels under different metabolic conditions. No such studies have been reported on dystrophic muscle.

Glycogen levels have variously been reported as low (Vignos and Warner, 1963; Hess, 1965), normal or slightly reduced (Collazo *et al.*, 1936; Hoagland, 1946; Chibisov and Sitnikov, 1973) or raised (Stengel-Rutkowski and Barthelmai, 1973). The actual level is probably not very important, since that of normal humans varies widely (Hultman, *et al.*, 1971). Muscle lactate was found to be normal (Collazo *et al.*, 1936; Hess, 1965). Glucose 6-phosphate was reduced, but normal when corrected for collagen (Hess, 1963). The most searching study is that of Stengel-Rutkowski and Barthelmai (1973), who found marked reduction in glucose 6-phosphate, phosphopyruvate, glycerol phosphate, lactate, malate, oxaloacetate and citrate, normal levels of fructose diphosphate and phosphogluconate, and slight reduction in pyruvate. These results imply that control of glycolysis was normal, and that the pentose phosphate pathway and citric acid cycle were functioning without impedance. The redox ratio of pyruvate:lactate was normal, that of glycerol phosphate:dihydroxy-acetone phosphate was somewhat reduced, and malate:oxaloacetate was very much reduced. This might imply increased lipogenesis via extra-mitochondrial citrate cleavage and esterification of glycerol phosphate, agreeing with the increased citrate lyase found by Niebrój-Dobosz (1971) and increased esterification found by West *et al.* (1977).

ATP and creatine phosphate

These substances are rapidly interconverted by creatine kinase and provide the source of immediate energy for contraction. ATP presumably in a separate compartment provides energy for membrane maintenance and for biosynthesis. Both have been generally found to be reduced in dystrophic muscle, as also has the ratio of ATP:ADP (Collazo *et al.*, 1936; Ronzoni *et al.*, 1958; Vignos and Warner, 1963; Berthillier *et al.*, 1967; Stengel-Rutkowski and Barthelmai, 1973), although Ronzoni *et al.* (1958) found ATP itself to have a normal level. The enzymes which govern the levels of ATP, and particularly the balance of ATP, ADP, AMP and IMP are generally also reduced in activity (Pennington, 1962; Heyck *et al.*, 1963; Kar and Pearson, 1973), and the effective available levels of ATP cannot really be determined, except that a reduced ATP:ADP ratio implies an overall deficiency. The very presence of any creatine phosphate at all suggests that contraction in surviving fibres is not limited by a serious long-term drain on this energy reserve, whatever may be the deleterious effect of overall ATP deficiency on membrane properties (Thomson *et al.*, 1975). The data deal only in global terms with a substance in constant flux, and thus few conclusions can be drawn.

Glucose Metabolism

The problems of metabolite flux crop up again here. It has already been noted that lactate production for a given glucose uptake is lower in dystrophic muscle and that hexokinase activity is regulated separately from that of enzymes of glycolysis; it is also clear that glucose metabolism and glycogen breakdown are separate. (Beloff-Chain *et al.*, 1971).

Glucose uptake and insulin. McCrudden (1918) found low blood sugars in all his cases of dystrophy and likening the fatty degeneration seen in them to that occurring in adrenalectomy, suggested that: '... the hypoglycaemia and fatty infiltration are due to impaired glucogenesis, the carbohydrate of the food being changed largely into fat instead of glycogen.' Adrenalin is released in response to muscle exercise and activity inhibits insulin release (Wright and Malaisse, 1968) so that normal (trained) subjects undergo both a reduction in plasma insulin levels and an increase in blood sugar when subjected to extremely hard exercise (Pruett, 1971). If Thomson *et al.* (1975) are right to supposing the muscle in active patients with dystrophy to be in an exhausted state, McCrudden's assessment of dystrophy as an endocrine disorder seems prophetic, even if for the wrong reason.

Glucose tolerances were found to be abnormal, probably because the mass of muscle was reduced (Van Bekkum and Querido, 1953; Ionasescu and Luca, 1965; Blietz and Paulman, 1966; Takagi *et al.*, 1970), but there were other peculiarities. Van Bekkum and Querido (1953) found glucose uptake to be associated with a much lower uptake of inorganic phosphate, and Ionesescu and Luca (1965) found a lower lactate production. Blietz and Paulmann (1966) showed that, independent of the degree of disability, the same larger dosage of insulin per kilogram body weight was necessary in dystrophic patients to give the same hypoglycaemic response suggesting that the effective musculature had fewer insulin receptor sites than normal. A similar phenomenon occurs in obese rats (Olefsky *et al.*, 1976).

Pathways of glucose utilization. The function of glucose uptake by muscle, *except* in severe exercise is chiefly to resynthesise glycogen. Glucose utilization is compartmentalized (Shaw and Stadie, 1959; Beloff-Chain *et al.*, 1971) and insulin affects only that compartment leading to glycogen synthesis. Under normal conditions glucose entry is slower than its phosphorylation by hexokinase (Walker, 1966) so that glucose does not accumulate.

Using [^{14}C−] glucose to label metabolic pathways of muscle we found that fructose was an unexpected major product in dystrophy (Ellis, 1965; Ellis and Eccleston, 1968; Ellis *et al.*, 1973). The labelling patterns of normal and dystrophic muscle were compared using labelled glucose, fructose, glucitol, glycerol, hexose phosphate, acetate, pyruvate, citrate, malate, glycine, glutamate and aspartate without revealing any other outstanding differences. Despite undoubted differences in flux rates the radioactivities (which roughly measure metabolite levels) were frequently similar in normal and dystrophic muscle. Attempts to quantify the fructose route have been unsuccessful so far although inhibition of glucitol formation inhibited fructogenesis (Ellis and Strickland, 1974) because the process apparently occurs with glucitol as a common hydrogenated intermediate (Ellis *et al.*, 1973). Glucose 6-phosphate appeared to dilute out the radioactivity of glucose products other than fructose (Strickland and Ellis, 1973) and was rapidly and normally metabolized.

As in diabetic muscle (Beloff-Chain *et al.*, 1971) dystrophic muscle yielded little lactate or glucose 6-phosphate as products of glucose metabolism (Ellis, 1965; J.M. Strickland and D.A. Ellis, unpublished). This suggested fructose to be an alternative to glucose 6-phosphate in glucose metabolism. Fructose metabolism is intact in dystrophic muscle (Canal *et al.*, 1959; Ellis *et al.*, 1973) so the explanation was sought at the hexokinase level where a changed mobility of each of the two bands (a and b of Katzen *et al.*, 1970) of isoenzyme II have been found (Strickland and Ellis, 1974, 1975; Ellis *et al.*, 1976) which may indicate a genetic lesion of this protein. Although the hexokinase system is complex and still ill-understood, it is probable that hexokinase II is a target of insulin action (Katzen, 1967; Katzen *et al.*, 1970; Bernstein and Kipnis, 1973; Edminson, *et al.*, 1973). Hexokinase II has not yet been shown to be attached to the muscle surface membrane at which the insulin action on glucose transport occurs, but it would be convenient if it were there.

Dystrophic muscle and certain other types of diseased muscle are more permeable to glucose; dystrophic is not noticeably more permeable to glucitol than normal, whereas muscle affected by polymyositis does appear to be more permeable to both sugars. (Table 1). The apparently selective increase in permeability to glucose in Duchenne dystrophy (as opposed to the general increase seen in myositis) probably allows fructose formation within the muscle (Pottinger, 1967). This seems to have become an adaptation in later life of a pathway which foetal muscle possesses but normal adult muscle probably lacks (Ellis *et al.*, 1973). If hexokinase and these

TABLE 1
Sugar Spaces in Muscle Disease
ml g^{-1} (fresh weight) (Mean and sample no.)

	Glucose	Fructose	Glucitol
Normal human	†0.074 (19)	0.033 (5)	0.20 (5)
Foetal (12-20 weeks)	*0.095 (6)	0.061 (4)	0.18 (6)
Duchenne dystrophy	*0.108 (15)	0.049 (6)	0.17 (5)
Polymyositis	†0.127 (7)	–	0.39 : 0.54
Adult dystrophy	0.119 (5)	0.056 (5)	0.31 (5)
Neurogenic muscle disease	0.097 (3)	0.023 (6)	

The glucose and fructose spaces were determined from the radioactivity of pieces of muscle equilbrated with [^{14}C] sugar which were then washed before extraction; glucitol spaces were determined without washing, and thus refer to total extracellular space in addition to any space permeable to glucitol. Glucose and fructose spaces are however intracellular permeability spaces. Methods of Ellis *et al.*, 1973.

*, †. the differences are significant: $p > 0.05$.

latter phenomena are found to be related a role in aetiology would await this enzyme. By diverting glucose to fructose, glyceraldehyde (Strickland and Ellis, 1973) and glycerol phosphate (West *et al.*, 1977) a plausible modern explanation of McCrudden's early suggestion would revolve around hexokinase II and its relationship to hormone action. A further consequence would be that ATP production from glucose would be reduced (West *et al.*, 1977) should this prove to be a necessary part of any aetiological theory. How inter-related are these various phenomena may be seen from the Deceptive Cycle (Fig. 1). Probably one of these is significant in aetiological terms, but which? Whichever effect one oberves can at least in theory arise as an expression of some other cause.

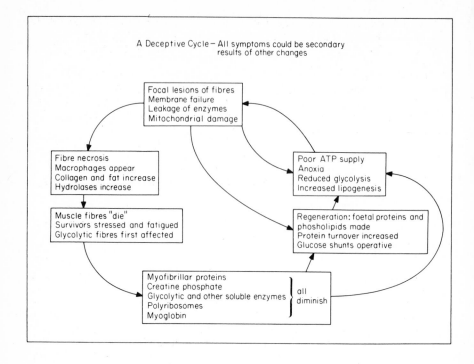

A Deceptive Cycle – All symptoms could be secondary results of other changes

References

Ahkong, Q.F., Fisher, D., Tampion, W. and Lucy, J.A. (1973). *Biochem. J.*, **136,** 147-155.

Aronson, S.M. and Volk, B.W. (1957). *Amer. J. Med.*, **22,** 414-421.

Audova, A. (1922). *Skand. Arch. Physiol.*, **44,** 1-19.

Baloh, R. and Cancilla, P.A. (1972). *Neurology (Minneap).*, **22,** 1243-1252.

Beckett, E.B. and Bourne, G.H. (1957). *Science*, **126,** 357-358.

Beloff-Chain, A., Chain, E.B. and Rookledge, K.A. (1971). *Biochem. J.*, **125,** 97-103.

Bernstein, R.S. and Kipnis, D.M. (1973). *Diabetes*, **22,** 923-931.

Berthillier, G., Gautheron, D. and Robert, J.M. (1967). *C.R. Acad. Sci. (Paris)*, **265,** 79-82.

Blietz, R.J. and Paulmann, F. (1966). *Hoppe-Seyler's Z. physiol. Chem.*, **347,** 35-51.

Blondin, G.A. and Green, D.E. (1967). *Proc. nat. Acad. Sci. (Wash.)*, **58,** 612-619.

Bonsett, C.A. (1963). *Neurology (Minneap.)*, **13,** 728-738.

Bonsett, C.A. (1969). 'Studies of Pseudohypertrophic Muscular Dystrophy' Thomas, Springfield.

Bourne, G.H. and Golarz, N. (1959). *Arch. Biochem.*, **85,** 109-114.

Brock, D.J.H. (1972). *In* 'The Biochemical Genetics of Man' (D.J.H. Brock and O. Mayo, eds) Academic Press, London, New York, pp.418, 443-444.

Bylund, A.C., Holm, J., Lundholm, K. and Scherstén, T. (1976). *Enzyme*, **21,** 39-52.

Canal, N. Manzini, B. and Saraval, A. (1959). *Minerva Med.*, **50**, 4386-4389.
Canal, N., Frattola, L. and Smirne, S. (1975). *J. Neurology*, **208**, 259-265.
Cao, A., Macciotta, A., Fiorelli, G., Mannucci, P.M. and Idéo, G. (1966). *Enzymol. biol. Clin.*, **7**, 156-166.
Chibisov, I.V. and Sitnikov, V.F. (1973). *Vopr. med. Khim.*, **19**, 321-325.
Collazo, J.A., Barbudo, J. and Torres, I. (1936). *Deut. med. Wschr.*, **62**, 51-54.
Davidenkova, E.F., Verzhbinskaya, N.A., Savina, M.V. and Schwartz, E.L. (1970). *Zh. Nevropatol. Psikiatr. im. S.S. Korsakova*, **70**, 1441-1445.
Debré, R., Marie, J. and Nachmansohn, D. (1936). *C.R. Acad. Sci. (Paris)*, **202**, 520-522.
Dhalla, N.S., McNamara, D.B., Balasubramanian, V., Greenlaw, R. and Tucker, F.R. (1973). *Res. Comm. Chem. Path. Pharmacol.*, **6**, 643-650.
DiMauro, S., Angelini, C. and Catani, C. (1967). *J. Neurol. Neurosurg. Psychiat.*, **30**, 411-415.
Diplock, A.T. and Lucy, J.A. (1973). *FEBS Letters*, **29**, 205-210.
Dreyfus, J.-C. and Schapira, G. (1960). *In* 'Enzymatische Regulationen in der Klinik'. Proc. 6th Int. Cong. Internal Med., Basel (1960), pp.145-181. (Schwabe, Basel/Stuttgart).
Dreyfus, J.-C. Schapira, G. and Schapira, F. (1954). *J. clin. Invest.*, **33**, 794-797.
Dreyfus, J.-C., Schapira, G., Schapira, F. and Demos, J. (1956). *Clin. Chim. Acta.*, **1**, 434-449.
Dreyfus, J.-C., Demos, J., Schapira, F. and Schapira, G. (1962). *CR Acad. Sci. (Paris)*, **254**, 4384-4386.
Dubowitz, V. (1974). *In* 'Disorders of Voluntary Muscle' 3rd ed. (J.N. Walton ed.) pp.310-359. Churchill Livingstone, Edinburgh and London.
Duma, D., Popoviciu, L., Marec, V., Serban, M., Pîrvu, M., Lazăr, T.C., Pop, R. and Băltescu, V. (1967). *Rev. Roumaine de Neurol.*, **4**, 121-128.
Edminson, P.D., Siebke, J.C. and Tjötta, E. (1973). *Biochem. biophys. Acta.*, **320**, 33-43.
Eggleston, L.V. and Krebs, H.A. (1974). *Biochem. J.*, **138**, 425-435.
Ellis, D.A. (1965). *In* 'Research in Muscular Dystrophy'. Proc. 3rd Symp. 1965. pp.198-207. Pitman Medical, London.
Ellis, D.A. and Eccleston, J.F. (1968). *In* 'Research in Muscular Dystrophy'. Proc. 4th Symp. 1968. pp.321-333. Pitman Medical, London.
Ellis, D.A. and Strickland, J.M. (1974). *Biochem. Soc. Trans.*, **2**, 131-133.
Ellis, D.A., Strickland, J.M. and Eccleston, J.F. (1973). *Clin. Sci.*, **44**, 321-334.
Ellis, D.A., Strickland, J.M. and Tye, J.E. (1976). *Biochem. Soc. Trans.*, **4**, 1054-1056.
Emery, A.E.H. (1964). *Nature, Lond.*, **201**, 1044-1045.
Folkers, K., Littarru, G.P., Nakamura, R. and Scholler, J. (1972). *Internat. J. Vit. Nutr. Res.*, **42**, 139-163.
Fröberg, S.O., Carlson, L.A. and Ekelund, L.-G. (1971). *In* 'Muscle Metabolism During Exercise' (B. Pernow and B. Saltin, eds.), pp.307-313. Plenum Press, New York and London.
Furakawa, T. and Peter, J.B. (1971). *Neurology (Minneap.)*, **21**, 920-924.
Furukawa, T. and Peter, J.B. (1972). *Arch. Neurol. (Chic.)*, **26**, 385-390.
Goldberg, D.M., Rider, C.C. and Taylor, C.B. (1976). *Clin. chim. Acta*, **71**, 89-93.
Gollnick, P.D., Ianuzzo, C.D. and King, D.W. (1971). *In* 'Muscle Metabolism During Exercise' (B. Pernow and B. Saltin, eds.), pp.69-85. Plenum Press, New York and London.
Goodfriend, T.L. and Kaplan, N.O. (1964). *J. biol. Chem.*, **239**, 130-135.

Górecka, A. (1974). *Neurol. Neurochir. Psychiat. Pol.*, **24**, 697-702.
Greville, G.D. and Tubbs, P.K. (1968). *Essays in Biochem.*, **4**, 189.
Grundman, E. and Beckmann, R. (1962). *Beitr. path. Anat.*, **127**, 335-350.
Harris, H. (1970). 'The Principles of Human Biochemical Genetics', pp.117-120; 156-160.
Hess J.W. (1965). *J. Lab. clin. Med.*, **66**, 452-463.
Heyck, M., Laudahn, G. and Lüders, C.-J. (1963). *Klin. Woch.*, **41**, 500-509.
Hoagland, C.L. (1946). *Adv. Enzymol.*, **6**, 193-230.
Holloszy, J.O., Oscai, L.B., Molé, P.A. and Don, I.J. (1971). *In* 'Muscle Metabolism During Exercise' (B. Pernow and B. Saltin, eds.), pp.51-61. Plenum Press, New York and London.
Hooft, C., de Laey, P. and Lambert, Y. (1966). *Rev. franc. Etudes. clin. biol.*, **11**, 510-518.
Horvath, B. (1958). *Neurology (Minneap.)*, **8**, suppl. pp.52-53.
Hughes, B.P. (1972). *J. Neurol. Neurosurg. Psychiat.*, **35**, 658-663.
Hultman, E. and Nilsson, L.H. (1971). *In* 'Muscle Metabolism During Exercise' (B. Pernow and B. Saltin, eds.), pp.143-151. Plenum Press, New York and London.
Huston, R.L., Weiser, P.C., Dohm, G.L., Askew, E.W. and Boyd, J.B. (1975). *Life Sci.*, **17**, 369-376.
Huvos, A.G. and Pruzanski, W. (1967). *Arch. Path.*, **83**, 234-240.
Idéo, G. and Cao, A. (1966). *Boll. Soc. ital. Biol. sper.*, **42**, 693-696.
Idéo, G., Maunucci, P.M., Spano, G., Cao, A. and Macciotta, A. (1966). *Boll. Soc. ital. Biol. sper.*, **42**, 691-693.
Ionasescu, V. and Luca, N. (1964). *Acta neurol. Scand.*, **40**, 47-57.
Ionasescu, V. and Luca, N. (1965). *Psychiat. Neurol.*, Basel, **149**, 375-386.
Ionasescu, V., Luca, N. and Vuia, D. (1967). *Acta neurol. Scand.*, **43**, 564-572.
Ionasescu, V., Zellweger, H. and Conway, T.W. (1971). *Arch. Biochem. Biophys.*, **144**, 51-58.
Ionasescu, V., Zellweger, H., McCormick, W.F. and Conway, T.W. (1973). *Neurology (Minneap).*, **23**, 245-253.
Ito, T. (1972). *Clinical Neurol. (Tokyo)*, **12**, 473-483.
John, H.A. (1976). *FEBS Letts.*, **64**, 116-121.
Kar, N.C. and Pearson, C.M. (1972a). *Proc. Soc. exp. Biol. Med.*, **141**, 4-6.
Kar, N.C. and Pearson, C.M. (1972b). *Clin. chim. Acta.*, **38**, 252-254.
Kar, N.C. and Pearson, C.M. (1972c). *Clin. chim. Acta.*, **38**, 183-186.
Kar, N.C. and Pearson, C.M. (1973). *Neurology (Minneap.)*, **23**, 478-482.
Kar. N.C. and Pearson, C.M. (1975). *Clin. chim. Acta.*, **65**, 153-155.
Katsantoni, A. (1976). *Clin. Genet.*, **9**, 371-373.
Katz, A.M. and Kalow, W. (1966). *Nature (Lond.)*, **209**, 1349-1350.
Katzen, H.M. (1967). Adv. Enzyme Regulation, **5**, 335-356.
Katzen, H.M., Soderman, D.D. and Wiley, C.E. (1970). *J. biol. Chem.*, **245**, 4081-4096.
Kiessling, K.-H., Piehl, K. and Lundquist, C.G. (1971). *In* 'Muscle Metabolism During Exercise'. (B. Pernow and B. Saltin, eds.), pp.97-101. Plenum Press, New York and London.
Kleine, T.O. (1970). *Clin. chim. Acta.*, **29**, 227-231.
Kleine, T.O. and Chlond, H. (1966). *Clin. chim. Acta.*, **13**, 407-411.
Kleine, T.O. and Chlond, H. (1967). *Clin. chim Acta.*, **15**, 19-33.
Krebs, H.A. (1972). *In* Essays in Biochemistry (P.N. Campbell and F. Dickens, eds.) Academic Press, London, **8**, 1-34.

Kunze, D. and Olthoff, D. (1970). *Clin. chim. Acta.*, **29**, 455-462.

Kunze, D., Reichmann, G., Egger, E., Leuschner, G. and Eckhardt, H. (1973). *Clin. chim. Acta.*, **43**, 333-341.

Kunze, D., Reichmann, G., Egger, E., Olthoff, D. and Dohler, K. (1975). *European J. Clin. Invest.*, **5**, 471-475.

Lilienthal, J.L., Zierler, K.L., Folk, B.P., Buka, R. and Riley, M.J. (1950). *J. biol. Chem.*, **182**, 501.

Lin. C.H., Hudson, A.J. and Strickland, K.P. (1972). *Life Sciences*, **11**, 355-362.

Lucy, J.A. and Dingle, J.T. (1964). *Nature (Lond.)*, **204**, 156-160.

Macciotta, A., Cao, A. and Scano, V. (1963). *Ann. ital. Pediat.*, **16, No. 3**, 1-135.

McComas, A.J. and Thomas, H.C. (1968). *J. neurol. Sci.*, **7**, 309-312.

McCrudden, F.H. (1918). *Arch. internal Med.*, **21**, 256-262.

Mahler, H.R., and Cordes, E.H. (1966). 'Biological Chemistry'. pp.397-401. Harper International, New York, Evanston and London.

Mawatari, S., Miranda, A. and Rowland, L.P. (1976). *Neurology (Minneap.)*, **26**, 1021-1026.

Millward, D.J., Garlick, P.J., Stewart, R.J.C., Nnanyelugo, D.O. and Waterlow, J.C. (1975). *Biochem. J.*, **150**, 235-243.

Miyoshi, K., Saijo, K., Kuryu, Y. and Oshima, Y. (1963). *Science*, **142**, 929-933.

Miyoshi, K., Saijo, K., Kuryu, Y. and Oshima, Y., Nakano, M. and Kawai, H. (1968). *Science*, **159**, 736-737.

Mokri, B. and Engel, A.G. (1975). *Neurology (Minneap.)*, **25**, 1111-1120.

Monckton, G. Nihei, T. (1966). *Ann. N.Y. Acad. Sci.*, **138**, 329-341.

Morgan, T.E., Cobb, L.A., Short, F.A., Ross, R. and Gunn, D.R. (1971). *In* 'Muscle Metabolism During Exercise' (B. Pernow and B. Saltin, eds.), pp.87-95. Plenum Press, New York and London.

Mosberg, G. (1930). *Klin. Wschr.*, **2**, 2051-2052.

Niebrój-Dobosz, I. (1971). *Neurol. Neurochir, Psychiat. Pol.*, **21**, 659-663.

Niebrój-Dobosz, I. and Hausmanova-Petruszewicz, I. (1965). *Acta med. Pol.*, **6**, 117-123.

Olefskey, J., Bacon, V.C. and Baur, S. (1976). *Metabolism*, **25**, 179-191.

Olson, E., Vignos, P.J., Woodlock, J. and Perry, T. (1968). *J. Lab. clin. Med.*, **71**, 220-231.

Ostenda, M. and Sluga, E. (1971). *Acta Neuropath. (Berlin)*, **18**, 173-189.

Pennington, R.J. (1962). *Proc. Assoc. clin. Biochemists*, **2**, 17-18.

Pennington, R.J.T. (1974). *In* 'Disorders of Voluntary Muscle' 3rd edn. (J.N. Walton, ed.), pp.488-516. Churchill Livingstone, Edinburgh and London.

Pernow, B. and Saltin, B. (1971). 'Muscle Metabolism During Exercise'. Plenum Press, New York and London.

Pette, D. (1971). *In* 'Muscle Metabolism During Exercise' (B. Pernow and B. Saltin, eds.), pp.33-49. Plenum Press, New York and London.

Pottinger, P.K. (1967). *Biochem. J.*, **104**, 663-668.

Pruett, E.D.R. (1971). *In* 'Muscle Metabolism During Exercise' (B. Pernow and B. Saltin, eds.), pp.165-175. Plenum Press, New York and London.

Reinhold, J.G. and Kingsley, G.R. (1938). *J. clin. Invest.*, **17**, 377-383.

Romero-Herrera, A.E. Lehmann, H., Tomlinson, B.E. and Walton, J.N. (1973). *J. med. Genet.*, **10**, 309-322.

Ronzoni, E., Wald, S., Berg, L. and Ramsey, R. (1958). *Neurology (Minneap.)*, **8**, 359-368.

Ronzoni, E., Berg, L. and Landau, W. (1961). *Res. Publ. Assoc. Res. Nerv. Dis.*, **38**, 721-729.

Rowland, L.P., Dunne, P.B., Penn, A.S. and Maher, E. (1968). *Arch. Neurol. (Chic.)*, **18**, 141-150.

Ruddle, F.H., Chapman, V.M., Chen, T.R. and Klebe, R.J. (1970). *Nature (Lond.)*, **227**, 251-257.

Ryman, B.E. (1974). *In* 'Molecular Variants in Disease' (D.N. Raine, ed.), pp.106-121. Royal College of Pathologists, London.

Saltin, B. and Karlsson, J. (1971). *In* 'Muscle Metabolism During Exercise' (B. Pernow and B. Saltin, eds.), pp.289-299. Plenum Press, New York and London.

Samaha, F.J. (1972). *Arch. Neurol. (Chic.)*, **26**, 547-550.

Samaha, F.J. and Gergely, J. (1969). *New Eng. J. Med.*, **280**, 184-188.

Schapira, F. (1968). *In* 'Homologous Enzymes and Biochemical Evolution' (N. Van Thoai and J. Roche, eds.), pp.151-164. Gordon and Breach, New York, London and Paris.

Schapira, G., Joly, M. and Dreyfus, J.-C. (1954). *C.R. Soc. Biol.*, **148**, 1056-1058.

Schapira, F., Dreyfus, J.-C. and Allard, D. (1968). *Clin. chim. Acta*, **20**, 439-447.

Schirmer, R.H. and Thuma, E. (1972). *Biochim. biophys. Acta*, **268**, 92-97.

Shaw, W.N. and Stadie, W.C (1959). *J. biol. Chem.*, **234**, 2491-2496.

Shepard, T.H., Gordon, L.H. and Wollenweber, J.E. (1965). *Nature (Lond.)*, **208**, 1107-1108.

Shields, R.P., Whitehair, C.K., Carrow, R.E., Heusner, W.W. and Van Huss, W.D. (1975). *Lab. Invest.*, **33**, 151-158.

Stengel-Rutkowski, L. and Barthelmai, W. (1973). *Klin. Wschr.*, **51**, 957-968.

Strickland, J.M. and Ellis, D.A. (1973). *Biochem. Soc. Trans.*, **1**, 735-742.

Strickland, J.M. and Ellis, D.A. (1974). *Biochem. Soc. Trans.*, **2**, 1125-1127.

Strickland, J.M. and Ellis, D.A. (1975). *Nature (Lond.)*, **253**, 464-466.

Susheela, A.K., Kaul, R.D., Sachedeva, K. and Naunihal, S. (1975). *J. neurol. Sci.*, **24**, 361-363.

Szent-Gyorgyi, A. (1967). *Proc. nat. Acad. Sci. (Wash.)*, **57**, 1642-1643.

Takagi, A., Shimada, Y. and Mozai, T. (1970). *Neurology (Minneap.)*, **20**, 904-908.

Takagi, A., Schotland, D.L. and Rowland, L.P. (1973). *Arch. Neurol. (Chic.)*, **28**, 380-384.

Takahashi, K., Ushikubo, S., Oimomi, M. and Shinko, T. (1972). *Clin. Chim. Acta*, **38**, 285-290.

Thomson, W.H.S. (1964). *Adv. Clin. Chem.*, **7**, 137-197.

Thomson, W.H.S., Sweetin, J.C. and Hilditch, T.E. (1975). *Clin. Chim. Acta*, **63**, 383-394.

Tollersund, S. (1971). *Acta vet. Scand.*, **12**, 365-374.

Tsukiyama, K. and Ueda, K. (1966). *Electromyography (Louvain)*, **6**, 77.

Tzvetanova, E. (1972). *Clin. Chem.*, **17**, 926-930.

Van Bekkum, D.W. and Querido, A. (1953). *J. clin. Invest.*, **32**, 1061-1064.

Vester, J.W., Sabeh, G., Newton, R.H., Finkelhor, H.B., Fetterman, G.H. and Danowski, T.S. (1968). *Proc. Soc. exp. Biol. Med.*, **128**, 5-8.

Vignos, P.J. and Lefkowitz, M. (1959). *J. clin. Invest.*, **38**, 873-881.

Vignos, P.J. and Warner, J.L. (1963). *J. Lab. clin. Med.*, **62**. 579-590.

Wahren, J., Ahlborg, G., Felig, P. and Jorfeldt, L. (1971). *In* 'Muscle Metabolism During Exercise' (B. Pernow and B. Saltin, eds.), pp.189-203. Plenum Press, New York and London.

Walker, D.G. (1966). *Essays in Biochem.*, **2**, 54-55.

Walton, J.N. and Gardner-Medwin, D. (1974). *In* 'Disorders of Voluntary Muscle' (J.N. Walton, ed.), pp.517-560. Churchill Livingston, Edinburgh and London.

Warner Kloepfer, H. and Emery, A.E.H. (1974). *In* 'Disorders of Voluntary Muscle' (J.N. Walton, ed.), pp.852-885.
Churchill Livingstone, Edinburgh and London.

West, D.P., Ellis, D.A. and Strickland, J.M. (1977). *J. Neurol. Sci.* 131-142.

Whorton, C.M., Hudgins, P.C. and Conners, J.J. (1961). *New Eng. J. Med.,* **265,** 1242-1245.

Wieme, R.J. and Lauryssens, M.J. (1962). *Lancet,* **i,** 433-434.

Williamson, J.R. (1965). *In* 'Control of Energy Metabolism' (B. Chance, R.W. Estabrook and J.R. Williamson, eds.), pp.333-346. Academic Press. New York and London.

Wright, P.H. and Malaisse, W.J. (1968). *Amer. J. Physiol.,* **214,** 1031-1034.

21 α-D-mannosidases in normal and atrophic muscle

R. RICHARD WALLACE · MAXWELL H.R. LEWIS

Department of Biochemistry, Queen's University of Belfast, BT7 1NN, U.K.

The presence of lysosomes in normal skeletal muscle has not been detected by light or electron microscopy. Many hydrolases which are associated with lysosomes in other tissues however, are found in muscle (Tappel *et al.*, 1962; Canonico and Bird, 1970; Wallace and Lewis, 1975) and display the latency characteristic of lysosomal enzymes. In muscle Pearce (1966) has suggested that these enzymes are associated with Golgi membranes or with the sarcoplasmic reticulum.

We have studied several glycosidases, known to be lysosomal in other tissues (Hultberg and Öckerman, 1972), in rat gastrocnemius and soleus muscle (Wallace and Lewis, 1975, 1977). Acidic α-D-mannosidase (EC 3.2.1.24) has long been recognized as a lysosomal hydrolase (Conchie and Hay, 1963; Hultberg and Öckerman, 1972), but Marsh and Gourlay (1971) presented evidence for the occurrence of an additional cytoplasmic enzyme activity in rat liver. This 'neutral' α-D-mannosidase has since been shown to be present in many other tissues and species (Suzuki *et al.*, 1969; Carroll *et al.*, 1972; Phillips *et al.*, 1974 a,b). In rat gastrocnemius and soleus muscle we have found both acidic and neutral α-D-mannosidases which differ markedly in their pH optima, thermolability and response to certain metal ions (Wallace and Lewis, 1977). Whereas the acidic activity was found to be membrane bound and exhibited latency, the neutral activity was cytoplasmic thereby facilitating partial separation of these activities by high speed centrifugation in an isotonic medium.

Gastrocnemius muscle from young adult male rats was removed and dissected free from surrounding connective tissue. It was then washed in 5 mM-Tris/HC1 buffer (pH 7.4, 4°C) containing 0.25-M sucrose, to remove blood and hair. The muscle was weighed, scissor-minced and suspended in 19 volumes of the same buffer. The highly fibrous nature of the muscle required an initial disruption in a Virtis homogenizer for three 15 s intervals over a 2 min period, followed by gentle homogenization in a Potter-

Elvehjem homogenizer. The muscle homogenate was filtered through four layers of gauze and the bulk centrifuged at 100,000 g for 30 min at 4°C. Following removal of the lipid layer, the supernatant was retained for subsequent assay of neutral α-D-mannosidase. The pellet was resuspended in the original volume of 5 mM-Tris/HCl buffer (pH 7.4, 4°C) containing 0.25-M sucrose. Both the original homogenate and the resuspended pellet were briefly rehomogenized in the presence of 0.2% Triton X-100 (v/v, final concn.) to solubilize the acidic activity.

The α-D-mannosidase activity of each fraction was measured fluorimetrically with 4-methylumbelliferyl-α-D-mannopyranoside (Öckerman, 1969). The standard reaction mixture contained 200 μl of this substrate, at suitable concentrations, dissolved in 0.15 M-citrate-phosphate buffer at the appropriate pH. Reactions were started by the addition of 50 μl of the relevant muscle preparation, diluted 1:1 (v/v) with distilled water, and incubated at 37°C in a shaking water bath. Incubation was normally for 20 min, but in kinetic studies this period was reduced to 10 min. Reactions were terminated by the addition of 3.0 ml of 0.2 M-glycine-NaOH buffer containing 0.1 M-Na$_2$CO$_3$ and 0.125 M-NaCl at pH 10.7. For studies with metal ions each enzyme source was preincubated at 4°C with an equal volume of the appropriate metal salt (ZnSO$_4$, CdCl$_2$ or CoSO$_4$) in distilled water and after 1 hour 50 μl was added to 200 μl of the buffered substrate. In all studies fluorescence was determined using a Zeiss ZFM4C spectrofluorimeter (activating wavelength 365 nm, fluorescing at 448 nm) and compared with that of 4-methylumbelliferone standards. The protein content of each preparation was determined by the method of Lowry et al. (1951) and related to bovine serum albumin standards. The activity of α-D-mannosidase was subsequently expressed as nmols of 4-methylumbelliferone released /mg protein/min.

The two pH optima (4.6-5.0 and 6.4-6.8) observed in assays of α-D-mannosidase in the original homogenate of rat gastrocnemius muscle confirmed our earlier findings (Wallace and Lewis, 1977). The acidic and neutral activities were located almost exclusively in the particulate and supernatant fractions respectively. The effect of various metal ions on these two activities was subsequently studied in the appropriate fraction at pH 4.8 or 6.6. Maximum activation (130%) of the acidic α-D-mannosidase was obtained in the presence of Zn^{2+} (0.5 mM) although, as reported previously (Wallace and Lewis, 1977), the pH profile was unaffected by this metal ion. Conversely the neutral activity was inhibited under similar conditions. This contrasting effect of Zn^{2+} has been previously observed in rat liver (Marsh and Gourlay, 1971; Dewald and Touster, 1973) but conflicting results have been reported (Suzuki and Kushida, 1973; Phillips et al., 1974 a,b) for rabbit, bovine and human liver. Our observations on the effect of Cd^{2+} on acidic and neutral α-D-mannosidase in gastrocnemius muscle are in general agreement with studies of this activity in other mammalian tissues (Suzuki and Kushida, 1973). The acidic activity in gastrocnemius muscle was halved in the presence of Cd^{2+} (10 mM) and maximum activation (380%) by Cd^{2+} (5 μM) of the neutral activity was observed. The effect of Co^{2+} on the two activities was similar to, but less marked than, that of Cd^{2+}. Both these metal ions caused a shift of the pH optimum of the neutral activity to 6.0-6.4, a further indication that Co^{2+} and Cd^{2+} stabilize the enzyme (Shoup and Touster, 1976). Our present findings also suggest that α-D-mannosidase activity in the particulate fraction is stimulated by Co^{2+} at pH 5.5-5.8. The existence of α-D-mannosidase with a pH optimum intermediate between the established acidic and neutral activities (Dewald and Touster, 1973; Phillips *et al.*, 1974b; Winchester *et al.*, 1976) requires further investigation in skeletal muscle

Interruption of the normal activity of the motor nerve to skeletal muscle, either by disease or experimental section of the nerve, causes the muscle to atrophy and results in increased levels of acid hydrolases (Weinstock and Iodice, 1969; Maskrey *et al.*, 1977). We have previously reported the effect on several glycosidases following denervation of rat gastrocnemius and soleus muscle (Wallace and Lewis, 1975). A similar procedure, including a 'sham' operation on the contralateral muscles, was adopted in the present study of α-D-mannosidases. It was established in separate experiments that a sham operation, in which the sciatic nerve was exposed but not damaged, does not appear to affect the enzyme activity. Throughout the present study α-D-mannosidase activity was assayed five days following denervation, at which stage in the atrophic process the wet weights of gastrocnemius and soleus muscles were approximately 80% and 70% respectively of the corresponding contralateral muscles.

We have observed no alteration in the pH optima of either acidic or neutral α-D-mannosidases following denervation, although a marked increase in the specific activity of the particulate fraction was obtained. Under our experimental conditions both acid and neutral α-D-mannosidases in denervated and contralateral gastrocnemius muscle appear to obey normal Michaelis-Menten kinetics. The apparent K_m value of 4-methylumbelliferyl-α-D-mannopyranoside, calculated from Lineweaver and Burk plots, was considerably lower for the neutral than for the acidic activity. Dewald and Touster (1973) reported a similar observation in studies on α-D-mannosidases in rat liver.

The K_m value of the activity in the particulate fraction from contralateral muscle, assayed at pH 4.8, is intermediate between those values reported for similar activity in rat liver (Dewald and Touster, 1973) and human liver and leucocytes (Desnick *et al.*, 1976). Although denervation did not affect the apparent K_m, the higher V_{max} values obtained were correlated with the observed increase of acidic activity in denervatd muscle.

Desnick et al. (1976) have reported that the apparent K_m of human liver acidic α-D-mannosidase is altered by Zn^{2+} and Co^{2+}. From our work the three metal ions studied appear to have no significant effect on the K_m of this activity in gastrocnemius muscle. However, in both denervated and contralateral muscles, the V_{max} was increased by Zn^{2+} and decreased in the presence of Cd^{2+} or Co^{2+}. Hultberg and Masson (1975) reported similar effects of Zn^{2+} and Co^{2+} on human liver acidic activity. Zn^{2+} inhibits the neutral activity in both denervated and contralateral muscle. In contrast the V_{max} of this activity in both preparations is significantly increased in the presence of Cd^{2+} or Co^{2+}. That binding between the neutral α-D-mannosidase and the fluorimetric substrate is more effective in the presence of certain metal ions is suggested by our observation that Co^{2+} markedly lowers the apparent K_m of neutral α-D-mannosidase in both normal and denervated gastrocnemius muscle.

Acknowledgements

We are grateful for financial support from the Eastern Health and Social Services Board of Northern Ireland.

Canonico, P.G. and Bird, J.W.C. (1970). J. Cell. Biol., **45**, 321-333.
Carroll, M., Dance, N., Masson, P.K., Robinson, D. and Winchester, B.G. (1972). Biochem. Biophys. Res. Commun., **49**, 579-583.
Conchie, J. and Hay, A.J. (1963). Biochem. J., **87**, 354-361.
Desnick, R.J., Sharp, H.L., Grabowski, G.A., Brunning, R.D., Quie, P.G., Sung, J.H., Gorlin, R.J. and Ikonne, J.U. (1976). Pediat. Res., **10**, 985-996.
Dewald, B. and Touster, O. (1973). J. Biol. Chem., **248**, 7223-7233.
Hultberg, B. and Masson, P.K. (1975). Biochem. Biophys. Res. Commun., **67**, 1473-1479.
Hultberg, B. and Öckerman, P.A. (1972). Clin. Chim. Acta, **39**, 49-58.
Lowry, O.H., Rosebrough, J.H., Farr, A.L. and Randall, R.J. (1951). J. Biol. Chem., **193**, 265-275.
Marsh, C.A. and Gourlay, G.C. (1971). Biochem. Biophys. Acta, **235**, 142-148.
Maskrey, P., Pluskal, M.G., Harris, J.B. and Pennington, R.J.T. (1977). J. Neurochem., **28**, 403-409.
Öckerman, P.A. (1969). Clin. Chim. Acta, **23**, 479-482.
Pearce, G.W. (1966). Ann. N.Y. Acad. Sci., **138**, 138-150.
Phillips, N.C., Robinson, D., Winchester, B.G. and Jolly, R.D. (1974a). Biochem. J., **137**, 363-371.
Phillips, N.C., Robinson, D. and Winchester, B.G. (1974b). Clin. Chim. Acta, **55**, 11-19.
Shoup, V.A. and Touster, O. (1976). J. Biol. Chem., **251**, 3845-3852.
Suzuki, I. and Kushida, H. (1973). J. Biochem. (Tokyo), **74**, 627-629.
Suzuki, I., Kushida, H. and Shida, H. (1969). Seikagaku, **41**, 334-341.
Tappel, A.L., Zalkin, H., Caldwell, K.A., Desai, I.D. and Shibko, S. (1962). Arch. Biochem. Biophys., **96**, 340-346.

Wallace, R.R. and Lewis, M.H.R. (1975). *Biochem. Soc. Trans.*, **3**, 1027-1030.
Wallace, R.R. and Lewis, M.H.R. (1977). *Biochem. Soc. Trans.*, **5**, 231-233.
Weinstock, I.M. and Iodice, A.A. (1969). *In* 'Lysosomes in Biology and Pathology' (Dingle, J.T. and Fell, H.B., eds.), vol. 1, pp.450-468., North-Holland, Amsterdam.
Winchester, B.G., van-de-Water, N.S. and Jolly, R.D. (1976). *Biochem. J.*, **157**, 183-188.

22 Hexokinase in human muscle disease

JENNIFER M. STRICKLAND · DAVID A. ELLIS · JUDITH E. TYE

Pathology Dept., Midland Centre for Neurosurgery and Neurology,
Holly Lane, Smethwick, Warley, West Midlands B67 7JX.

Tracer experiments with [^{14}C] Glucose have shown there to be an increase in the production of fructose from glucose in muscle from patients with Duchenne dystrophy (Ellis *et al.*, 1973). Glucose is converted to fructose by the sorbitol pathway:−

$$
\begin{array}{ccc}
\text{NADPH} \quad \text{NADP} & & \text{NAD} \quad \text{NADH} \\
\text{Glucose} \longrightarrow \text{Sorbitol} & & \longrightarrow \text{Fructose} \\
\text{Aldose} & & \text{Sorbitol} \\
\text{Reductase} & & \text{Dehydrogenase} \\
\text{(polyol-NADP oxidoreductase)} & & \text{(L-iditol-NAD oxidoreductase)} \\
\text{EC. 1.1.1.21} & & \text{EC. 1.1.1.14}
\end{array}
$$

The activities of these two enzymes aldose reductase and sorbitol dehydrogenase, which in normal muscle are barely detectable, are raised considerably in muscle from patients with Duchenne dystrophy (Ellis *et al.*, 1973).

It is possible that glucose is being diverted through this shunt because of inability of the muscle to metabolise glucose through normal pathways, the first step of which is the phosphorylation of glucose to glucose − 6 − phosphate by hexokinase:−

$$
\begin{array}{c}
\text{ATP} \quad \text{ADP} \\
\text{Glucose} \longrightarrow \text{Glucose} - 6 - \text{phosphate} \\
\text{Hexokinase} \\
\text{(ATP − D-hexose 6 phosphotransferase)} \\
\text{EC. 2.7.1.1.}
\end{array}
$$

The total activity of hexokinase in muscle from patients with Duchenne dystrophy compares well with that of normal muscle (Ronzoni *et al.*, 1961; Heyck *et al.*, 1963; Davidenkova *et al.*, 1970). Since hexokinase has three isoenzymes, and the total activity is a summation of the activities of the isoenzymes, it is possible for the activity of one or more of the isoenzymes to vary without necessarily affecting the total activity. It is with this in mind that we have examined the isoenzymes of hexokinase by electrophoresis.

The three isoenzymes of hexokinase (Types I, II and III) are present in all tissues in varying degrees. Type I is the chief isoenzyme of brain and has a K_m of 10^{-5} M; Type II predominates in rat muscle, is insulin-responsive, and has a K_m of 10^{-4} M; Type III is substrate-inhibited and has a K_m of 10^{-6} M (Katzen, 1967).

Fig. 1. shows the isoenzyme patterns observed in muscle from various states of health and disease. The methods for extraction, electrophoresis and staining for all tissues have been given previously (Strickland and Ellis, 1975; Ellis *et al.*, 1976). The complement and distribution of isoenzymes in the male and female groups of the normal controls appears similar,

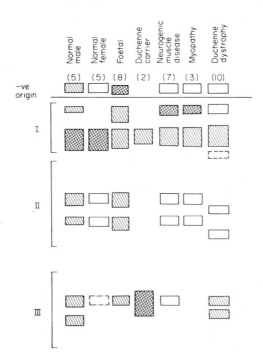

Fig. 1. Hexokinase isoenzyme patterns of human muscle in health and disease. Figures in parenthesis refer to the number of cases. Activity of each band is shown by density of shading.

although the apparent quantity of the isoenzymes clearly differs. Males have similar activity in all isoenzymes, whilst in females there is a predominance of Type I. This was the case in all the controls studied regardless of the site of muscle biopsy, with the exception of the only two cervical muscle samples from females, whose isoenzyme activities resembled those of the males (not illustrated, but see Ellis *et al.*, 1976).

The electrophoretic positions of the isoenzymes from muscle in two confirmed female carriers of Duchenne dystrophy do not seem to differ significantly from the normal. However there is an unusually large amount of Type III isoenzyme in these carriers. The Type II isoenzymes of the Duchenne dystrophy cases have different mobilities to those of all other cases, normal or diseased. Other muscle diseases vary considerably in the activity of each isoenzyme band, but Duchenne dystrophy and Becker dystrophy (not illustrated, but see Strickland and Ellis, 1975) are the only cases which show differing mobilities of Type II isoenzymes. The neurogenic muscle disease group and the myopathic group both contain several different disease states, and the patterns are a summary of a series of results. A fuller exposition has already been given (Ellis *et al.*, 1976).

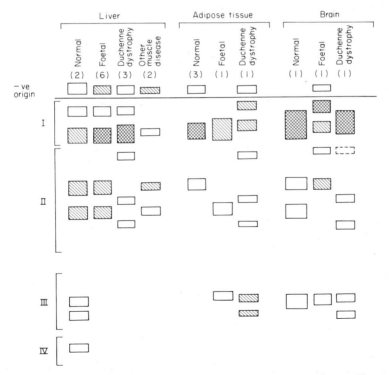

Fig. 2. Hexokinase isoenzyme patterns of human tissues in health and disease. Figures in parenthesis refer to the number of cases. Activity of each band is shown by density of shading.

The abnormal Type II bands are not only seen in the muscle from Duchenne patients, as they also appear in the liver, brain and adipose tissue (Fig. 2). The abnormal bands in brain may be of little metabolic significance, since the brain relies almost exclusively on Type I, and any other isoenzymes will be of minor importance. Differences in Type II isoenzyme will have more effect in muscle, because although there are adequate amounts of Type I present in Duchenne dystrophic muscle, it is known that muscle relies more on Type II for its glucose metabolism (Katzen *et al.*, 1970).

Muscle from Duchenne dystrophy does not resemble foetal muscle in its isoenzyme bands suggesting that the muscle is not reverting to a foetal type of glucose metabolism; furthermore no resemblance is seen in other tissues between isoenzyme patterns from cases with Duchenne dystrophy and foetal isoenzymes. Since the abnormal isoenzyme bands have been seen only in Duchenne and Becker dystrophy (the X-linked recessive dystrophies) it is quite possible that these isoenzymes are the expression of genetic constitution rather than a result of diseased and astrophying cells.

References

Davidenkova, E.F., Verzbinskaya, N.A., Savina, M.V., Schwartz, E.I. (1970). *Zh. Nevropat. Psikiat*, **70**, 1441-1445.

Ellis, D.A., Strickland, J.M., Ecclestone, J.F. (1973). *Clin. Sci.*, **44**, 321-334.

Ellis, D.A., Strickland, J.M., Tye, J.E. (1976). *Biochem. Soc. Trans.*, **4**, 1054-1056.

Heyck, H., Laudahn, G., Luders, C-J. (1963). *Klin. Wschr.*, **41**, 500-509.

Katzen, H.M. (1967). *Adv. Enzyme Regulation*, **5**, 325-356.

Ronzoni, E., Berg, I., Landau, W. (1961). *Res. Publs. Ass. Res. nerv. ment., Dis.*, **38**, 721-729.

Strickland, J.M., Ellis, D.A. (1975). *Nature*, **253**, 464-466.

23 Mitochondria and sarcoplasmic reticulum fragments isolated from slow and fast contracting muscles of the cat

SALLY E. KITCHEN · W.B. VAN WINKLE* · G.S. CRUICKSHANK
G. SPIEGEL† AND ELEANOR ZAIMIS

Department of Pharmacology, Royal Free Hospital School of Medicine, 8 Hunter Street, London WC1N 1BP, U.K.

In skeletal muscle, there is considerable evidence to support the hypothesis of Ebashi (1961) that sequestration of calcium by the sarcoplasmic reticulum is involved in the relaxation phase of the muscle. On the other hand, mitochondria isolated from many sources, e.g. liver, kidney and heart, can also accumulate considerable amounts of calcium (Carafoli and Lehninger, 1971). We therefore decided to measure the calcium sequestering properties of mitochondria isolated from a slow and from a fast contracting muscle of the cat and to compare them with those of the sarcoplasmic reticulum fragments.

Mitochondria were isolated from the soleus (slow) and tibialis (fast) muscles of the cat by the method of Bullock *et al.* (1970); their yield in the 10,000 g sediment from the soleus was 10 mg protein per g wet wt. muscle. This represented 18% of the total mitochondrial fraction in the muscle as measured by the activity of a mitochondrial marker, succinate dehydrogenase (E.C.1.3.9.9.1;) (Pennington, 1961). For the tibialis the corresponding yield was 8.7 mg mitochondrial protein per g wet wt. muscle and this represented 11% of the total muscle mitochondrial fraction. Sarcoplasmic reticulum fragments were isolated by the method of Ash *et al.* (1972). The yield of SRF from the soleus muscle was 1.3 mg, and from the tibialis muscle 1.8 mg, protein per g wet wt. muscle.

Calcium uptake was measured by a millipore filtration technique using $^{45}CaCl_2$ (Ash *et al.*, 1972). For mitochondrial Ca^{2+} uptake the medium contained 100 mM-KC1, 10 mM-$MgCl_2$, 20 mM-tris-maleate buffer pH 7.0, 5 mM-Na_2 succinate, 5 mM-K phosphate pH 7.0, 2.5 mM-Na_2 ATP, 0.1 mM $^{45}CaCl_2$ and 0.2–0.25 mg protein per ml. Incubation temperature was 30°C. For sarcoplasmic reticulum Ca^{2+} uptake, the medium contained

---

* *Present address: Department of Cell Biophysics, Baylor College of Medicine, Houston, Texas, U.S.A.*
† *Present address: Department of Chemistry, Washington University, St. Louis, Missouri, U.S.A.*

100 mM-KC1, 10 mM-MgCl$_2$, 20 mM-tris-maleate buffer pH 6.8, 5 mM-Na oxalate, 2 mM-MgATP, 0.1 mM ^{45}CaCl$_2$ and 15 μg protein per ml. Incubation temperature was 37°C. Addition of azide (an inhibitor of the mitochondrial electron transport chain and of mitochondrial ATPase) to the medium reduced by over 90% Ca^{2+} uptake by mitochondria but uptake by sarcoplasmic reticulum was unchanged. Clearly, there was little cross-contamination between the two fractions.

Sarcoplasmic reticulum fragments isolated from the tibialis took up Ca^{2+} at a significantly faster rate than those from the soleus. In addition, in the absence of the chelating agent oxalate and at a calcium concentration of about 10^{-5} M Ca^{2+} binding by fragments from tibialis was greater than by those from soleus. However, since there is no specific marker enzyme for the sarcoplasmic reticulum it is not possible to be absolutely sure whether the lower Ca^{2+} accumulation by soleus fragments is due to a less pure preparation or to a lower activity of the Ca^{2+} transport system in the sarcoplasmic reticulum. Martonosi and Halpin (1971) showed that the ATPase of the sarcoplasmic reticulum is associated with Ca^{2+} transport. Analysis of our sarcoplasmic reticulum proteins by SDS-acrylamide gel electrophoresis (Weber and Osborn, 1969) revealed that the soleus muscle contained relatively less ATPase protein than tibialis.

For both soleus and tibialis muscles the rate of Ca^{2+} uptake per mg mitochondrial protein was significantly less than that per mg sarcoplasmic reticulum protein even allowing for the different incubation temperatures. When a comparison of the two muscles was made, the results showed that Ca^{2+} uptake per mg mitochondrial protein was greater for the soleus than for the tibialis although when expressed per unit of succinate dehydrogenase activity there was no difference between the two preparations.

It is concluded that sarcoplasmic reticulum fragments take up and bind Ca^{2+} but both processes are significantly faster in preparations isolated from the tibialis muscle than from the soleus. Mitochondria isolated from either muscle take up Ca^{2+} but a slower rate than sarcoplasmic reticulum fragments. Both these organelles could be involved in the relaxation phase of muscles. The fact that the accumulation of Ca^{2+} is significantly faster in the fragments isolated from tibialis could explain the differences between the rates of relaxation of the two muscles.

From our results with the isolated mitochondria it is difficult to quantify their contribution to the relaxation phase. The fact remains that mitochondria of either muscle do take up calcium and that soleus contains more mitochondria than tibialis. We would like to suggest that the mitochondrial calcium uptake may become significant under certain physiological conditions such as an increase in the amount of circulating adrenaline. Adrenaline and other β-adrenoceptor stimulant substances are well known to speed up the relaxation of the slow soleus muscle (Bowman and Zaimis, 1958).

References

Ash, A.S.F., Besch, H.R., Harigaya, S. and Zaimis, E. (1972). *J. Physiol. (Lond.)*, **224**, 1-19.

Bowman, W.C. and Zaimis, E. (1958). *J. Physiol. (Lond.)*, **144**, 92-107.

Bullock, G.R., Carter, E.E. and White, A.M. (1970). *FEBS Letters*, **8**, 109-111.

Carafoli, E. and Lehninger, A.L. (1971). *Biochem. J.*, **122**, 681-690.

Ebashi, S. (1961). *J. Biochem. (Tokyo)*, **50**, 236-244.

Martonosi, A. and Halpin, R.A. (1971). *Arch. Biochem. Biophys.*, **144**, 66-77.

Pennington, R.J. (1961). *Biochem. J.*, **80**, 649-654.

Weber, K. and Osborn, M. (1969). *J. Biol. Chem.*, **244**, 4406-4412.

24 The use of quantitative histochemical techniques in studies on normal and dystrophic muscle fibres

KENNETH HOWELLS · CHRISTOPHER J. BRANFORD WHITE

Department of Biology, Oxford Polytechnic, Headington, Oxford. OX3 0BP. United Kingdom.

The past twenty years has seen a great increase in the application of histo-chemical techniques to studies of normal and diseased muscle fibres. As a result of the specificity and accuracy of localization of modern histochemical procedures these methods are becoming increasingly valuable to the clinician in the diagnosis and assessment of neuromuscular disorders.

The histochemical localization of oxidative enzymes in skeletal muscle fibres has revealed considerable differences in staining intensity between individual fibres within the same muscle, and these variations have been used in early classifications of muscle fibres into 'types' (Dubowitz, 1956; Stein and Padykula, 1960; Romanul, 1964). Because of the present wide clinical usage of histochemical methods for myofibrillar and intermyo-fibrillar ATPases in studies on human muscle fibres, localization of oxida-tive enzymes also plays an important confirmatory role. A great advantage of oxidative enzyme histochemistry is that the procedures used can be adapted to give quantitative results obviating reliance on visual assessment of staining intensity. This can be done using microdensitometric methods or by microscope cytophotometry, usually using sections assayed for succinic dehydrogenase activity with tetrazolium salts as electron acceptors. The first cytophotometric measurements of this enzyme in muscle using frog (Glasz-Moerts *et al.*, 1968), and mouse (Goldspink, 1969) muscle fibres revealed an inverse relationship between the enzyme concentration and fibre size. This was confirmed by further studies on rat (Goldspink and Waterson, 1971) and hamster (Howells and Goldspink, 1974a) muscle fibres from physiologically fast and slow muscles. These techniques have also been used to study the effect of inanition (Goldspink and Waterson, 1971) and the progression of hamster dystrophy (Howells and Goldspink, 1974b) on muscle fibre growth and development. The quantitation possible with cytophotometric and microdensitometric methods was confirmed by elution of deposited tetrazolium formazan, parallel biochemical determina-

281

tions and examination of the specificity of the reaction (Jones *et al.*, 1963; Cabrini *et al.*, 1969; Goldspink, 1969; Butcher, 1970; Eadie *et al.*, 1970; Atlman, 1971; Howells *et al.*, 1977). They can therefore form a valuable adjunct to studies on muscle fibre form and function. In addition computer-aided evaluation of the cytophotometric data and comparison with that obtained from parallel histological and quantitative histochemical prepara-tations, make it possible to gain much fuller details of muscle fibre growth and development and the effect of factors controlling these processes.

Materials and methods

Muscles from normal and dystrophic hamsters were quickly excised, immersed in 10% polyvinyl alcohol (to minimize ice crystal formation during subsequent freezing and thawing) and frozen at their *in vivo* resting lengths in liquid Freon pre-cooled to a viscous fluid with liquid nitrogen. They were then stored on a bed of dry ice, and groups of muscles quickly mounted in Ames O.C.T. Embedding Medium (Miles Laboratories, Indiana, U.S.A.) after which they were re-frozen in liquid Freon. By this means it was found possible to freeze the muscles at their resting lengths and so obtain valid fibre size distributions. Transverse sections 6μm in thickness were cut on a Cambridge rocking rotary microtome in a Bright

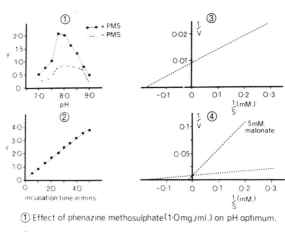

① Effect of phenazine methosulphate (1·0 mg./ml.) on pH optimum.

② Effect of incubation time on Nitro BT formazan deposition.

③ Lineweaver & Burke determination of K_m.

④ Competitive inhibition by malonate.

Fig. 1. Cytophotometric determination of Nitro Blue Tetrazolium (Nitro BT) diformazan deposition in muscle fibre sections incubated for SDH activity. These studies agree closely with microdensitometric studies by Butcher (1970) using neotetrazolium chloride, and indicate that SDH activity as determined by cytophotometric methods can give very similar results to those obtained by biochemical techniques.

cryostat. The temperature inside the cryostat was −30°C. and the microtome knife was cooled further with dry ice. The sections were mounted on coverslips, brought to room temperature and air dried for 10 minutes prior to incubation. Sections were incubated for succinic dehydrogenase activity using the method of Wattenburg and Leong (1960) and phenazine methosulphate (PMS) was added to give a final concentration of 1mg/ml. The pH of the incubation medium was 7.8. Control sections were incubated in the presence of malonate (Butcher, 1970). Histochemical and histological preparations were also made from adjacent sections.

Cytophotometric readings of SDH activity were made on a Leitz MPVI microscope photometer fitted with an RCA 1P21 photomultiplier. Illumination was provided by a ribbon filament lamp with constant voltage supply; and monochromasy of this light source was effected by a Schott VERIL S200 graduated interference line filter. The output from the photometer, after amplification, was displayed on a Pye Scalamp galvanometer and also transferred to a paper tape puncher for computing analysis. The two wavelength method of Patau (1952) was used. For each absorbance reading, four measurements are made, two at each wavelength. At each wavelength, absorbance was measured with the object in the measuring area, and also a reference reading was taken on the same portion of the same muscle fibre in the control section (incubated in the presence of malonate). Six such absorbance readings were made on each muscle fibre, three at points on the periphery of and three at points in the centre of the fibre. The means of

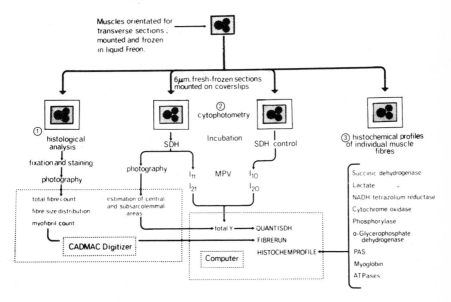

Fig. 2. Experimental scheme.

these two sets of readings were taken. The area of each measuring field was 1.5 × 1.5 μm. The fibres to be measured were taken from over the whole cross-sectioned area of the muscle so as to cover the whole range of fibre diameters present in the muscle. Fifty fibres per muscle were sampled and each fibre was photographed for determination of fibre area, and to quantify the central and peripheral areas in the case of fibres showing a visible subsarcolemmal ring of intense staining.

Computer aided data analysis

An interactive graphic system comprising: CADMAC Digitizer/Plotter, Tetronix 611 storage display unit, PD11/20 computer was used. Three programmes were displayed:

(i) *Quantisdh*. Each muscle fibre selected for cytophotometry was photographed and prints made at set magnifications. The outline of the fibre was plotted on the Digitizer and each fibre was assigned an identification number. Cytophotometric data of diformazan deposition (Y), is fed in and the programme displays:

  (a) a scale representation of the fibre cross section, with central and peripheral areas if present
  (b) mean central and peripheral Y values
  (c) total fibre Y, central and peripheral Y
  (d) fibre area and central and peripheral areas
  (e) a plot of total fibre Y against fibre area.

(ii) *Fibrerun*. The Digitizer data on muscle fibre area is combined with histological results to give:

  (a) fibre size distributions
  (b) myofibril numbers
  (c) myofibrillar density
  (d) a plot of myofibril number against fibre size.

Work is currently in progress to extend this program to include myofibril size distributions.

(iii) *Histochemprofile*. The staining intensity of the identified fibres for selected histochemical reactions is assessed visually on a 1-4 scale and is presented in this form.

Results

Two main sets of results are provided by this study; information on the muscle as a whole as indicated by the fifty fibres sampled (Fig. 3), and analysis of individual muscle fibres. From Fig. 3, the normal hamster biceps showed a linear increase in SDH activity with increasing fibre size up to 2000 μm^2., above which SDH concentration decreased. This was also seen in the dystrophic muscle fibres, but a marked decrease in enzyme activity was present in all the fibres, being most noticeable in the larger ones. In Fig. 4, the data collected for a small fibre in the hamster soleus is shown. Using the various histochemical criteria for classification of fibres into types, the information could, for example, be very useful in studies on human muscle fibres, where fibre typing is widely used.

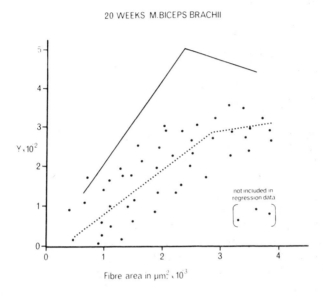

Fig. 3. Total Nitro Blue Tetrazolium diformazan deposition (Y) in arbitrary units plotted against muscle fibre area. Previous histological studies (Howells and Goldspink, 1974c) have shown that by 20 weeks of age the dystrophic hamster biceps has lost approximately 25% of its total fibre complement and the mean muscle fibre area is 40% lower than that of the normal biceps. − Normal (data points not shown); . . . . Dystrophic.

At present this experimental method is limited by the memory storage available in the computer; it is hoped shortly to put the system on-line to an ICL 1905 computer, and thus to expand analysis of the data. With automatic analysis of results from different muscles (which at present is not on these computer programs), and a more comprehensive summation of the properties of individual fibres to provide more detailed information on a given muscle, this technique should more than justify itself. Although we have used microscope photometry for this study, quantitative histochemical preparations are equally amenable to microdensitometric analysis. Preliminary investigations using a Vickers M85 microdensitometer have indicated that the latter method will give comparable results, and it does permit more rapid aquisition of data.

FIBRERUN

HISTOCHEMPROFILE

QUANTISDH

M. SOLEUS R412 N HAMSTER 20 WEEKS

FIBRE IDENTIFICATION 21

21 FIBRE AREA 1450	21 HISTOCHEMPROFILE
21 MYOFIBRIL No 1312	SDH 4
21 MYOFIBRIL DENSITY 1.10	NADHTR 4
21 DENSITY CENTRAL AREA ONLY 2.43	LDH 3
21 SDH CONTENT Y	CYTOX NOT DONE
CENTRAL AREA 595 SUBSARCO AREA 855	AGLYPIDEH 1
CENTRAL MEAN Y 0.33 SUBSARCO 0.63	PHOSPHORYLASE 1
CENTRAL TOTAL Y 91 SUBSARCO 247	PAS NOT DONE
FIBRE TOTAL Y 338	OILRED O NOT DONE
	ATPASE 4.3 4
	ATPASE 9.4 1

Fig. 4. Reconstruction of computer display on data collected from one muscle fibre; in this case a small fibre from a 20 week normal hamster soleus.

Acknowledgements

Part of this work was financed by grants from the Muscular Dystrophy Group of Great Britain to one of the authors (K.H.). We are grateful to Mr. A. Brown of the Department of Computation, Hull University, and Mr. T. Fox of the Computing Centre, Oxford Polytechnic for expert help with the computer programming.

References

Altman, F.P. (1971). *Histochemie*, **27**, 125-136.
Butcher, R.G. (1970). *Exp. Cell Res.*, **60**, 54-60.
Cabrini, R.L., Vinuales, E.J. and Itoiz, M.E. (1969). *Acta Histochem*, **34**, 287-291.
Dubowtiz, V. (1957). *J. Neurol. Neurosurg. Psychiat.*, **28**, 516-523.
Eadie, M.J., Tyrer, J.H., Kukums, J.R. and Hooper, W.D. (1970). *Histochemie*, **21**, 170-180.
Glasz-Moerts, J.J., Diegenback, P.C. and Van der Stelt, A. (1968). *Proc. Kon. Ned. Akad. Van. Wet. C. Biol. Med. Sci.*, **71**, 337-383.
Goldspink, G. (1969). *Life Sci.*, **8**, 791-808.
Goldspink, G. and Waterson, S. (1971). *Acta Histochem*, **40**, 16-22.
Howells, K.F. and Goldspink, G. (1974a). *Histochemie*, **38**, 195-201.
Howells, K.F. and Goldspink, G. (1974b). *Histochem. J.*, **6**, 523-530.

Howells, K.F. and Goldspink, G. (1974c). *J. Anat.*, **117**, 385-396.
Howells, K.F., White, C.J.B. and Goldspink, G. (1977). *Leitz Sci. Tech. Information*, **9,** in press.
Jones, G.R.N., Maple, A.J., Aves, E.K., Chayen, J. and Cunningham, G.J. (1963). *Nature (Lond.)*, **197,** 568-569.
Patau, K. (1952). *Chromosoma*, **5,** 341-362.
Romanul, F.C.A. (1964). *Arch. Neurol.*, **11,** 355-371.
Stein, J.M. and Padykua, H.A. (1964). *Am. J. Anat.*, **110,** 103-115.
Wattenburg, L.W. and Leong, J.L. (1960). *J. Histochem. Cytochem.*, **8,** 296-306.

25 Enzyme histochemical observations on benign sex-linked recessive muscular dystrophy (Becker type)

HANS H. GOEBEL

Division of Neuropathology, University of Göttingen

Introduction

Precise classification of the type of muscular dystrophy is of vital importance for the patient's prognosis as well as for the genetic implications for other members of the family. Among the slowly evolving and progressive neuromuscular disorders of older children, adolescents and young adults, differential diagnostic evaluation has to consider entities such as juvenile spinal muscular atrophy (Kugelberg-Welander), autosomal recessive limb girdle dystrophy, occasionally facio-scapulo-humeral dystrophy, congential myopathies of late infantile or juvenile onset and benign sex-linked muscular dystrophy of the Becker type. Sporadic cases of any of these disorders are much more difficult to diagnose than familial cases. In addition, a very young boy with a progressive myopathy who is an only diseased member of his family, poses the problem of the differential diagnostic aspects of Duchenne's versus Becker's dystrophy.

In order to perceive the entire spectrum of the benign sex-linked muscular dystrophy of the Becker type, precise investigations utilizing modern enzyme histochemical techniques can be helpful. Since the report on two families described by Becker (1962) did not entail morphological studies by biopsy or at autopsy, such findings obtained by a later biopsy from one of the original patients are presented here.

Clinical data

The boy (subject 7 of Fig. 3; Becker, 1962) has always been a frail and somewhat weak child compared to his school mates. He was noted to have a peculiar way of running. He experienced a normal motor development. When 10 years old (Becker, 1962) no muscle atrophy was noted but both his calves were slightly enlarged and firm. There was a limited dorsal flexion of both his feet. Running and walking were not impaired but he was unable to hop stairs on one foot. When climbing stairs, he spread his legs wide apart.

289

For the past 2-3 years he had experienced increasing difficulties in climbing stairs or getting up from a squatting position, physical exertion was occasionally associated with muscle ache. Examination revealed a thin, (166 cm tall) 22-year-old man weighing 60 Kg. His proximal limb muscles appeared atrophic, their strength was reduced, but muscle tone appeared normal. He climbed stairs slowly and was only able to rise from a squatting position twice consecutively. Slight hypertrophy of both calves was present. His deep tendon reflexes were either weak or negative but no pathological reflexes or any other neurological deficits were encountered. His intellectual performance was within normal limits.

Laboratory data

Creatine phosphokinase levels were 160, 120 and 100 mU/ml (normal up to 50 mU/ml). No abnormalities were noted in his electrocardiogram. Electromyographic tracings taken from his left quadriceps and left anterior tibialis muscles were compatible with a myopathy comprising short units 2-3 msec. and amplitudes between 500 and 1800 μV. These small units were found intermingled with normal units of 4-5 msec. and amplitudes of about 1000 μV. The interference pattern was rarified. Bizarre polyphasic units were more obvious in the tibialis muscle with amplitudes between 600 and 1200 μV. Muscle biopsy was obtained from the left biceps muscle at the age of 22 years.

Morphology

Light microscopical observations revealed surprisingly mild changes at the age of 22 years. A broadened spectrum of fibre diameters (Fig. 1) involving both atrophic and hypertrophic fibres of both types (Fig. 2) is shown. Calculations using the ATPase preparation after alkaline preincubation gave the following numerical distribution of type I- and type II-fibres which are approximately within normal limits.

	Type I-fibres	Type II-fibres
Distribution	43%	57%
Mean fibre diameter	52,5 μ	53,55 μ
Standard deviation	17,15	21,07
Variability coefficient	326	393
Atrophy factor	1023	1368
Hypertrophy factor	209	254

Myofibres were round, in places separated by increased endomysium but no necrosis, phagocytosis, or regeneration of myofibres were encountered. The opaque fibres and groups of necrotic or regenerating fibres typical of Duchenne's dystrophy and also depicted in Becker's muscular

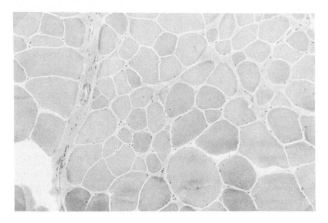

Fig. 1. Enlarged spectrum of myofibre diameter, endomysial thickening and some numerical increase of internal muscle fibre nuclei represent the myopathic features. Trichrome; × 210.

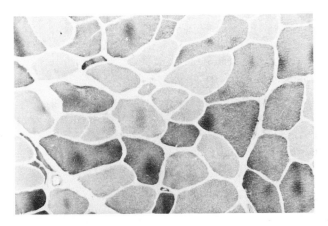

Fig. 2. Type I (light) and type II (dark) myofibres are well differentiated. Atrophic fibres belong to both types. ATPase, pH 9.3; × 215.

dystrophy (Dubowitz and Brooke, 1973) were also absent. Type II-fibres differentiated well into IIA- and IIB-fibres, though type IIB-fibres outnumbered IIA-fibres by almost 100%. Several angular fibres were present belonging to both fibre types. Some of them gave strong reactions for NADH-tetrazolium reductase and menadione linked α-Glycerophosphate dehydrogenase. Other hallmarks of neurogenic atrophy such as group atrophy or fibre type grouping were absent.

Electron microscopic investigation revealed no specific findings. Nonspecific pathological observations entailed focal loss of myofilaments, increase of lipid droplets and lipofuscin, folding and reduplication of muscle basal lamina and pentad formation in atrophic myofibres.

Comment

It is rare to have the opportunity to apply newly developed diagnostic techniques to tissues from cases described earlier of unidentified diseases which have later gained a wide-spread recognition. Becker's benign sex-linked muscular dystrophy is an example of such a well established entity reported about 20 years ago (Becker and Kiener, 1955). Since enzyme histochemical studies had not been performed on biopsies from any member of the families described by Becker (1962) the opportunity for such morphological investigations appeared both timely and promising. Indeed, the enzyme histochemical and histological alterations in the biceps muscle at the age of 22 years in Becker's muscular dystrophy turned out to be rather mild. This may reflect one end of the morphological spectrum in Becker's muscular dystrophy. It also emphasises the need for further studies on other members of originally described families. Although fibres reacting strongly to tests for oxidative enzyme activity might indicate a neurogenic component in our patient's biopsy, the remainder of the pathological muscle changes appeared myopathic.

Acknowledgements

I am grateful for clinical and electromyographic details provided by H. Steuber, M.D. and F. Duensing, M.D., both from the Department of Neurology, University of Göttingen. Assistance in preparing the histograms by Mrs. I. Fehrensen and in photography by Mr. H.J. Zobel is very much appreciated. This study was in part supported by a grant from the Volkswagenstiftung.

References

Becker, P.E. (1962). *Rev. Canad. Biol.*, **21**, 551-566.
Becker, P.E. and Kiener, F. (1955). *Arch. Psychiat. Nervenkr.*, **193**, 427-448.
Dubowitz, V. and Brooke, M.H. (1973). Muscle biopsy: A modern approach. W.B. Saunders Corp., London-Philadelphia-Toronto.

26 The use of animal models in the study of human neuromuscular diseases

A ROUND TABLE DISCUSSION ORGANISED BY R.L. WATTS

Department of Biochemistry, Guy's Hospital Medical School, London, S.E.1. 9RT.

The title of this discussion, in using the word 'models' of human disease, may be thought to imply a very simple relationship between disrupted function in the animal and in the human. A true *model* should reflect all the observable features of its original. First, therefore, we have to examine whether this is true in specific cases. We have to consider the clinical picture, the pathology and any experimental findings in the animal in the context of the possible human diseases of which it may be a model. At the same time, we have to remember that the chances of finding a perfect model for any human disease are remote. It may be that some of us are depressed at this thought, for instance because findings with the animal, such as encouraging results with drug-testing, cannot simply be applied in man. However, in the deeper context of understanding life processes, and this includes disease processes, the fact is that the differences, once we appreciate them, are one of the main strengths of models.

It is probably the geneticist in me that stands up to say that a series of slightly different disruptions of the same function can provide a ringful of keys to the locked doors of understanding that function. I look back at the power of this approach in genetics to my student days when Beadle and Tatum had shown that a series of mutations in the mould *Neurospora* disrupted its growth by their effects on a series of steps in a biosynthetic pathway, and thus made possible the birth of the one gene-one enzyme hypothesis (Beadle, 1945; Bonner, 1946; Horowitz and Leupold, 1951). The power of this concept was not lessened by the fact that it predated an understanding of the structure of DNA and its role in heredity, and its proposers did not fail to note that not all genes would be found to determine the structure and specificity of enzymes. More recently, both their method and their wisdom have again been illustrated, for the almost unbelievably detailed things we now know (Gilbert *et al.*, 1974; Dickson *et al.*, 1975) about the *lac* operon in *E. coli* and how it works rest upon the use of mutations that disrupt its function (Monod *et al.*, 1962).

293

In the human muscular dystrophies, the pointers at present (Edwards, 1977; Brooks and Emery, 1977) suggest that some of our difficulties of understanding may arise because the mutations are in an unusual kind of gene. Maybe this is true. Maybe we have a genetic problem to solve, among others. But not by genetic techniques alone; the comparison of effects of mutations within an organism is just one approach. We have a different approach — the comparison of related disruptions of the same function in a series of organisms. We are going to consider here a number of these in man and animals that are genetically determined and also some that are brought about by experimental techniques. Each of them will have its own special messages for us and will offer us particular chances for the future. But all of them, taken together, offer us a way into the two inextricably joined mysteries that we pursue, the mysteries of normal function in muscle acting under nervous control, and the disfunction of these systems in man that all of us would like to be able to alleviate.

References

Beadle, G.W. (1945). *Physiol. Rev.*, **25**, 643-663.
Bonner, D. (1946). *Cold Spring Harbor Symp. Quant. Biol.*, **11**, 14-24.
Brooks, A. and Emery, A.E.H. (1977). Seventh Symposium on Current Research in Muscular Dystrophy. Abstract 2.
Dickson, R.C., Abelson, J., Barnes, W.M. and Reznikoff, W.S. (1975). *Science*, **187**, 27-35.
Edwards, J.H. (1977). Seventh Symposium on Current Research in Muscular Dystrophy Abstract 1.
Gilbert, W., Maizels, N. and Maxam, A. (1974). *Cold Spring Harbor. Symp. Quant. Biol.*, **38**, 845-855.
Horowitz, N.H. and Leupold, U. (1951). *Cold Spring Harbor Symp. Quant. Biol.*, **16**, 65-74.
Monod, J., Jacob, F. and Gros, F. (1962). *Biochem. Soc. Symp. (Cambridge Eng.)*, **21**, 104-132.

The dystrophic mouse (129Re-dy)

HEATHER STEPHENS

Departments d'Anatomie et de Pharmacologie, Faculte de Medecine, Université de Montréal, Montréal, Quebec, Canada. H3C 3J7.

Dystrophia muscularis, the first genetically determined animal model for muscular dystrophy to be discovered, appeared as a spontaneous mutation in a colony of inbred mice (strain 129Re) at the Jackson Laboratory, Bar Harbor, Maine (Michelson *et al.*, 1955). The disease is characterized by muscular weakness, particularly of the hindlimbs, which cannot support the animal in either a climbing or a hanging position, and, when the animal is suspended by the tail are clasped together, instead of held splayed as a normal mouse. In the early stages, one or both hindlimbs are dragged following stress. Later the hind limbs are dragged all the time and become completely paralysed. Also in response to stress the animal makes characteristic 'gasping' motions, nodding the head while the mouth gapes, and it may paw its mouth; these movements probably result from its difficulty in breathing. Occasional seizures occur in younger animals, when the mouse hurtles round the cage for a few seconds then collapses and lies inert for a few seconds before recovery. Other features include a defective growth pattern, inflammation of the skin, a scruffy coat, and eye defects resulting in late opening of one or both eyes during postnatal development. From about 8 or 10 weeks the body weight declines, there is pronounced kyphosis and the heart is affected as well as the diaphragm. Most mutant animals that survive to this stage die between 3 and 6 months of age, often of pneumonia. Neither sex normally breeds.

The disease shows autosomal recessive inheritance although the theoretical 25% dystrophic animals is seldom recovered from matings of heterozygotes, probably because they are less viable than littermates during foetal and early postnatal life. The gene has been located on chromosome 10. The gene is commonly maintained by test-mating of sibs of dystrophic animals. There is no known method of carrier detection apart from this. In some laboratories stocks are raised by ovarian transplant from *dy/dy* females into ovarectomized non-dystrophic females, which can either be mated to normal males to produce all heterozygous offspring or artificially inseminated with *dy/dy* sperm to produce all dystrophic litters. At the Jackson laboratory, some litters were produced by artificial insemination of hormone-treated young dystrophic females (Wolfe and Southard, 1962).

Many of the histopathological correlates of muscle degeneration are similar to those found in other forms of animal and human muscular dystrophy and may be a non-specific response common to several forms of muscle injury. They include variation in fibre size and shape, fibre splitting, haphazard fibre distribution, internal nuclear rowing and amyloidosis. Features characteristic of dystrophic muscle in the mouse include the absence of pronounced fibre hypertrophy, the preferential involvement of type I fibres in muscular atrophy, abortive regeneration, and partial replacement of necrotic fibres by interstitial and to a small extent by adipose tissue (West and Murphy, 1960; Susheela *et al.*, 1968).

On the basis of the histological abnormalities, Pearce and Walton (1963) suggested that the human disease most closely resembled by murine dystrophy was dystrophia myotonica. There is also a resemblance in physiological phenomena, for Sandow and Brust (1962) showed that, although contraction time was normal, relaxation was delayed. However, myopathies found in man and mouse differ in various respects. The dystrophic mouse is unique among all known myopathies in having an extensive peripheral nerve abnormality, which consists of large amyelinated areas in the cranial nerves (Biscoe *et al.*, 1975) in the ventral cervical and lumbosacral roots and in the mixed spinal nerves (Bradley and Jenkinson, 1975) Bradley (page 301). There are resemblances to human myopathies in the elevation of some muscle enzymes, such as the NADP+-linked dehydrogenases and the acid hydrolases (McCaman, 1963, Pennington, 1964) and the reduced level of AMP deaminase (Pennington, 1963) but these may be non-specific effects of muscle damage. The characteristic extreme elevation of serum creatine kinase levels seen in human dystrophies is not found in the mouse (Dreyfus *et al.*, 1966; Watts *et al.*, Chapter 28).

In homozygotes, the *dy* gene seems to have an effect on many systems with respect to alterations in enzyme levels, nutrient and drug transport and turnover rates (Stephens, Chapter 29). There are also diverse biological effects. The thymus of older dystrophic mice weighs more than that of control animals (de Kretser and Livett, 1976). The histological architecture of the thymus is disrupted, and this is often accompanied by stimulation of phagocytic reticular cells (Stephens, 1976). Although the large arteries do not appear to be abnormal, the microvasculature is dilated as compared with control animals (Stephens and Sandborn, 1976). The percentage of total area occupied by vascular lumen in sections of a number of tissues is shown in Table 1. This marked vasodilation may reflect an imbalance in vasomoter regulation, since the abnormality of the peripheral nervous system affects the sympathetic component (Biscoe *et al.*, 1975). Alterna-

TABLE 1
Degree of vascularization in tissues of control and dystrophic mice
(Values are mean ± standard deviation)

Tissue	% Area occupied by Vascular Lumen	
	Control	Dystrophic
Oesophagus:		
mucosa	6.80 ± 4.17	10.57 ± 1.37
musculature	3.45 ± 0.50	5.41 ± 2.24
Thymus:	2.25 ± 0.25	6.27 ± 2.14
Dorsal root of peripheral nerve from lumbar spinal cord:	1.72 ± 0.84	4.39 ± 0.87
Liver: excluding sinusoids	2.25 ± 0.27	6.21 ± 2.14
sinusoids	14.61 ± 1.23	20.43 ± 5.26

tively, the vasodilation may be a response to elevated histamine levels due to the increased number of mast cells in several tissues (Bois, 1964). The lumen of the oesophagus is also dilated, the adrenals often hypertrophied and the liver depleted of glycogen stores, perhaps as a reaction to stress (Stephens, 1976).

There has as yet been no major breakthrough in the search for the primary biochemical lesion behind the muscular dystrophies. Murine muscular dystrophy, like other myopathies, has multisystem involvement. It remains to be determined whether these changes are secondary to some other primary disorder yet to be uncovered, or whether they reflect a generalized membrane disorder.

References

Biscoe, T.J., Caddy, K.W., Pallot, D.J. and Pehrson, U.M. (1975). *J. Neurol. Neurosurg. Psychiat.*, **38**, 391-403.
Bois, P. (1964). *Am. J. Physiol.*, **206**, 338-340.
Bradley, W.G. and Jenkinson, M. (1975). *J. Neurol. Sci.*, **25**, 249-255.
de Kretzer, T.A. and Livett, B.G. (1976). *Nature (Lond.)*, **263**, 683-684.
McCaman, M.W. (1963). *Am. J. Physiol.*, **205**, 897-901.
Michelson, A.M., Russell, E.S. and Harman, P.J. (1955). *Proc. Natl. Acad. Sci.*, **41**, 1079-1084.
Pearce, G.W. and Walton, J.N. (1963). *J. Path. Bact.*, **86**, 25-33.
Pennington, R.J. (1963). *Biochem. J.*, **88**, 64-68.
Pennington, R.J. (1974). *In* 'Disorders of Voluntary Muscle', Walton, J.N. (ed.). 488-516.
Sandow, A. and Brust, M. (1962). *Am. J. Physiol.*, **202**, 1126-1127.
Stephens, H. (1976). Ph.D Thesis, Université de Montréal.
Stephens, H. and Sandborn, E. (1976). *In* 'Microcirculation Vol.2. Transport Mechanisms. Disease States', J. Grayson and W. Zingg (eds.), 330-332.
Susheela, A.K., Hudgson, P. and Walton, J.N. (1968). *J. Neurol. Sci.*, **7**, 437-463.
West, W.T. and Murphy, E.D. (1960). *Anat. Rec.*, **137**, 279-295.
Wolfe, H.G. and Southard, J.L. (1962). *Proc. Soc. Exptl. Biol. Med.*, **109**, 630-633.

Discussion

W.G. BRADLEY

In 1972 and subsequently we reported on the abnormalities of the peripheral nervous system of dystrophic mice of the *dy/dy* and *dy2J/dy2J* strain (Bradley and Jenkison, 1972, 1973, 1975). In the posterior and anterior spinal roots and in the cranial nerve roots, as well as in the proximal limb plexuses to a lesser extent, many of the axons of up to 8 μm diameter are crowded together without Schwann cell enwrapment. The nerve appears as if arrested at the foetal stage. The physiological effects of this have recently been reported (Huizar *et al.*, 1975). We have also shown that there is a decrease in the amounts of slow flowing protein, and an increase in the amount of fast flowing protein in axonal transport (Bradley and Jaros, 1973), and this has since been confirmed (Komiya and Austin, 1974; Jablecki and Brimijoin, 1974).

My colleague, Mrs. Evelyn Jaros has recently completed quantitative electron microscopic and autoradiographic analysis of the peripheral nervous system in murine muscular dystrophy. The abnormality of the lumbosacral nerve roots is present at birth, when the number of myelinated fibres is reduced to about half of normal. In the adult the number of myelinated fibres is only 1 or 2% of normal. The total number of Schwann cells is reduced to about ⅔ of normal throughout life, and the rate of division of the Schwann cells, as indicated by the labelling index following tritiated thymidine injection, is relatively normal in the dystrophic mouse. It thus seems likely that the gross decrease in the number of myelinated fibres is in major part due to a deficiency of Schwann cell enwrapment and myelination rather than due to a deficiency of the number of the Schwann cells.

More peripheral parts of the nervous system also show abnormalities in the dystrophic mouse. Despite original uncertainty, it does appear that there is a mild loss of myelinated nerve fibres in the motor nerve. The anterior horn cells however are normal in number and structure (Papapetropoulos and Bradley, 1972). In the peripheral nerves, there is evidence of Schwann cell and myelin abnormalities. The internodal length is shortened, the myelin sheath thinner, and the nodal gap considerably elongated compared with normal (Bradley *et al.*, 1977). There is evidence of abnormal Schwann cell behaviour, including more than one myelinated axon in a Schwann cell, and the retraction of Schwann cell cytoplasm from the nodes of Ranvier, as well as a reduction in the labelling index during Wallerian degeneration.

There is clearly developmental and continuing abnormality of the Schwann cells in murine muscular dystrophy. We interpret this as indicating that murine dystrophy is a multi-system disease, and not one entirely restricted to the skeletal muscle. It is not likely that these abnormalities are either the cause of or the response to skeletal muscle degeneration, since abnormalities of the peripheral nerves such as these are not seen in human or other animal muscle degenerations.

References

Bradley, W.G. and Jarose, E. (1973). *Brain*, **96**, 247-258.

Bradley, W.G., Jaros, E. and Jenkinson, M. (1977). *J. Neuropath. Exp. Neurol.* **36**, 797-806.

Bradley, W.G. and Jenkison, M. (1972). *Lancet*, **ii**, 384.

Bradley, W.G. and Jenkison, M. (1973). *J. neurol. Sci.*, **18**, 227-247.

Bradley, W.G. and Jenkison, M. (1975). *J. neurol. Sci.*, **25**, 249-255.

Huizar, P., Kuno, M. and Miyata, Y. (1975). *J. Physiol.*, **248**, 231-246.

Jablecki, C. and Brimijoin, F. (1974). *Nature (Lond.)*, **250**, 151-153.

Komiya, Y. and Austin, L. (1974). *Exp. Neurol.*, **43**, 1-12.

Papapetropoulos, T.A. and Bradley, W.G. (1972). *J. Neurol. Neurosurg. Psychiat.*, **35**, 60-65.

D.C. Watts: Further evidence of liver involvement in the 129Re-*dy* mouse has been found in measurements made by Andy Johns, Phil Mason and me of liver enzyme levels. The activities per g. wet weight of tissue (or per whole liver) of glucose-6-phosphate dehydrogenase (G6PD) and 6-phosphogluconate dehydrogenase were both about 200% higher in dystrophics. These enzymes are also elevated in dystrophic mouse muscle (M.W. McCaman, *Science* **132**, 621-622, 1960). There could be a whole-body switch to a more reducing metabolism involving NADP$^+$-linked enzymes, related, in turn, to the increased deposition of lipid. No differences were found in liver G6PD isoenzymes patterns.

Branford White: Is anything known of the organization of collagen fibrils in the basement membrane of the endplate region, or if this is changed in the dystrophic mouse?

Professor Bradley: This had not been looked at. The molecular structure of basement membranes is as yet undetermined.

Vrbova: Which part of the vascular bed shows the increase in volume? Is the blood pressure abnormal in dystrophic mice?

Stephens: The dilation is in the smaller vessels. It is very difficult to measure the blood pressure of a mouse. Bond and Leonard (*Proc. Soc. Exp. Biol. Med.,* **100**, 189-191, 1959), reported no differences in the total blood volume per unit body weight or in erythrocyte and plasma volumes in the dystrophic mouse.

Bradley: (Answering a question on axonal packing). The total number of axons in the dorsal roots in dystrophic mice is normal. The Schwann cells have a basement membrane which is patchy in appearance.

Neerunjun: Our discussion of the dystrophic mouse has been entirely about one of the mouse models, 129Re-*dy*, the first to be discovered. For completeness, we ought to note the existence of at least two other kinds of dystrophic mice. The first, C57B1-*dy*2J (*Life Science,* **9**, 137, 1970), is the result of a mutation on chromosome 10, like *dy*. The disease is milder and these mice have been used quite widely. The other, *myd* (myo-dystrophy) results from a mutation on chromosome 8; the severity of the disease is very like that caused by *dy*, except that the hindlimbs do not become paralysed, and the histological findings are very similar. So far as I know, no other tissues have been reported to be affected. (Lane, *et al., J. Hered.* (1976), **67**, 135).

The dystrophic chicken as an experimental model

E.A. BARNARD

Department of Biochemistry, Imperial College, London, S.W.7.

The chicken is not a species that immediately springs to mind for common laboratory use in the study of some pathological state, but I would like to draw attention to the experimental advantages of these animals for the study of muscular dystrophy. The disease is inherited as a single Mendelian autosomal trait. Strains with hereditary dystrophy have become available by breeding at the University of California, Davis and selected, e.g., for various ages of onset of clinical symptoms (Asmundson and Julian, 1956). Thus, line 304 has particularly early onset, the first symptoms appearing within the first 3 weeks of age. The main features of the disease are:
(i) a muscle weakness which spares the grossly red muscles and largely affects the white muscles, the fast twitch, 'type II' fibres being affected first;
(ii) an initial hypertrophy of the most affected muscles, and atrophy at the late stages;
(iii) progressive changes in structure in the affected muscles, including formation of a wide range of fibre sizes and shapes, with some fibre splitting, as well as vacuolization, inflammatory cell invasion and infiltration by adipose and connective tissue;
(iv) modifications of muscle fibre type, as shown by histochemical enzyme staining patterns and overall muscle enzyme contents, e.g., an increase in high-oxidative fibres and lower glycogenolytic activities;
(v) selection of the white muscles, and those proximal to the mid-line, for the histopathological changes mentioned;
(vi) an increase in blood plasma creatine phosphokinase (CPK), progressive with the disease, and reaching extremely high levels (eventually >15,000 mU/ml, compared to about 300 in the normal chicken).

Data on these changes are given by Julian and Asmundson (1963), Cardinet *et al.* (1972) and Julian (1973). These and other investigators of this disease have pointed out the similarity of many of its features to muscular dystrophies in man.

Measurement of progress of chicken muscular dystrophy

A unique feature of this species is the ease of applying a 'performance test', i.e. a test of muscular disability in the living animal as shown in an unequivocal performance which can be scored quantitatively. This is the Flip Test (Asmundson, Kratzer and Julian, 1966) in which the fully dystrophic bird, when placed on its back, is seen to be unable to right itself.

A bird must use its wings to rise from this position, and weakness or stiffness in the large white muscles controlling the wing elevation is readily perceived in the righting performance. For obvious anatomical reasons, an equivalent Flip Test is not applicable in a dystrophic mammal. In the test, the bird is placed on its back five times and allowed to rise. A normal bird invariably scores a Flip Number of five out of five successful attempts, rising in a rapid, co-ordinated movement. As dystrophy develops, the chicks have increasing difficulty, struggling up fewer and fewer times, and eventually will score 0/5. The progression of the Flip Number with age, in chickens homozygous for dystrophy, is shown in Fig. 1. The unbroken line shows that (in the 304 birds, bred for early onset) a highly significant difference from the normals is apparent at day 10 *ex ovo* and thereafter.

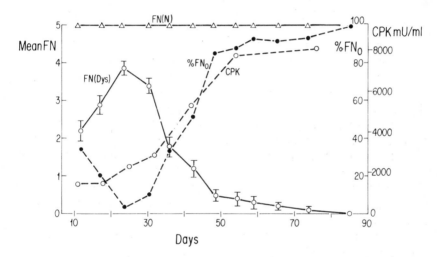

Fig. 1. Flip Number (FN) and plasma CPK values in chickens. Mean FN of dystrophic chickens, O—O (S.E.M. is shown; 50-82 animals per point), or of normals, Δ–Δ. %FN$_0$ = percentage of population of dystrophic chickens flipping 0 out of 5 attempts (●---●). Mean CPK activity (in milli-Units per ml plasma) from dystrophic chickens, O---O. Age in days *ex ovo*. (From Bhargava *et al.*, 1977).

Normal chicks (top line) show 100% performance from day 10 onwards. Up to about day 25, the dystrophic chickens improve in performance as their muscles grow. A peak Flip Number below the maximum value of five is reached by the dystrophic population, and thereafter their performance declines until the Flip Number is zero for all of them.

Despite the apparent crudity of the method of measurement, the Flip Number is an astonishingly reliable guide to the progress of the disease. Different observers, testing (blind) the same individual birds with developing dystrophy (after a suitable recovery interval) find identical values, and each individual bird shows a steady progression in Flip Number along the general form of the curve shown, without aberrations. Care is taken, to administer the test with all environmental and operational factors constant, and this is simple to do. Three different measures of the distribution of disability within a group of affected birds of the same age are useful in practice; (a) the mean Flip Number for the population, with its standard error, (b) Flip Number 0 (%), the percentage totally failing, i.e. with a zero score and (c) Flip Number 100 (%), the percentage showing no detectable disability, i.e. scoring five out of five. When small populations are being compared and more sophisticated expressions of the distribution of Flip Number values are both unjustified and too cumbersome, plotting of these three parameters reveals any changes clearly. The comparison between the mean Flip Number and Flip Number 0 (%) for the same population changing with age (Barnard *et al.*, 1976) is shown in Fig. 1. An example of the trend of Flip Number 100 (%) for this population is seen in Fig. 2, Chapter 27.

A second, independent measure of the progress of the disease in the chicken, as for some human and other dystrophies, is the level of CPK in the blood. At a given age, there is less variation in plasma CPK level either between birds of one of the inbred lines, or day to day, than in other species. The course of the CPK rise corresponds well with changes in Flip Number, (Fig. 1), supporting the use of this parameter as an index of muscle damage. It is presumed that the great increase in CPK in the blood is due to its leaking from muscle cells rendered abnormal in some way by the dystrophic process. Even at the earliest stages, the circulating CPK is elevated significantly in the dystrophic line, showing that the defect is expressed from hatching, and probably before. There is little change in plasma CPK in normal chickens; a population of 52 normal birds showed over the period 11-60 days a mean value of 340 with a standard error of 22mU/ml. At day 11, CPK in line 304 dystrophic chickens was 1700 mU/ml, compared to 300 mU/ml in related non-dystrophic (line 200) chickens. The steep rise to about 8000 mU/ml in the dystrophic birds occurs between days 30 and 50, when the major muscle damage obviously occurs. Subsequently the level continues to rise much more slowly.

Other quantitative measures of the disease stage are also possible. In the original work on this condition, the performance was measured by the 'exhaustion score', i.e. the number of times the bird could rise from the supine position in trials continued until it failed (Chung *et al.*, 1960; Asmundson *et al.*, 1966). After a few weeks of age normal birds give an average exhaustion score of 20 or more, but dystrophic chickens rarely exceed four. This has the advantage of giving finer gradations than the Flip Number score out of five, but the individual variation of the birds is greater, so comparisons are not necessarily more accurate, and it has the disadvantage that the procedure itself is so rigorous that it affects the course of the dystrophy (Entrikin *et al.*, 1977). Prolonged exercise also affects the CPK output and similar effects are well known in humans. The exhaustion score has recently been used by Entriken *et al.* (1977) to show a positive effect of diphenylhydantoin in the dystrophic chicken.

Another criterion is the wing apposition measurement. The wings of dystrophic chickens show an increasing resistance with age to being raised to touch each other, whereas the normals always show complete flexibility. The distance in cm between the raised wings in such a trial increases from 0 to about 12 over the period in which the Flip Number declines to 0, in the dystrophic birds. This criterion has been used by Chou *et al.*, (1977) to show an improvement in these birds produced by penicillamine treatment. Like those workers, our laboratory has found that wing apposition values are reproducible and provide a useful additional check on the course of the disease. Since wing flexibility loss seems due to stiffness at the tendons, it may not reveal changes in overall muscle strength, and it seems desirable for it not to *replace* measurements of the Flip Number. A number of plasma enzymes besides CPK have been examined and do not show sufficient differences with dystrophy to be useful for gauging effects of treatment (Bhargava, Barnard and Hudecki, 1977). The release of muscle pyruvate kinase in the blood, however, while less striking than plasma CPK changes in the dystrophic state, may offer a useful independent check on the muscle damage. There are further possible quantitative criteria, which, however, require invasive tissue sampling, unlike the others. Mean fibre diameter in an afflicted muscle (Linkhart *et al.*, 1975) makes use of the characteristic fibre hypertrophy; a better guide would be furnished by a comparison of histograms of the fibre size distribution. The dystrophic chicken, after about 4 weeks, develops an unusual elevation in sarcoplasmic acetylcholine-sterase and butyrylcholinesterase in the fast-twitch muscles (Wilson *et al.*, 1973; Entrikin *et al.*, 1977) which may also be used as a supplementary guide.

Advantages of the chicken for experimental study of muscular dystrophy

A number of favourable features can be recognized:
(1) Selective breeding has provided eggs 100% homozygous for dystrophy. This greatly facilitates experimental design. Moreover, the new homozygous line 413 has been bred (by the group at Davis, California) so that it is closely related genetically to a control line 412 which lacks the dystrophy gene.
(2) The progress of the disease can be monitored quantitatively in a non-destructive manner, by the Flip Number, wing apposition and CPK criteria defined above.

(3) Since the flip test is sensitive to quite early changes, major effects can be measured over a few weeks (Fig. 1). This contrasts, for example, with the long periods needed for survival times in dystrophic mice. (4) In the bird, where some muscles are pure in fibre type, investigation at the physiological, tissue and cellular levels of the progress and selectivity of the disease process is facilitated. The adjacent and anatomically similar posterior latissimus dorsi (Type II fibres; affected early) and anterior latissimus dorsi (Type I fibres; unaffected until very late) are useful for comparisons within the same animal. (5) The accessibility of the chick embryo to manipulation, in contrast to the mammalian embryo, renders feasible many new types of study on the determinants of the dystrophic processes. (6) Several enzymes, e.g. soluble acetylcholinesterase of muscle (Wilson *et al.*, 1968; Wilson *et al.*, 1973), remain present in the dystrophic chicken as their isoenzymes of embryonic type, but disappear from the normal, fast-twitch muscles after hatching. Such isoenzymic series in development easily studied in the chick, offer biochemical probes for the processes controlled by the gene defective in inherited dystrophy.

Conclusion

Though no exact equivalent in another animal can reasonably be expected, it seems useful to seek inherited conditions in animals which possess features in common with a human dystrophy that are amenable to experimental study. The chicken dystrophy appears to fit this requirement. In the search for chemotherapeutic agents effective on the human disease, a process which can be expected to play an increasing part in dystrophy research, the chicken is of interest since it offers the opportunity to measure the effects of controlled treatments on the affected musculature. An example is given by Barnard and Barnard (Chapter 27) of positive effects of anti-serotonin drugs on dystrophy, discovered and evaluated by the use of this model.

References

Asmundson, V.S. and Julian, L.M. (1956). *J. Hered.*, **47**, 248-250.
Asmundson, V.S., Kratzer, F.H. and Julian, L.M. (1966). *Ann. New York Acad. Sci.*, **138**, 49-58.
Barnard, P.J. and Barnard, E.A. (1977). *This volume.* pp. 319-329.
Barnard, E.A., Bhargava, A.K. and Hudecki, M.S. (1976). *Nature*, **263**, 422-424.
Bhargava, A.K., Barnard, E.A. and Hudecki, M.S. (1977). *Exptl. Neurol.*, **55**, 583-602.
Cardinet, G.H., Freedland, R.A., Tyler, W.S. and Julian, L.M. (1972). *Am. J. Vet. Res.*, **33**, 1671-1684.
Chou, T., Hill, E.J., Bartle, E., Wooley, K., Le Quire, V., Olson, W., Roelofs, R. and Park, J.H. (1975). *J. Clin. Invest.*, **56**, 842-849.

Chung, C.S., Norton, V.E. and Peters, H.A. (1960). *Am. J. Human Genet.*, **12,** 52-66.
Entrikin, R.K., Swanson, K.L., Weidoff, D.M., Patterson, G.T. and Wilson, B.W. (1977). *Science,* **195,** 873-875.
Julian, L.M. (1973). *Am. J. Pathol.,* **70,** 273-276.
Julian, L.M. and Asmundson, V.S. (1963). In *Muscular Dystrophy in Man and Animals* (Bourne, G.H. and Golarz, M.N., eds.) pp.458-498, Hafner, New York.
Linkhart, T.A., Yee, G.W. and Wilson, B.W. (1975). *Science,* **187,** 549-551.
Wilson, B.W., Linkhart, S.G. and Nieberg, P.A. (1973). *J. Exp. Zool.,* **186,** 187-192.
Wilson, B.W., Montgomery, W.A. and Asmundson, V.S. (1968). *Proc. Soc. Exptl. Biol. Med.,* **129,** 199-206.

At the end of Professor Barnard's paper, a film that he had made to illustrate the Flip Test was shown. A dystrophic chicken, placed on its back, was seen to beat its wings rapidly, but was unable to get up. A normal chicken was able to return to an upright position immediately it was released.

Discussion:

R.L. Watts: I noticed in the film that the operator took very great care in turning the chicken upsidedown. Is this important to the result of the Flip Test?

Barnard: Care in inversion is not necessarily important. It is part of the endeavour to standardize conditions.

Neerunjun: How long does the effect of the drug in improving the course of the disease persist after treatment is stopped?

Barnard: There is a relapse after a few days without treatment.

Neerunjun: Has pectoral muscle biopsy been looked at during improvement? You might find reappearence of Type II fibres, for example, or regenerative activity.

Barnard: Autopsy specimens have been examined histologically and by enzyme histochemistry, but so far not in an exhaustive series. Subjective assessment of these indicated improvement occurs in the muscle of treated animals.

Hamster muscular dystrophy

J.S. NEERUNJUN

Muscle Research Unit, Department of Paediatrics and Neonatal Medicine, Hammersmith Hospital, London W.12.

A myopathy affecting both skeletal and cardiac muscle of the Syrian hamster was first reported by Homburger *et al.* (1962). Breeding data have indicated that the disease is transmitted by an autosomal recessive gene. After mating homozygous diseased animals with unrelated normal hamsters, the mutant gene can be recovered in the F_2 generation. This approach has enabled several myopathic lines to be established (see Table 2).

The disease affects both males and females and the affected animals breed to produce homozygous dystrophic offspring, although less well than normal animals. Clinically, the disease is mild. The myopathic animals are of normal weight and do not show paralysis of either fore- or hindlimbs.

TABLE 2
Onset of muscular dystrophy and cardiomyopathy in different strains of hamsters

Year of origin	Strains of dystrophic hamsters	Age of onset of muscular dystrophy (days)	Age of onset of cardiomyopathy (days)
1962	BIO 1.50	21	30-40
1962	BIO 14.6	50-90	30-40
1970	BIO 40.54	30-50	30-40
1971	UM-X 7.1	10-20	30
1974	BIO 8262	5-10	40

However, muscle weakness can be demonstrated by causing the animals to swim and observing their hindlimbs. In normal hamsters, these are kept in a parallel position and tread water until exhaustion whereas, in dystrophic animals within a short time the hindlimbs flap sideways because of weakness in the adductor muscles. As compared to normal hamsters, which live for about 700 days, myopathic animals live for only about 200 days. Severely affected animals appear cyanotic and oedematous. Death occurs from congestive heart failure.

Histologically, skeletal muscle is abnormal early in the disease, showing variation in fibre size and fibres with internal nuclei. Later, fibres are seen undergoing degeneration, regeneration and splitting, sometimes accompanied by proliferation of connective tissue and fatty infiltration. Histochemical studies (Johnson and Pearce, 1971) have shown an impairment in the differentiation and development of Type II fibres. The cardiac lesions consist of focal myolysis, hyalinisation and secondary calcification.

Muscle lactate and malate dehydrogenase, aldolase and creatine kinase (CPK) levels are similar in normal and myopathic hamsters (Homburger *et al.*, 1966). However, the serum levels of these enzymes are increased in myopathic animals. Serum CPK level is markedly elevated in 20-25 day old myopathic hamsters, reaches extremely high levels between 26 an 120 days of age and then slowly declines, but always remains above normal up to 200 days of age (Eppenberger *et al.*, 1964).

Attempts to settle the long-lived debate as to whether the muscular dystrophies are primary myopathies or not have been made using this model. Reinnervation, allowed to take place between parabiotically coupled normal and diseased animals (BIO 14.6 strain; age 60 days) did not result in an increase in the number of internal nuclei in a normal muscle when the donor animal was dystrophic, nor in any slackening of the progressive increase in numbers of internal nuclei in diseased muscle when the donor animal was normal (Johnson and Montgomery, 1976). Muscle transplant experiments between normal and diseased animals (Jasmin and Bokdawala, 1970; Neerunjun and Dubowitz, 1974) also gave no indication of a neurogenic origin for hamster dystrophy.

Dhalla *et al.* (1975) have pursued the hypothesis that failure of mechanisms for the control of calcium concentrations in muscle might be responsible for its abnormal performance in the dystrophic hamster. Their biochemical investigations of diseased muscle from the UM-X 7.1 (early onset) strain have suggested the presence of defective membrane systems. In the sarcolemma, the activities of three ATPases (Ca^{2+}-activated, Mg^{2+}-activated and $Na^+ + K^+$-activated) were elevated in older animals, although only the first was elevated at 60 days, when light microscopy already showed extensive muscle fibre degeneration. However, ouabain inhibition of the $Na^+ + K^+$-activated enzyme was demonstrably lower at this stage. In the mitrochondria, rates of respiration and phosphorylation, which were lower at 60 days, did not differ from those of controls at 150 days. Calcium uptake was reduced, as it was in the sarcoplasmic reticulum. In the latter, however, calcium binding and the activity of Ca^{2+}-stimulated ATPase did not differ from control values. It was concluded that the relatively weak contraction of dystrophic muscle could result from the low level of intracellular calcium stores resultant from the membrane disturbances found.

Various agents have been used to treat the heart and skeletal muscle lesions. Verapamil, which is a calcium antagonist, prevents the cardiomyopathy completely but has no effect on skeletal muscle. On the other hand, α- and β-adrenergic blockers or a low calcium diet seem to reduce the development and/or severity of both heart and skeletal muscle lesions. It has been suggested (Jasmin and Bajusz, 1975) that the adrenergic blockers act by improving the microcirculation.

References

Dhalla, N.S., Singh, A., Lee, S.L., Anand, M.B., Bernatsky, A.M. and Jasmin, G. (1975). *Clin. Sci. Molec. Med.*, **49**, 359-368.

Eppenberger, M., Nixon, C.W., Baker, J.R. and Homburger, F. (1964). *Proc. Soc. Exp. Biol. Med.*, **117**, 465-468.

Homburger, F., Baker, J.R., Nixon, C.W. and Whitney, R. (1962). *Medicina Experimentalis*, **6**, 339-345.

Jasmin, G. and Bajusz, E. (1975). *In* 'Recent Advances in Studies on Cardiac

Structure and Metabolisms' eds. Fleckenstein, A. and Rona, G. University Park Press, Baltimore. **6,** 219-229.
Jasmin, G. and Bokdawala, F. (1970). *Rev. Canad. Biol.,* **29,** 197-201.
Johnson, M.A. and Montgomery, A. (1976). *J. Neurol. Sci.,* **27,** 201-215.
Johnson, M. and Pearce, A.G.E. (1971). *J. Neurol. Sci.,* **12,** 459-472.
Neerunjun, J.S. and Dubowitz, V. (1974). *J. Neurol. Sci.,* **23,** 521-536.

Discussion

Howells: I wonder whether the genetic disease in hamsters should be called a dystrophy, since the physiological properties are very similar for normal and dystrophic hamsters and since the skeletal muscle as a whole is very little affected by the time the animals die from the cardiomyopathy.
Neerunjun: Most skeletal muscles are involved by the time of death. There is much variation between strains in the time of onset of recognizable changes in both heart and skeletal muscle, and as to which is seen earlier, as I showed in the slide (Table 2). It is a common feature of muscular dystrophies that physiological parameters of muscle are not grossly abnormal, and the hamster shares a number of histological and biochemical abnormalities with other dystrophies. The least dystrophy-like feature in the hamster is perhaps the low incidence of fibre atrophy.
Branford White: Can variation in the levels of glycolytic enzymes be considered an important factor in the muscular dystrophies when there is so much difference among the human and animal diseases in the extent to which aldolase, for example, diverges from the normal? Why do you think these differences occur?
Neerunjun: I mentioned this feature of difference in the extent to which enzyme levels are abnormal because I think it is striking. At present, I have no explanation to offer for it.

Film: The myasthenic dog

A.C. PALMER

School of Veterinary Medicine, Cambridge.

Myasthenia in the dog affects both large and small breeds, of both sexes, especially between the age of nine months and two years. It can be congenital, and is sometimes associated with mediastinal tumours, including thymomas. Onset of the condition may be related to the treatment of a non-specific febrile illness with streptomycin or corticosteroids (Fraser *et al.*, 1970).

Clinical manifestations include lowered tolerance to exercise, difficulty in eating and swallowing, drooping of the facial features and progressive shortening of the stride of the forelimbs. Rest and anticholinesterase drugs lead to remission of clinical signs (Palmer and Barker, 1974). Because of its large content of striated muscle, the oesophagus is usually dilated, but not in congenital cases (Jenkins *et al.*, 1976).

Decrement of muscle action potentials after repeated nerve stimulation is reduced with anticholinesterases (Fraser *et al.*, 1970). Ultrastructurally, there is widening of secondary synaptic clefts (Zacks *et al.*, 1966). In one case, miniature endplate potentials were absent.

Immunological studies are in progress.

The film illustrated the disease in three dogs, a retriever, an alsatian and a Jack Russell terrier, in the last of which it was congenital. The retriever was seen flagging, particularly in forelimb movement, as a result of exercise, and showed difficulty in feeding and the characteristic facial drooping. It was seen restored to full activity after resting, and within minutes of receiving an injection of prostigmine. The other two dogs showed similar signs, except that, in the alsatian, the hindlimbs were more than usually affected.

References

Fraser, D.C., Palmer, A.C., Senior, J.E.B., Parkes, J.D. and Yealland, M.F.T. (1970). *J. Neurol. Neurosurg. Psychiat.*, **33**, 431-437.

Jenkins, W.L., Van Dyke, E. and McDonald, C.B. (1976). *J. S. Afr. Vet. Assoc.*, **47**, 59-62.

Palmer, A.C. and Barker, J. (1974). *Vet. Rec.*, **95**, 452-454.

Zacks, S.I., Sheilds, D.R. and Steinberg, S.A. (1966). *Ann. N.Y. Acad. Sci.*, **135**, 79-97.

The A2G-*adr* mouse

R.L. WATTS

Department of Biochemistry, Guy's Hospital Medical School, London SE1 9RT.

The *adr* (arrested development of the righting-response) mutation was first noticed early in 1975 in a stock colony of A2G mice by an animal house technician who reported that a 'white dystrophic' mouse had appeared. The effects of the mutation are, in fact, quite different from those of the *dy* gene in strain 129Re.

The film *showed normal and mutant mice at four ages: 10 days, when the righting response is about to appear in normal mice, and at 3½, 12 and 38 weeks, to follow the progress of the inherited disease.*

In the 10 day old litter, all the mice are slow to get up when turned on their backs. As soon as normal littermates resist inversion the affected animals can be distinguished. When turned on their backs they kick rapidly a number of times and flex their spines repeatedly before succeeding in righting themselves. As they get older, they also drag their hindlimbs stiffly for a few seconds after inversion or other handling. 129Re-*dy* mice can get up normally from their backs until prevented by muscle weakness which occurs late in the progress of the dystrophy. On the other hand, their hindlimbs are always too weak for them to climb up the walls of their plastic cage, while A2G-*adr* mice can do this easily and can also sit on their haunches in order to rub their noses. (Mice of all ages were seen performing these movements in the film.)

The growth curves followed by the two mutants are quite different. The A2G strain normally grows to a body weight 15-20% greater than that of 129Re, the males being 30% heavier than the females. For the first few weeks, mutant (*adr*) mice of both sexes grow rapidly and, although their body weight is less than that of littermates, they are not reliably distinguished on this basis. They then suddenly stop growing normally, and put on very little weight after 8 weeks of age; their body shape becomes shortened, so that they are very noticeably different from littermates by 10 weeks. (See Fig. 1, Chapter 28).

Normal mice of the A2G strain, including those heterozygous for *adr*, breed from the age of 5 weeks and a pair may produce 7-9 litters of average size 5.8. There is very good survival of the litters. This makes it relatively easy to produce *adr* homozygotes, in contrast to the problems of poor breeding and litter survival encountered in raising 129Re-*dy* homozygotes from test-mating of sibs. The A2G-*adr* females are also capable of bearing small litters. Male *adr* homozygotes have not been found to breed when tested in pen-matings with a mixture of normal and *adr* females.

It is assumed that *adr* is inherited as an autosomal recessive. The ratio of *adr/adr* to normal offspring in carrier × carrier matings, the number of such matings found among sib × sib matings and the sex ratio of affected animals are consistent with this mode of inheritance (Chapter 28). The muscle of normal and affected mice has been examined histologically and histochemically by Jean Watkins who will describe what she found in a moment. Briefly, muscle in *adr* mice showed abnormalities consistent with the general concept that the mutation causes *arrested development*, but these did not have the features of either a primary myopathy or of a neuropathy (Chapter 28).

Richard von Witt and I have looked at the levels of plasma creatine kinase (CPK), which we have recently examined in detail in 129Re-*dy*. In the *adr* mutant, we found a lowered plasma CPK, in contrast to the consistently raised level in *dy* mice (Chapter 28). Since a lowered plasma activity level of an enzyme cannot quite so readily be explained as a raised one by invoking membrane changes, we shall have to wait until we have some data on tissue CPK levels before we do more than note this finding as a difference from the dystrophic mouse.

During normal muscle contraction (see Fig. 2), ADP is rephosphorylated via respiratory processes or from phosphocreatine via the CPK reaction. In severe exercise, when phosphocreatine is exhausted, the adenylate kinase reaction becomes important. The removal of AMP via AMP deaminase ensures that ADP levels are kept below those inhibitory to muscle function (Watts and Watts, 1974). The IMP produced may build up until, during rest, ATP is available for the completion of the AMP cycle. It is hence of interest to measure nucleotide levels in normal and diseased muscle, and this we have done in collaboration with Dr. John Griffiths and Zubaidah Rahim at St. Bartholomews Medical College. Freeze-clamped samples were taken from resting muscle and after the mice had exercised by swimming for 30 minutes.

The results are quite·simple; ATP and ADP concentrations changed very little on a percentage basis in control or *adr* muscle after exercise; in control muscle AMP did not change, and IMP went up slightly after exercise; in *adr* muscle both AMP and IMP were significantly increased by exercise. It seems likely that the control mice were not really fatigued by 30 minutes swimming, while the *adr* mice were; this is being investigated further. The build up in *adr* muscle of both IMP and AMP is consistent with our finding (Chapter 28) of lower levels of AMP deaminase in *adr* than in control muscle.

References

Watts, R.L. and Watts, D.C. (1974). *In* Chemical Zoology, vol. VIII (eds. Florkin and Scheer) Academic Press, 369-446.

Discussion

Watkins: I have made cryostat sections of muscles from hind and fore-limbs and from the back of control and affected mice ranging in age from two weeks to 28 weeks and examined them histologically and histo-chemically. All the differences that I found between *adr* and control muscles could be seen regardless of the site from which the muscle was obtained.

It was difficult to obtain satisfactory transverse sections of muscle from young *adr* mice. Fig. 2a shows fibres cut obliquely and the occurrence of spaces between them in the gastrocnemius from a 3 week old affected mouse. This can be compared with Fig. 2b, showing control muscle of the same age; both are stained for succinate dehydrogenase (Nachlas *et al.*, *Histochem. Cytochem.*, **5**, 420-436, 1957). In more mature muscle, the difference between the rounded shape of fibres in the *adr* and the clearly polygonal shape in controls was more pronounced. Nuclei in *adr* muscle appeared vesicular many with prominent nucleoli.

When the sections were stained for ATPase at pH 9.4 (Dubowitz and Brooke 'Muscle Biopsy: a Modern Approach' p.32 1973. W.B. Saunders) fibre types could be distinguished and counted in both control and *adr* muscle (Figure 2c a and d). However, when the sections were stained for succinate dehydrogenase (Fig. 2e and f) or other oxidative enzymes, fibre types could not be distinguished in *adr* muscle.

Ward: I have seen the same picture of rounded fibre shape and fibre separation in rodent skeletal muscle sectioned after electrical stimulation.

Bradley: A similar appearance is seen in oedematous muscle, or in muscle that has been heavily used.

D.C. Watts: Dr. Rebello, Mrs. Watkins and I have looked at lipid components in muscle from 129Re-*dy*, A2G-*adr* and controls of each strain. Six animals were used in each group. We measured:

(a) Total triglycerides and their fatty acid components
(b) Cholesterol
(c) Cholesterol esters
(d) Total phospholipids and their fatty acid components

No differences were found between the controls of the two strains. In 129Re-*dy* muscle, apart from the phospholipids, all lipids showed significantly (p 0.005-0.001) raised levels, whereas in A2G-*adr* muscle, all levels were the same as in the controls.

The composition of the phospholipid fraction differed from that of the controls in both mutants. The palmitic acid content of the phospholipids was lower than in controls (p0.00-0.001) and the linoleic acid content higher than in controls (p 0.01-0.005) in both mutants. In A2G-*adr*, the stearic acid content was also higher (p 0.001)

We conclude that these differences indicate membrane composition changes associated with the two diseases. We note that, in Duchenne muscular dystrophy, raised palmitic acid and lowered linoleic acid contents have been found (Kunze *et al.*, *Clin. Chem. Acta*, **43**, 333-341, 1973), changes in the opposite direction to those we have seen in the mouse mutants.

Changeux: The mutant mice appeared in the film to show fine tremor. Has the cerebellum been investigated?

R.L. Watts: We have no-one in our group able to do this, and my attempts to persuade brain-oriented people that it might be interesting have so far failed. If you are making an offer to look at the *adr* mouse, we should be very happy to accept. However, the mice do not appear to us to show any tremor.

The peripheral nerves have not been examined either, but Dr. Heather Stephens is hoping to do this shortly.

Fig. 2. Transverse section of gastrocnemius muscle from A2G mice. Sections (a) affected and (b) control are from 3 week old mice, stained for succinate dehydrogenase; sections (c) affected and (d) control are from 12 week old animals, stained for ATPase at pH 9.4; sections (e) and (f) are as (c) and (d), but stained for succinate dehydrogenase. All magnifications are the same; the bar represents 20 microns.

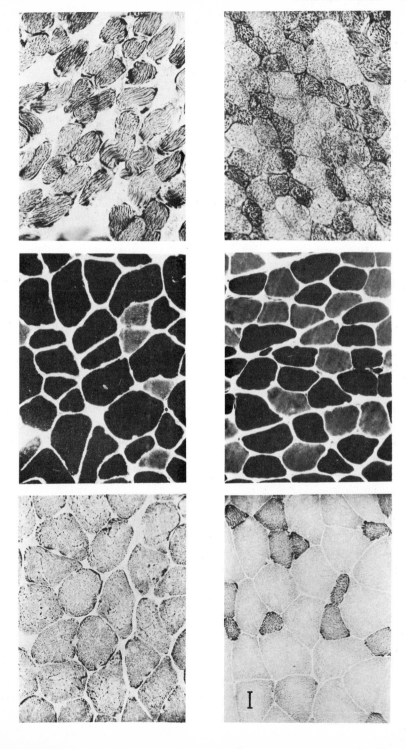

Experimental (Non-Genetic) models of human myopathy and neuropathy

W.G. BRADLEY

Muscular Dystrophy Research Laboratories, Newcastle General Hospital, Newcastle upon Tyne.

A considerable number of experimental neuropathies and myopathies have been studied in animals, and an adequate review of them would fill a book. In addition to the inherited diseases of animals, some of which have been discussed above, there have been extensive series of reports on the degeneration of skeletal muscle due to toxins, vitamin and other deficiencies, and a number of traumata including the injection of toxic substances, crush lesions, cold and heat lesions, etc. (Blaxter, 1974; Kakulas, 1974). These studies have been very useful for the elucidation of the basic processes of degeneration and regeneration in skeletal muscle. The central point about such experimental models is that they begin with skeletal muscle which is inherently normal. It is against such studies that the degeneration and regeneration seen in inherited diseases must be compared.

The vascular theory of muscular dystrophy, which held the field for a period, produced a number of ischaemic models of muscle damage both by aortic ligation and the injection of vasoactive substances (Mendell *et al.*, 1971), and also the pharmacological combination of serotonin and imipramine (Parker and Mendell, 1974). These ischaemic models were mainly directed towards supporting the vascular theory. When no vascular abnormalities were discovered in the muscular dystrophies, these models were largely forgotten (Bradley, 1977).

Similarly the neural theory of the aetiology of muscular dystrophy produced an increased interest in the effect of nerve upon muscle (McComas *et al.*, 1971; Bradley, 1974; Bradley *et al.*, 1975). Many diseases produce progressive denervation of the skeletal muscle in man with characteristic pathological and electrophysiological changes. These include peripheral neuropathies and motor neuron disease. Similarly in a disease like Duchenne muscular dystrophy, there are characteristic pathological changes which appear to be specifically due to skeletal muscle degeneration. However in a number of the chronic neuromuscular diseases of man, such as the juvenile and adult onset spinal muscular atrophies, limb girdle and facioscapulohumeral muscular dystrophy, and the Becker type of X-linked muscular dystrophy, the changes both electromyographically and pathologically appear to be a combination both of myopathy and denervation (Chapter 3).

Are we seeing in such chronic human neuromuscular diseases evidence of multi-system involvement, as I have suggested in murine muscular dystrophy above (page 316), are we studying simply the effect of chronic denervation of muscle producing degeneration of the skeletal muscle, or are we seeing the chronic effect of skeletal muscle abnormality in a retrograde fashion upon the motor nerves? All these interpretations are theoretically possible. Intuitively, I think that the multi-system involvement is the most likely explanation. However our uncertainty would be considerably less if we had models of chronic denervation and chronic myopathy in experimental animals. The inherited diseases of animals present the same intrinsic problem as that experienced in man, namely that the skeletal muscle and nerve may be the subject of multi-system involvement. The only answer is to study an animal in which the skeletal muscle is intrinsically normal at the start of the experiment, and investigate the effects either of a chronic neuropathy, or of a chronic myopathy in this experimental setting.

There have been many studies of the effect of acute denervation on skeletal muscle, sectioning the nerve and studying the muscle at intervals thereafter. Similarly there have been many studies of the effect of traumata upon the skeletal muscle. However in all of these studies, the insult has been applied at one moment, and the effect studied with increasing time thereafter. Human muscle diseases are however different in that they are chronic and progressive, the insult being applied slowly and repeatedly. I will briefly describe two attempts which we have made to produce animal models in which this chronic progressive insult occurs.

The first attempt was to produce chronic progressive denervation of the skeletal muscle in rat, and was only partially successful. Irradiation of the lumbar spine of rats produces chronic progressive neurological dysfunction 120 to 220 days later. This is due mainly to generation of the anterior and posterior roots, there being little change in the spinal cord (Bradley *et al.*, 1977). Evidence from the histological staging of the axonal degeneration in the peripheral nerves, and from the time of onset of electrophysiological evidence of denervation, suggest that the spinal root degeneration and the subsequent denervation of the muscle progresses for at least six weeks, and perhaps longer. This however is still relatively acute, for the ideal model is one in which denervation progresses for more than a year. In the muscle from these animals, there was fibre type dedifferentiation, random angulation and atrophy of the fibres, an increase in the number of internal nuclei, slight increase in endomysial fibrosis, and a number of minor myofibrillary alterations. There was however almost no acute necrosis, phagocytosis or regeneration (Fewings *et al.*, 1977).

If the lumbar radiation radiculopathy model in the rat is a good one, then it indicates that a necrotising myopathy, such as that seen in Duchenne dystrophy, is not likely to arise from chronic denervation, though the other changes encountered clearly can so arise.

The second model to be described investigated the capacity of inherently normal skeletal muscle to regenerate after multiple episodes of necrosis, such as occur in Duchenne muscular dystrophy. Is normal muscle able to regenerate itself adequately after many such episodes, and is there perhaps a reduced regenerative capacity in Duchenne dystrophy which explains the progressive loss of muscle fibres? Bupivicaine produces acute necrosis of skeletal muscle fibres with rapid regeneration occurring within the basement membranes (Jirmanova and Thesleff, 1972). Studies with W.J.K. Cumming have indicated that in the rat there is very rapid degeneration and regeneration, and that the muscle has fully recovered by 28 days with the exception of internal nuclei which persist. We have subjected the rat E.D.L. muscle to up to twelve monthly episodes of necrosis and studied the changes one month and six months after these episodes. The muscle is able to maintain its normal weight and normal muscle fibre area for up to three such monthly necrotic episodes. After six or twelve episodes, there is progressive loss of these parameters, though the total number of muscle fibres remains unchanged. The number of muscle nuclei increase to about six months, and thereafter remain constant. It appears that repeated episodes of necrosis can impair the eventual capacity of the muscle to recover, and the evidence suggests that this is due to inadequate synthesis of muscle fibre protein, and not due to an inability of the satellite cells to divide. Further study of this model is however required.

Conclusions

All studies of muscular dystrophy are in the end aimed at understanding and being able to treat human diseases. The genetically inherited animal models of muscle degeneration are of great help in this aim, since they provide material from all parts of the body which is easily available, and can be studied at any age and by any form of preparation. However, as in man, the genetically inherited models have some drawbacks in that all systems are potentially affected by the underlying biochemical abnormality. Non-genetic models such as those outlined here, avoid this drawback, and add another string to the bow of the experimenter.

References

Blaxter, K.L. (1974). *In* Disorders of Voluntary Muscle. Ed. J.N. Walton, 3rd edition, pp.908-916, Churchill Livingstone, Edinburgh.

Bradley, W.G. (1974). *Nature,* **250,** 285-286.

Bradley, W.G. (1977). Pathogenesis of human muscular dystrophies. 5th International Scientific Meeting of the Muscular Dystrophy Association. Ed. L.P. Rowland, *Excerpta Medica,* 672-677.

Bradley, W.G., Fewings, J.D., Cumming, W.J.K. and Harrison, R.M. (1977). *J. neurol. Sci.,* **31,** 63-82.

Bradley, W.G., Gardner-Medwin, D. and Walton, J.N. (1975). Recent Advances in Myology, *Excerpta Medica,* Amsterdam.

Fewings, J.D., Harris, J.B., Johnson, M.A. and Bradley, W.G. (1977). *Brain,* **100,** 157-183.
Jirmanova, I. and Thesleff, S. (1972). *Z. Zellforsch.,* **1931,** 77-97.
Kakulas, B.A. (1974). *In* Disorders of Voluntary Muscle, Edit. J.N. Walton, 3rd edition, pp.908-916, Churchill Livingstone, Edinburgh.
McComas, A.J., Sica, R.E.P. and Campbell, M.J. (1971). *Lancet,* **i,** 321-325.
Mendell, J.R., Engel, W.K. and Derrer, E.C. (1971). *Science,* **172,** 1143-1145.
Parker, J.M. and Mendell, J.R. (1974). *Nature,* **247,** 103-104.

Discussion:

R.L. Watts: If you cause injury to the muscle at monthly intervals twelve times, the later part of the experiment must be performed towards the end of a rat's lifespan. Would the regenerative capacity of the muscle be much lessened if the first rather than the twelfth injury was received at this stage?
Bradley: This has not so far been tested.
Barnard: Can the changes in the irradiated animals really be considered to be progressive?
Bradley: In that physiological changes preceded clinical signs, the defect was progressive.
Neerunjun: Do you think the role of macrophages as a source of nuclei in muscle regeneration appears likely, if satellite cells were not damaged?
Bradley: There is some evidence that cells other than muscle satellite cells may be involved in regeneration.

27 An approach to the chemotherapy of muscular dystrophy: retardation of symptoms in genetically dystrophic chickens and hamsters

PENELOPE J. BARNARD · ERIC A. BARNARD

Department of Biochemistry, Imperial College, London, S.W.7.

We have very little idea what causes the multiple set of pathological changes that constitutes muscular dystrophy, apart from the fact that (for the commoner forms in man and in animals) it is determined by a defective gene. This does not mean, however, that it is profitless to seek any drug therapy of these disorders. In many other pathologies, effective drugs can be found prior to an understanding of the basic mechanisms of the pathogenesis. Consideration of the symptoms can give clues to possible ameliorative processes even without such fundamental understanding, and development of drugs for these purposes can be on a basis that is far from random trial. In the present state of knowledge the minimum requirements for the chemotherapy of muscular dystrophy are two-fold: (i) to identify factors likely to affect the development of the disease, and of a type that can be acted upon by drug treatments; and (ii) a system for following objectively and reproducibly the progress of the disease. The purpose of such studies is only in the longer term that some treatment useful in human dystrophic patients will be developed. The immediate findings of any factor in the pathology that responds to a foreign compound can give tangible evidence on the processes occurring, and can lead to new and more effective approaches to arresting them.

Choice of Drugs

We shall describe here the use of serotonin antagonists as anti-dystrophic drugs. We were led to these compounds by evidence that has accumulated for some years that a deficiency developing in the local vascular supply or degree of oxygenation of skeletal muscle aids the development of muscular dystrophy (Ashmore and Somes, 1968; Cazzato, 1968; Demos *et al.*, 1968; Hathaway *et al.*, 1970; Mendell *et al.*, 1971). Nervous control of the local vasculature to vertebrate skeletal muscle is mediated by noradrenaline or serotonin. The involvement of one of these neurohormones in the patho-

319

genesis is also rendered a plausible possibility by the observation that they can, in rats, themselves induce muscle damage when injected locally (Selye, 1967; Mendell *et al.*, 1971). In the rat model introduced by W.K. Engel and colleagues (Mendell *et al.*, 1971; Mendell *et al.*, 1972; Parker and Mendell, 1974), muscle lesions similar to those characterizing human Duchenne dystrophy were reported to be produced by aortic ligation together with injection of one of these bioamines, both procedures being required. Moreover, Gordon and Dowben (1966) found twice as much serotonin in the spleens of dystrophic mice as in normal mice, and muscle lesions have been induced by serotonin in normal mice (O'Steen, J.L. Barnard and Yates, 1967). An additional circumstantial suggestion arises from the fact that mast cells of hamsters and mice are rich in serotonin (but not adrenalines) and they extensively infiltrate the muscle in those strains which are genetically dystrophic (Nixon *et al.*, 1962; Walter and O'Steen, 1963; Bois, 1964; Selye, 1965). For these reasons, therefore, we have tested anti-serotoninergic and anti-adrenergic compounds in dystrophic animals.

Use of a test system for monitoring chemotherapy of dystrophy

The most useful system would be an animal line that inherits dystrophy in a form as close as possible in causation and course to human (say Duchenne) dystrophy, and that permits quantitative assessment of the progress of the disease, by as many independent methods as possible. One of us dicusses elsewhere in this Volume (Chapter 26) the merits of the dystrophic chicken homozygote for such assessments. As described there, the Flip Test on the chicken provides a measure of the strength of muscles affected by the disease. For example, in homozygous lines 304 or 413 of the University of California (Davis) stock, muscle weakness appears with regularity during the first 4 weeks of life, and histopathology typical of human Duchenne dystrophy develops (Holliday *et al.*, 1965; Julian, 1973; Linkhart *et al.*, 1976).

As a second criterion of muscle damage, the elevation of the plasma creatine phosphokinase level (CPK) can be used. The large increase in plasma CPK, found in the human (Dreyfus *et al.*, 1958; Munsat *et al.*, 1973) and hamster (Homberger *et al.*, 1966) dystrophies, occurs in the dystrophic chicken, too. A close correlation has been shown in these dystrophic chickens between the rise of plasma CPK with age of the animal and its development of muscular weakness as measured by Flip Number (Barnard *et al.*, 1976), as illustrated elsewhere in this Volume (Chapter 26). The availability of the chicken model, with the advantages noted, is an important factor in facilitating chemotherapy trials of the type discussed here. We have established the course of the muscle weakness (by the Flip Number scored out of 5) and the plasma CPK rise in the 304 and 413 line chickens, and found these to be fully reproducible patterns, such that changes due to drug treatment can be monitored unambiguously.

We have also used dystrophic hamsters. These do not have the advantage of the chicken of offering a readily quantitated 'performance test' of muscle weakness, but it nevertheless seems important to check that a therapeutic effect seen with the dystrophic bird is extendable to the mammal. The only quantitative measure of the progress of the disease so far established for these animals is the blood CPK level. Since, as in the chicken, this reaches very high levels, changing from about 100 mU/ml serum in the normal hamster to about 6000 mU/ml in the dystrophic hamster at 10 weeks of age, it is very difficult to repress this rise and an agent which does so significantly and continually is presumed to be retarding the muscle damage. While this needs further detailed investigation to determine the extent of the effect on the muscles themselves CPK depression serves as a useful screening device in the mammal, since drugs that cannot exert this effect can be taken to have little or no therapeutic value in dystrophy.

Drug treatments

Three drugs of diverse structure, in use as antagonists of serotonin, have been used; cyproheptadine and methysergide most extensively (Fig. 1), and, in trials now under way, hydroxindasole. Chickens were injected twice-daily intraperitoneally with either or both cyproheptadine and methysergide at doses well below those eliciting any toxic symptoms in normal chickens. Hamsters were injected intraperitoneally at longer intervals, with cyproheptadine or hydroxindasole. Lower doses were given when the animals were very young. The control ('untreated') dystrophic animals were given water injections similarly. Measurements of the Flip Number (this volume Chapter 26) and of blood CPK were done in a completely blind fashion with respect to the status of the animals.

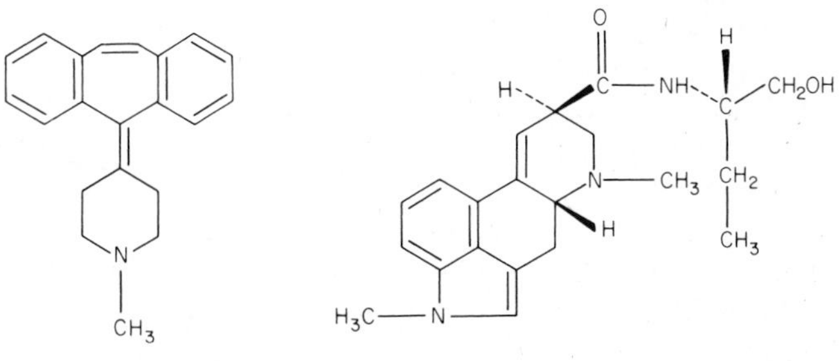

Fig. 1. Cyproheptadine (C, left) and methysergide (M).

Effects of drug treatment of dystrophic chickens

By regular treatment (Barnard *et al.*, 1976) with cyproheptadine or methysergide, or with both drugs in combination, the onset of clinical symptoms of dystrophy in the affected chickens is significantly delayed and the magnitude of the disability, when it does develop, is reduced. The mean Flip Numbers are shown for several treatment regimes in Figs. 2 and 3, where a postponement is clearly seen of the decline which occurs with the untreated dystrophic chickens. A difference between the methysergide-treated and untreated dystrophic chickens continued throughout the remaining period of the study; thus, at day 60 *ex ovo*, 80% of the treated chickens retained the unimpaired ability to rise from the supine, whereas only 6% of the untreated ones had such ability at that stage.

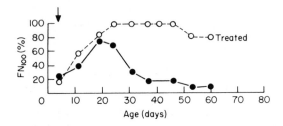

Fig. 2. Effect of a treatment with methysergide on the Flip Test of muscle weakness of dystrophic chickens. The percentage of the population (of about 30 birds throughout) whose performance remained at 100%, FN_{100}, i.e. scoring 5 out of 5 successful consecutive righting attempts, is plotted (broken line). The solid line shows the same variable plotted for water-injected control dystrophic chickens. Dosage started where marked (arrow), and was initially 12.5 mg kg^{-1}, increasing in steps to 31 mg kg^{-1} at day 45 and constant thereafter.

With cyproheptadine, at a low dose regime (for the chicken), substantial improvement in the Flip Number was shown (Fig. 3). A medium level dose (12mg kg^{-1}d^{-1}) extended the period of this effect, but the performance still declined sharply after day 55. The latter decline was postponed further by a combination of higher doses of cyproheptadine and methysergide (Figs. 2 and 3). For the latter case, all the treated animals remained at a passing level (Flip Number = 4-5) up to day 60, whereas all of the untreated birds were below this level from about day 30. Beyond day 65 (at the same dose levels) performance fell off, but these later stages, when the untreated animals are severely dystrophic, have not yet been studied with sufficient numbers to know how far the relief can be maintained. Constant dosing was always needed to maintain the effects illustrated. Likewise, the percentage of the population totally failing the Flip Test (i.e. having Flip Number = 0), showed, for the animals treated with these drugs (at medium or higher doses) a pronounced difference from the untreated dystrophics (Fig. 4).

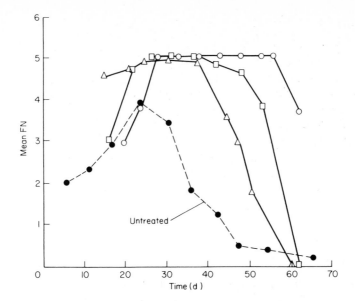

Fig. 3. Mean Flip Number (FN) of cyproheptadine-treated or untreated (●, n=50-82 animals) dystrophic chickens. Low dosage regime (Δ, n=12) was 2.4 mg kg⁻¹ d⁻¹ at days 3-16, 6.0 at days 17-43 and 8.0 at day 44 onwards. Medium dosage (□, n=9) was 12.0 mg kg⁻¹ d⁻¹ from day 3 onwards. A combined treatment (○, n=27) was also given, with cyproheptadine at 8.0 mg kg⁻¹ d⁻¹ at days 3-10, 12 at days 11-30, 17.5 at days 31-52, and 23 at day 53 onwards, plus methysergide at 12.5 mg kg⁻¹ d⁻¹ at day 3-15, 20 at days 10-30, 41 at days 31-45, and 52 onwards. The standard error of the mean FN was in the range 0.1-0.3 units for the untreated birds, and 0.2-0.7 units for the treated birds. From Barnard *et al.* (1976).

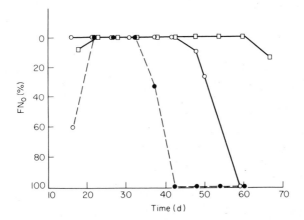

Fig. 4. Percentage of the population of dystrophic chickens having Flip Number=0, when untreated (●, n=15), or treated with cyproheptadine (○ dose low or medium, see Fig. 3; n=21) or treated with both drugs (□, doses as stated for Fig. 3; n=27). From Barnard *et al.* (1976).

Using the criterion of CPK release, the drug-treated animals also showed a smaller change than the untreated birds (Fig. 5). The tendency to stabilize at a plateau of about 2,500 mU per ml plasma in the treated dystrophic birds, compared with about 8,500 in the untreated dystrophics, is seen more clearly for the treatment with the two drugs combined. The treated dystrophic birds always showed a lower CPK level than the untreated ones of the same age, but there was considerable fluctuation in the values up to about day 30, tending to obscure any effect, but after that stage those animals (the great majority of those treated with medium or higher doses) which improved in the Flip Test showed CPK level differences that were invariably significant at P<0.001, for all of the treatments (n=57, cyproheptadine + methysergide treatment, e.g., up to day 60). Plasma enzymes other than CPK showed little equivalent effect (Bhargava *et al.*, 1977). Alkaline phosphatase was (at ages greater than 20 d) about 30% higher in dystrophic than normal chickens (n=66, P<0.02), and did not show a consistent reduction when the drug treatments were effective. Glutamate oxaloacetate transaminase was 40% higher in the dystrophic chickens (n=66, P<0.001) and showed no significant change with the drug treatment, nor did lactate dehydrogenase (which was the same in normals and dystrophics). Blood serotonin was 1.55 μg/ml in normal, compared to 2.03 μg/ml in dystrophic, birds (n=35, P<0.001), and was changed towards the normal level by 8-39% according to the drug treatment received (Bhargava *et al.*, 1977).

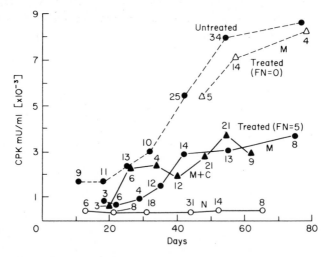

Fig. 5. Comparisons of plasma CPK activity (mean mU/ml plasma). ●--●, Untreated dystrophic chickens. M-treated chickens (those passing Flip Test, i.e. FN=5, ●—●; *or those failing* flip test, i.e. FN=0; Δ--Δ--) ▲, (C+M) − treated chickens (with FN=5; too few in this group had FN=0 to be plotted). Doses as in Fig. 3 (data for all dose levels pooled). O—O, Normal, untreated chickens. The number of animals used is indicated next to each point. From Bhargava *et al.* (1977).

Tests with adrenergic antagonists

1-(3',4'-dichlorophenyl)-2-isopropylaminoethanol (DCI) had a small or zero effect in tests on small numbers of chickens over the 6-75 day period, and α-methyldopa had no effect at all, on the symptoms of dystrophy (Bhargava *et al.*, 1977). The doses used were 1/20th of the mammalian LD50. Since nothing like the effect of the serotonin antagonists was seen with these compounds, it seemed more profitable to explore the anti-serotoninergic system in more depth.

Effect of drugs on dystrophic hamsters

Hamsters of the AA strain (derived from BIO.14.6 line), homozygous for dystrophy, were used. The serum CPK in these animals rises sharply over the first 8-10 weeks of life, to about 6000 mU/ml, and remains high, although fluctuating (Fig. 6). With cyproheptadine given at 12 mg $kg^{-1}d^{-1}$ this rise is moderated in some, but not all animals, but at 40 mg kg^{-1}, given twice-weekly, CPK output is rapidly reduced to near the initial level (Fig. 7). With hydroxindasole a similar effect was obtained. The untreated dystrophic hamsters show considerable variations in their serum CPK levels from day to day and between individuals, and the course of the drug effect on each animal is therefore plotted, due to the small numbers so far available. The curve for the hydroxindasole effect shown in Fig. 8 is representative of the pattern obtained in all of the treated animals; the sharp initial rise in CPK output can be countered by subsequent administration of hydroxinda-sole at levels of the order of 10 mg kg^{-1} given twice-weekly.

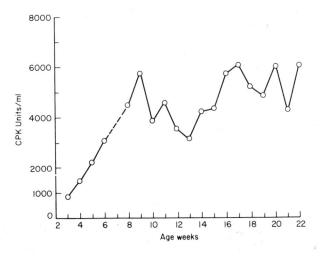

Fig. 6. The rise in the serum CPK of the untreated dystrophic hamsters as a function of age. Each point is the mean for 11 animals.

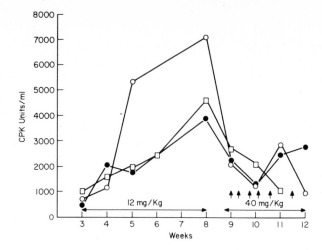

Fig. 7. Examples of the response of invidual dystrophic hamsters to cyproheptadine. The response is measured by the decline of the elevated serum CPK (compare Fig. 6). At 12 mg kg^{-1} (given on each day marked by an arrow, little effect is ever seen. At 40 mg kg^{-1}, even when started late (as here), a marked decline in serum CPK is induced. Note that for the hamster the LD$_{50}$ of this drug is >80 mg kg^{-1}.

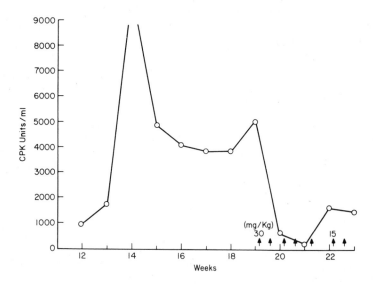

Fig. 8. An example of the response of the dystrophic hamster serum CPK to hydroxindasole. In this case the drug treatment was withheld until a late stage (19 weeks), but an effect is still provoked. Dosage was 30 mg kg^{-1} at each point marked by an arrow.

Conclusions

The finding of these anti-dystrophic effects with 3 compounds of diverse structure, having in common only their pharmacological action as antagonists of serotonin, suggests strongly that serotonin plays some role in the pathogenesis of this disease. That the same effect is found in a mammalian form of dystrophy as in the dystrophic bird argues likewise that a general factor in dystrophy is involved. Of course, there is a need now for much more extensive testing, especially in the mammal where the project is at an early stage, as well as the monitoring of the histopathological picture throughout the treatments. The latter can provide an additional assessment of the progress of muscle damage or its repair.

It has been found necessary to maintain the treatment or the animals regress rapidly. This suggests a continual action of serotonin somewhere in the development of the overt symptoms of this disorder. While the dystrophic chickens have a higher serotonin level than the normals, it seems doubtful that it is the circulating serotonin level *per se* that is responsible. This elevation is not great. As a working hypothesis, we assume, instead, that some site of serotonin action in the muscle or its micro-vasculature differs between the normal and the dystrophic animal, such that antagonism of serotonin is helpful. In humans with carcinoid tumours producing large amounts of circulating serotonin, a myopathy can indeed develop, but only after about 10 years. In the studies of this myopathy (Berry *et al.*, 1974; Swash *et al.*, 1975) it was found that it can, indeed, be corrected by the drugs used here.

We do not know if the effect seen with the dystrophic animals has its origin in an action on local blood flow in the muscles. Methysergide, it is known, can exert a marked vasodilator action, but it can also constrict veins (Aellig, 1975). Agents such as serotonin which increase the total blood flow can simultaneously cause a stagnation of the circulation through certain capillaries of skeletal muscle (Vetterlein and Schmidt, 1975). It is possible that a very localized impairment of the blood flow in muscle occurs in the dystrophy, and is countered by the anti-serotonin compounds we have used. However, the vascular hypothesis of dystrophy aetiology has been questioned (Paulson *et al.*, 1974; Bradley *et al.*, 1975). Alternatively, it is possible that in genetically dystrophic animals a membrane alteration has occurred such that serotonin can act directly on the muscle cells in a deleterious fashion. In this connection, Patten *et al.* (1974) have shown on normal rat muscle a direct effect of serotonin, which can be blocked by methysergide and by cyproheptadine. Such an alternative site of action of serotonin in the muscle is possibly indicated by the work of Wright *et al.* (1973), who in a fluorescence microscope examination of muscle biopsy samples from human Duchenne patients demonstrated an abnormal accumulation of catecholamine-related substances in the muscle fibres themselves, and in the vasomotor plexus surrounding the small muscle arterioles. This phenomenon was not seen in muscle from normal subjects.

Much further investigation will be needed to determine whether a therapeutic effect applicable to human dystrophies has been indicated here. Such studies seem worthwhile, since the drugs used have been chronically administered in man for other conditions (e.g. migraine) without effects that would preclude their use, and the doses effective in the chicken and hamster are at a level below that of chronic toxicity in the species concerned.

Acknowledgements

The work reviewed was generously supported by the Muscular Dystrophy Association of America. The Eastwood Muscular Dystrophy Research Facility at Imperial College was founded with the invaluable help of the W. and JB Eastwood Company (Bilsthorpe, U.K.), and is maintained with their aid and that of the Muscular Dystrophy Group of Great Britain. We thank Dr. B.W. Wilson, University of California (Davis) for the supply of chickens, and Merck, Shape and Dohme, West Point, Pa., U.S.A., for the donation of the cyproheptadine and hydroxindasòle. For the previously unpublished portions of this work, very expert assistance was rendered by Mrs. Joan Lyles and Mr. David Green.

References

Aellig, W.H. (1975). *Triangle*, **14**, 39-46.
Ashmore, C.R. and Somes, R.G. (1968). *Proc. Soc. Exp. Biol. Med.*, **128**, 103-107.
Barnard, E.A., Bhargava, A.K. and Hudecki, M.S. (1976). *Nature*, **263**, 422-424.
Berry, E.M., Maunder, C. and Wilson, M. (1974). *Gut*, **15**, 34-38.
Bhargava, A.K., Barnard, E.A. and Hudecki, M.S. (1977). *Exp. Neurol.*, **55**, 583-602.
Bois, P. (1964). *Am. J. Physiol.*, **206**, 338-340.
Bradley, W.G., O'Brien, M.D., Walder, D.N., Murchison, D., Johnson, M. and Newell, D.J. (1975). *Arch. Neurol.*, **32**, 466-473.
Cazzato, G. (1968). *Europ. Neurol.*, **1**, 158-179.
Demos, J., Treumann, F. and Schroeder, W. (1968). *Revue Fr. Etud. Clin. Biol.*, **13**, 467-483.
Dreyfus, J.C., Schapira, G. and Schapira, F. (1958). *Ann. N.Y. Acad. Sci.*, **75**, 235-249.
Gordon, P. and Dowben, R.M. (1966). *Am J. Physiol.*, **210**, 728-732.
Hathaway, P.W., Engel, W.K. and Zellweger, H. (1970). *Arch. Neurol.*, **22**, 365-378.
Holliday, T.A., Asmundson, V.A. and Julian, L.M. (1965). *Enzymol. Biol. Clin.*, **5**, 209-216.
Homberger, F., Nixon, C.W., Eppenberger, M. and Baker, J.R. (1966). *Ann. N.Y. Acad. Sci.*, **138**, 14-27.
Julian, L.M. (1973). *Am. J. Pathol.*, **70**, 273-276.
Linkhart, T.A., Yee, G.W., Nieberg, P.S. and Wilson, B.W. (1976). *Develop. Biol.*, **48**, 447-457.

Mendell, J.R., Engel, W.K. and Derrer, E.C. (1971). *Science*, **172**, 1143-1145.

Mendell, J.R., Engel, W.K. and Derrer, E.C. (1972). *Nature*, **239**, 522-524.

Munsat, T.L., Baloh, R., Pearson, C.M. and Fowler, W. (1973). *J. Am. Med. Ass.*, **226**, 1536-1543.

Nixon, C.W., Whitney, R., Baker, J.R. and Homberger, F. (1962). *Fed. Proc.*, **21**, 313.

O'Steen, W.K., Barnard, Jr., J.L. and Yates, R. (1967). *Anat. Rec.*, **157**, 380.

Parker, J.M. and Mendell, J.R. (1974). *Nature*, **247**, 103-104.

Patten, B.M., Oliver, K.L. and Engel, W.K. (1974). *Arch. Neurol.*, **31**, 347-349.

Paulson, O.B., Engel, A.G. and Gomez, M.R. (1974). *J. Neurol. Neurosurg. Psychiat.*, **37**, 685-690.

Selye, H. (1965). 'The Mast Cells'. 488pp. Butterworth, Washington, D.C.

Selye, H. (1967). *Science*, **156**, 1262-1263.

Swash, M., Fox, K.P. and Davidson, A.R. (1975). *Arch. Neurol.*, **32**, 572-574.

Vetterlein, F. and Schmidt, G. (1975). *Arch. Int. Pharmacodyn.*, **213**, 4-16.

Walter, B.E. and O'Steen, W.K. (1963). *Proc. Soc. Exp. Biol. Med.*, **113**, 183-185.

Wright, T.L., O'Neill, J.A. and Olson, W.H. (1973). *Neurology*, **23**, 510-517.

28 A new mouse mutant with abnormal muscle function: comparison with the 129Re-dy mouse

R.L. WATTS · JEAN WATKINS · D.C. WATTS

Department of Biochemistry, Guy's Hospital Medical School, London SE1 9RT.

Introduction

A colony of 129Re-*dy* mice has been maintained and investigated by our research group since 1965. Early in 1975, abnormal animals were observed in a stock animal house colony of strain A2G albino mice. We decided to maintain and investigate this new mutation, and our colony was set up early that summer. We report here some preliminary findings with the mutant, which we have provisionally called *adr* (arrested development of righting response).

Biological features of the mutant

Up to the age of 4-6 weeks, *adr* mice grow almost as fast as littermates, and cannot be instantly distinguished in a litter, as *dy* mice often can be, on the basis of size alone. Their weight gain stops relatively suddenly at 8-10 weeks, after which their body shape becomes progressively shortened and distorted (see Fig. 1). However, they can be unequivocally detected from the age of 10-14 days by their inability to right themselves rapidly when turned on their backs; by this age, normal littermates have developed a righting-response so rapid that it is almost impossible to invert them at all. After handling, *adr* mice may drag their hindlimbs stiffly for a few seconds, a movement resembling the leg-dragging shown by stressed 129Re-*dy* mice. In the new mutant, the cause does not appear to be muscle weakness; *adr* mice can climb actively up their box walls, which dystrophic mice are never able to do. The occasional tetanic seisures seen in young dystrophic mice have not been observed in the new mutant. The usual lifespan is 7-8 months, but a number of affected animals have lived far longer. Several female *adr* mice have produced small litters, but males have not been found to breed. Neither sex of 129Re-*dy* mice normally breeds.

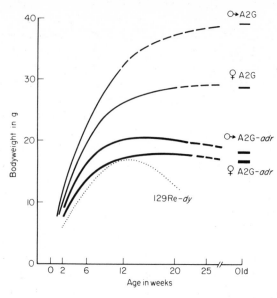

Fig. 1. Growth curves for A2G mice. Male and female controls are shown by fine lines, male and female affected (*adr*) mice are shown by heavy lines. The dotted curve shows body weights of 129Re-*dy* mice for comparison. Control 129Re mice, for which the sex difference in body weight is very small, follow a growth curve slightly above that for female A2G.

Inheritance pattern

The A2G-*adr* colony was organized on the assumption that *adr* was an autosomal recessive mutation, and the data collected so far are consistent with this.

In matings between siblings of affected animals, theoretically 4/9 of the pairs will both be carriers (heterozygotes). In 16 test matings, 11 carrier pairs were found.

Provided that the sizes of the sibships are not too small, 25% of the offspring of carrier pairs will be affected (homozygous recessive). In a total of 230 mice (from sibships of at least 10), 61 affected mice were found.

The sex ratio should approximate to 1:1. Of the 61 affected mice scored above, 36 were female, 25 were male.

Histological and Histochemical features of the mutant

Cryostat sections of various limb and back muscles were examined after staining with haematoxylin and eosin and with a series of enzyme-specific stains. As with 129Re-*dy* mouse muscle (Susheela *et al.*, 1968) the normal polygonal shape of fibres in transverse section was replaced by a rounded contour, but there appeared to be space between the fibres rather than massive infilling with connective and fatty tissue as in dystrophic muscle. The range of fibre diameters was no wider than normal; the small atrophied and large hypertrophied fibres characteristic of dystrophic muscle were not seen. However, in muscle from 3 week old *adr* mice, the average fibre diameter was below that of controls, resembling that of foetal muscle. The central nuclei which are seen in various myopathies were very rare, but nuclei were often vesicular with prominent nucleoli.

When sections were stained for ATPase at pH 9.4 (Dubowitz and Brooke, 1973) a checkerboard appearance like that in control muscle was seen. The percentage of Type II fibres was the same as in controls at 2 and 3 weeks of age, but the increase in type II fibres seen in older control muscle did not occur. When sections were stained for succinate dehydrogenase (Nachlas *et al.*, 1957) or other oxidative enzymes, differential staining of fibres was virtually absent from *adr* muscle.

All the differences observed from the normal appearance of muscle and its developmental changes suggest that in *adr* mice the process of muscle differentiation is arrested at a stage normally reached early in postnatal life. In developing muscle from the rat, aged 1-14 days, Dubowitz (1965) has observed differentiation of fibre types earlier by ATPase than by oxidative enzymes. Since fibre type has been shown to depend upon the type of nerve innervating the fibre (Romanul and van Der Meulen, 1966; Dubowitz and Newman, 1967) we suggest that in the *adr* mutant, a block occurs at a late stage in the nerve-muscle interactions which underlie muscle differentiation.

Enzymes levels in plasma and muscle

(a) Creatine kinase in plasma
Following previous conflicting reports on levels of creatine kinase (CPK) (Dreyfus *et al.*, 1966) we have investigated it in detail in plasma of 129Re-*dy* mice (Watts and Von Witt, unpublished). In normal mice 5 weeks old, CPK levels 6-10 times those in adult plasma were found. By 7 weeks the levels were only 3× that of the adult, which was reached by 11-12 weeks of age. CPK levels in dystrophic plasma were found to be at the top of or above the normal range throughout these age-dependent changes, but rarely exceeded the normal values by more than 200%. In a preliminary investigation of A2G-*adr* mice, the same developmental pattern was found, but CPK values for mutant mice were at the bottom of or below the normal range.

(b) AMP deaminase in muscle
Pennington (1963) reported levels of AMP deaminase in whole leg muscle of 129J-*dy* mice to be 60% of control values at 3-4 weeks, falling to 26% in older animals. Levels of the enzyme in A2G-*adr* mice measured separately on homogenates of soleus (red) muscle and the white part of the gastro-

cnemius (Table 1). In the former, comparable levels to the control values found by Pennington in 129J mice were found in both control and *adr* mice. In the white muscle, however, control levels 3-4 times higher were found, while in the mutant animals, values were about 35% of controls. AMP deaminase was found by Kendrick-Jones and Perry (1965) to increase rapidly after birth in rabbit leg muscle; hence, the reduced level found in *adr* mice is consistent with the hypothesis that the mutation causes developmental arrest.

TABLE 1

AMP deaminase levels in muscle of control and mutant mice (μmole NH$_3^+$/min/ mg protein). Values from Pennington (1963) recalculated for comparison.

Age (weeks)	A2G (mean value for 3-5 mice)				129Re		129Re (Pennington, 1963)	
	White muscle		Red muscle					
	control	*adr*	control	*adr*	control	*dy*	control	*dy*
3-4	10.17	3.53	3.13	3.25	–	–	2.94	1.76
6-8	9.61	3.76	2.51	3.23	–	–	–	–
12-20	–	–	–	–	1.84	0.55	2.53	0.66

References

Dreyfus, J.C., Schapira, E., Demos, J., Rosa, R. and Schapira, G. (1966). *Ann. N.Y. Acad. Sci.*, **138,** 304-314.

Dubowitz, V. (1965). *J. Neurol. Neurosurg. Psychiat.*, **28,** 516-524.

Dubowitz, V. and Brooke, M.H.(1973). 'Muscle Biopsy: A Modern Approach'. W.B. Saunders, London, Philadelphia, Toronto.

Dubowitz, V. and Newman, D.L. (1967). *Nature (Lond.),* **214,** 840-841.

Kendrick-Jones, J. and Perry, S.V. (1965). *Biochem. J.,* **103,** 207-214.

Nachlas, M.M. Tsou, K-C, de Souza, E., Cheng, C-S and Seligman, A.M. (1957). *J. Histochem. Cytochem.,* **5,** 420-436.

Pennington, R.J. (1963). *Biochem. J.,* **88,** 64-68.

Romanul, F.C.A. and Van Der Meulen, J.P. (1966). *Nature (Lond.),* **212,** 1369-1370.

Susheela, A.K., Hudgson, P. and Walton, J.N. (1968). *J. Neurol. Sci.,* **7,** 437-463.

Acknowledgements

Financial support for this research from the Muscular Dystrophy Group of Great Britain and from the Endowment Fund of Guy's Hospital is gratefully acknowledged.

29 Absorption and distribution of [2−14C] sodium barbital in normal and dystrophic mice

HEATHER R. STEPHENS* · DENIS NADEAU**   EDMUND B. SANDBORN
Départements d'Anatomie et de Pharmacologie, Faculté de Médecine,
Université de Montréal, Montréal, Quebec Canada H3C 3J7

In recent years the hypothesis that the muscular dystrophies may be due to an inherent defect in membrane structure has surplanted the concept of a strictly myogenic pathogenesis (Moore, 1975) or the alternate neurogenic (McComas et al., 1970) or vascular theories (Démos et al., 1970). Abnormalities of membrane function and in enzyme properties have been described in many tissues, in addition to those found in skeletal muscle, the tissue most visibly affected in human and animal dystrophies (Rowland, 1976). These findings suggest that the muscular dystrophies may be multisystem diseases.

Previous studies have indicated that there is increased uptake of nutrients by skeletal muscle tissue in dystrophic mice. The rate of entry of 14-C creatine into dystrophic muscle exceeded that found in normal animals (Fitch and Rahmanian, 1969) as did the concentrative uptake of α-aminoisobutyric acid (Baker, 1964). There is elevated incorporation of L-[U-14C] leucine into proteins of muscle subcellular fractions, which was more pronounced as the disease progressed (Srivastava, 1968). Time course experiments have revealed that in dystrophic mice the two major soluble muscle proteins, creatine kinase and adenylate kinase, initially incorporated two to three times more labelled amino acid relative to the initial size of the amino acid pool (Kitchin and Watts, 1973). This label was then lost equally rapidly and the final plateau value was much less than in normal mice. In addition another study on dystrophic mice has shown that there is enhanced incorporation of glycine into nucleic acids and proteins in muscle of dystrophic mice particularly in older mice (Coleman and Ashworth, 1959).

*Present address: Jerry Lewis Muscle Research Centre, Department of Paediatrics and Neonatal medicine, Hammersmith Hospital, Du Cane Road, London W12 OHS.

**Present Address: NIEHS/NIH, P.O. Box 12233, Research Triangle Park, N.C. 27709.

If there was a generalized membrane dysfunction in tissues of the dystrophic 129 ReJ mouse, then one might expect alterations in the pattern of drug absorption and distribution. In the present study we have analysed the time course of [2-^{14}C] sodium barbital uptake after oral administration with a gavage needle in normal and dystrophic mice. We have examined the levels of this narcotic drug recuperated from the gastrointestinal tract as well as plasma and tissue concentrations of the drug at various times after drug administration.

Methods

Normal and dystrophic 129 ReJ male mice were obtained from the Jackson Laboratory, Bar Harbor, Maine. Prior to each experiment the animals, 3 months of age, were deprived of food but not water for approximately 20 h. [2-^{14}C] sodium barbital (specific activity 2.24 mCi/mmol; New England Nuclear, Boston, Massachusetts) was diluted with unlabelled sodium barbital (Fisher Scientific Company) in normal saline before administration into the stomach with a gavage needle. Both normal and dystrophic mice were given the drug at a dosage of 200 mg/kg (71.67 μCi) body weight. If the dystrophic mice regurgitated after oral administration of the drug they were discarded from the experiment. At various time intervals after the administration of sodium barbital the mice were weighed and then killed by decapitation. A plasma sample was collected at this time.

The stomach and intestine, including the colon, were removed after ligation of the oesophagus and pylorus, homogenized (Polytron PT-10, Brinckman Instruments) in 5 ml of normal saline, and aliquots of 0.5 to 0.7 ml were kept for determination of radioactivity. The rate of absorption of sodium barbital was estimated by measuring the percentage of the dose recovered from the organs at various time intervals after drug administration. Immediately after decapitation the adrenal glands, brain, heart, kidney, liver, fore- and hindlimb skeletal muscle, pancreas, salivary glands, spleen, testes, testicular fat and thymus were removed from each normal and dystrophic mouse, weighed, and kept for estimating [2-^{14}C] sodium barbital. After removal of the above mentioned tissues the carcass of each mouse was minced with scissors and homogenized in a Waring blender for 5 min in 75 to 100 ml of normal saline. The homogenates were further processed with the Polytron apparatus and aliquots of 0.3 to 1.0 ml were used for counting. All tissue specimens and homogenates were digested in Protosol (New England Nuclear), and 10 ml of Aquasol (New England Nuclear) were added to each sample before counting in a Tri-Carb liquid Scintillator counter (Packard Instuments). The results were analysed with a student's t test.

Results

Preliminary time course experiments over a 24 h period showed that the sodium barbital was more rapidly removed from the gastrointestinal tract of the dystrophic mice than that of the normal animals. This resulted in initially (5-60 min) higher plasma levels of the drug, and consequently enhanced tissue concentrations. During the last 20 h of the time period studied the initially higher plasma and tissue levels of sodium barbital were reversed and less drug was recuperated in the dystrophic mouse. The percentage of the drug recovered from the gastro-intestinal tract of normal and dystrophic mice at 15 and 60 min, and 12 h is shown in Table 1. At 15 min significantly greater amounts of the drug were retained in the stomachs of normal mice. This difference was no longer apparent at 60 min or 12 h.

TABLE 1

Percentage of the dose of barbital recovered from the gastrointestinal tract and the carcass after oral administration of 200 mg/kg sodium barbital in 3 month old normal and dystrophic mice

		Percentage of the dose recovered		
Time of sacrifice after drug administration		15 min	60 min	12 h
Stomach	Dystrophic	$13.9 \pm 1.5^*$ (6)	11.0 ± 1.7 (4)	0.9 ± 0.9 (5)
	Normal	33.1 ± 3.9 (8)	27.9 ± 5.8 (7)	1.6 ± 0.6 (8)
Intestine	Dystrophic	9.6 ± 1.7	$9.6 \pm 1.6^*$	2.4 ± 1.1
	Normal	10.6 ± 1.1	6.6 ± 0.6	4.6 ± 0.5
Carcass	Dystrophic	$56.4 \pm 3.3^*$	$62.2 \pm 5.6^*$	26.7 ± 3.2
	Normal	40.4 ± 3.5	42.8 ± 5.1	46.0 ± 8.6

All values are mean $\pm$ SE. Numbers in parentheses refer to the numbers of animals.
  * $P < 0.05$

Significantly more of the sodium barbital was recovered in the intestine of dystrophic mice at 60 min but there was no difference at 12 h. The concentration of the drug in the plasma of dystrophic mice was significantly greater at 60 min but significantly less at 12 h than in the normal mice (Table 2). Table 2 illustrates the concentrations of the drug in adipose, tissue, brain, heart, kidney, liver, fore- and hindlimb muscle, spleen and thymus at 15 and 60 min and 12 h. At 15 min in all tissues of the dystrophic mice, except for the spleen, higher levels of sodium barbital were present. At 60 min barbital concentrations were significantly higher in the dystrophic tissues, whereas at 12 h during the elimination phase of the drug there were significantly lower concentrations of the drug in tissues of diseased mice. Similarly at 15 and 60 min there was a significantly greater percentage of the barbital dose recovered in the remaining tissues of the carcass of the dystrophic mice but less of the drug remained in these diseased animals

TABLE 2

Plasma and tissue distribution of barbital after oral administration of 200 mg/kg sodium barbital in 3 month old normal and dystrophic mice.

Tissues	Groups of mice	Barbital concentration (μg barbital/ml of plasma or /g of tissue)		
		15 min	60 min	12 h
Plasma	Dystrophic	217.1 ± 36.8 (6)*	217.0 ± 27.8* (4)	58.3 ± 6.1* (5)
	Normal	159.1 ± 15.8 (8)	161.1 ± 9.0 (7)	152.7 ± 29.2 (8)
Muscle (Hindlimbs)	Dystrophic	158.3 ± 15.8*	147.1 ± 13.0*	45.9 ± 4.0*
	Normal	96.0 ± 9.7	98.9 ± 13.6	86.9 ± 14.0
Muscle (Forelimbs)	Dystrophic	151.5 ± 21.4	147.9 ± 13.9*	45.4 ± 7.1
	Normal	110.1 ± 14.7	90.5 ± 14.0	86.8 ± 17.1
Heart	Dystrophic	169.4 ± 20.2*	170.3 ± 14.3*	47.8 ± 9.6*
	Normal	118.8 ± 11.0	110.7 ± 14.1	107.3 ± 17.5
Kidney	Dystrophic	186.2 ± 20.3*	182.6 ± 15.5*	58.8 ± 8.4
	Normal	128.2 ± 10.5	120.3 ± 13.9	125.3 ± 30.6
Liver	Dystrophic	165.8 ± 21.9	171.4 ± 15.1*	48.7 ± 5.6*
	Normal	143.1 ± 13.4	119.7 ± 10.1	104.7 ± 15.8
Brain	Dystrophic	99.3 ± 15.0*	131.6 ± 13.2*	38.5 ± 3.5
	Normal	67.1 ± 6.0	92.8 ± 11.9	71.8 ± 14.4
Adipose tissue	Dystrophic	103.2 ± 22.7	220.7 ± 61.9*	51.5 ± 17.0
	Normal	66.8 ± 11.8	59.0 ± 15.7	79.5 ± 18.4
Spleen	Dystrophic	162.6 ± 26.0	160.8 ± 18.7*	62.5 ± 9.4
	Normal	191.0 ± 9.0	104.1 ± 13.5	109.2 ± 23.4
Thymus	Dystrophic	207.2 ± 40.4*	229.2 ± 25.3*	50.7 ± 10.1
	Normal	88.4 ± 14.7	102.1 ± 16.4	90.2 ± 13.4

All values are mean ± SE. Numbers in parentheses refer to the number of animals. *P<0.05 or less.

at 12 h (Table 1). Tissue/plasma ratios were calculated from the results of Table 2. These values were consistently higher at 15 and 60 min and at 12 h in the dystrophic mice. The tissue/plasma ratios were significantly higher in the thymus of the diseased animals at 60 min and 12 h.

Discussion

Our data indicate that there is an increased rate of gastric emptying in the dystrophic mice. Thus absorption of the barbital from the intestine of these animals would be facilitated. Consequently the initial plasma and tissue concentrations (the latter being a reflection of the former) would be enhanced in comparison with those of the controls. The more rapid gastric emptying may be due to the atrophied condition of this organ in dystrophic animals or perhaps to deficient regulation of the smooth muscle contraction in the pylorus. The rapid absorption of the barbiturate observed in the dystrophic mouse may also be a reflection of the dilated micro-vasculature found in most organs and particularly within the digestive tract (Stephens and Sandborn, 1976). This could result in a relatively increased circulation in these organs with a massive shunt mechanism therein, and, in addition, an increased capillary surface area. In addition to a more rapid gastric emptying and the dilated micro-vasculature present in tissues of the dystrophic mice, the higher tissue/plasma ratios in these animals appear to be responsible in part for the significantly higher tissue uptake of the sodium barbital. The skeletal muscle tissue, both fore- and hindlimbs, of the dystrophic mouse exhibits the same pattern of rapid initial distribution and diminished retention of barbital, characteristic of other tissues. If murine muscular dystrophy were a primary myopathy, one might expect that if there were changes in drug kinetics, they should be expressed mainly within skeletal muscle. Our results indicate that this does not appear to be the case. Moreover, the tissue/plasma concentration ratios, throughout the entire time period studied, tend to be higher for all tissues of the dystrophic mice as compared with the normal animals. Thus our results suggest that there might be a membrane abnormality in all tissues of the dystrophic mouse. Although the levels of the drug remaining in tissues of the diseased animal at 12 h are lower than those of the control, there does not appear to be any difference in the actual excretion rate of the barbiturate. Since the drug is distributed more rapidly in the dystrophic mouse it follows that it would be excreted sooner. Since sodium barbital is not metabolized by mouse tissues, the excretion rate of the drug should not be complicated by alterations in metabolic rates (Dorfman and Goldbaum, 1947).

The phenomenon of more rapid tissue absorption of the barbiturate seemed to be more consistent as the disease progresses in older mice (Stephens, 1976). The altered absorption of sodium barbital in many tissues, including skeletal muscle, supports the concept that a generalized membrane disorder may be involved in the pathogenesis of murine muscular dystrophy. Although it remains to be established that such a phenomenon as the one reported in this paper is relevant to man, our results do suggest that drug administration to patients with muscular dystrophy may require special attention (Grob, 1976).

Acknowledgements

We wish to thank Dr. Claude Marchand, Département de Pharmacologie, Université de Montréal, who provided the facilities for this project and graciously donated the [2-^{14}C] barbital. This research was supported by grants from the Muscular Dystrophy Association of Canada, the Université de Montreal and the Sandborn Foundation.

References

Baker, R.D. (1964). *Texas. Rep. Biol. Med. Suppl.*, **22,** 880-886.
Coleman, D.L. and Ashworth, M.E. (1959). *Am. J. Physiol.*, **197,** 839-841.
Démos, J., Place, T. and Chereau, H. (1970). *Excerpta Med., Int. Congr., Ser.*, **199,** 408-411.
Dorfman, A. and Goldbaum, L.R.G. (1947). *J. Pharmacol. Exp. Ther.*, **90,** 330-337.
Fitch, C.C. and Rahmanian, M. (1969). *Proc. Soc. Exp. Med.*, **131,** 236-239.
Grob, D. (1976). *Ann. Rev. Pharmacol. Toxicol.*, **16,** 215-229.
Kitchin, S. and Watts, D. (1973). *Biochem. J.*, **136,** 1017-1028.
McComas, A.J., Sica, R.E.P. and Currie, S. (1970). *Nature*, **226,** 1263-1264.
Moore, M.J. (1975). *J. Neurol. Sci.*, **24,** 77-93.
Rowland, L.P. (1976). *Arch. Neurol.*, **33,** 315-321.
Srivastava, U. (1968). *Can. J. Biochem.*, **46,** 35-41.
Stephens, H.R. (1976). Murine muscular dystrophy — a multisystemic disorder. Ph.D. Thesis. Université de Montréal, Quebec, Canada.
Stephens, H. and Sandborn, E.B. (1976). *In* Microcirculation Vol.2. Transport Mechanisms. Disease States J. Grayson and W. Zingg (eds.). Plenum Press, New York, pp.330-332.

30 Increased endocytosis in skeletal muscle of dystrophic mice causing lysosomal activation

R. LIBELIUS · I. JIRMANOVÄ · I. LUNDQUIST · S. THESLEFF

Department of Pharmacology, University of Lund, Sweden and Institute of Physiology, Czechoslovak Academy of Sciences, Prague

During studies on the binding *in vitro* of a cobra α-neurotoxin (*Naja naja siamensis)* to cholinergic receptors in mouse skeletal muscle, it became apparent that apart from a specific irreversible binding to cholinergic receptors the toxin was alto taken up intracellularly (Libelius, 1974). Such intracellular uptake of toxin was found to be stimulated by cationic proteins like protamine at $+37°C$ but blocked at $+4°C$, and it was suggested that it occurred by endocytosis (Libelius, 1975). It was also shown that extracellular tracers, like horseradish peroxidase could be used to study endocytosis in skeletal muscle. As for the toxin, protamine was found to stimulate the intracellular uptake of horseradish peroxidase as determined chemically, and observed ultrastructurally (Jirmanová *et al.,* 1977). In addition to internalization of horseradish peroxidase into numerous vesicles, membrane limited bodies (probably secondary lysosomes) and vacuoles, protamine was also found to cause segmental autophagic vacuolation with progressive muscle fibre degeneration (Jirmanová *et al.,* 1977).The interpretation that protamine induced vacuoles were of an autophagic type, was supported by recent findings that protamine *in vitro* at $+37°C$ within 1 hour of incubation caused an increase in the total acid phosphatase enzyme activity. The formation of numerous lysosomes (acid phosphatase positive) in the interfibrillar space adjacent to the Golgi region in extensor digitorum longus muscles from the mouse was also observed (Libelius and Lundquist, 1977). Protamine also caused proliferation of tubular and vesicular profiles originating from the transverse t-system. The overall ultrastructural features of this protamine induced myopathy i.e. lysosomal activation, t-tubule proliferation and autophagic vacuolation resemble changes observed in human and animal dystrophy and other degenerative muscle diseases (Schutta *et al.,* 1969; Engel and Macdonald, 1970; Schotland, 1970; Malouf and Sommer, 1976). Several lysosomal enzymes in skeletal muscle have been found to be increased in muscular dystrophy (cf. Weinstock and

Iodice, 1969). Since endocytotic activity has been found to activate the lysosomal system in a variety of other cell types (Warburton and Wynn, 1976), it seemed worth-while to examine endocytosis in dystrophic muscles.

Endocytosis *in vitro* was measured by the uptake of the two different extracellular tracers, ^{3}H-inulin and horseradish peroxidase, in extensor digitorum longus and soleus muscles from homozygous dystrophic mice of the Bar Harbour 129 strain and their unaffected littermates. After incubation in the presence of tracer the muscles were washed for 4 hours at +4°C in excess of tracer-free solution in order to clear the extracellular space of the tracers. Endocytosis *in vivo* was studied using horseradish peroxidase injected i.v. as tracer, and examination of the muscles for their content of the tracer 2 hours after injection by chemical (Lundquist and Josefsson, 1971) or morphological techniques (Graham and Karnovsky, 1966). In addition to the administration of horseradish peroxidase i.v., some dystrophic extensor digitorum longus muscles were soaked in the tracer solution to achieve a good labelling of the transverse t-tubules for ultrastructural examination.

The uptake *in vitro* of ^{3}H-inulin and horseradish peroxidase was found to be increased in both types of muscles from dystrophic mice as compared with littermate controls. For both tracers the increased uptake was more pronounced in the extensor muscle, which was also more affected by the disease than the soleus muscle. It was also noted that the uptake of horseradish peroxidase was relatively higher than that of inulin, possibly resulting from the ability of the peroxidase to bind to cellular membranes and thereby to be internalized by 'mixed' endocytosis (cf. Jacques, 1969). Horseradish peroxidase injected i.v. in the mouse was found to have a distribution—elimination curve with peak values in both types of muscles at about 2 hours after the injection (Libelius and Lundquist, unpublished results). Dystrophic muscles removed 2 hours after an i.v. injection of the peroxidase and thereafter washed *in vitro* in a Krebs solution for 4 hours at +4°C to reduce extracellularly bound tracer, were found to contain more peroxidase than control muscles from littermates which were treated identically. Although some of this peroxidase was likely to be extracellularly located, the difference observed between dystrophic and control muscles can be ascribed to an increase in intracellular tracer, as supported by our morphological findings.

Two hours after a single injection of the tracer, accumulations of peroxidase positive structures of varying sizes were identified at the light microscopic level in both types of dystrophic muscles, but not in controls. Ultrastructural examination of these peroxidase positive fibres showed that it was contained in intracellular membrane limited bodies of diverse size and appearance. These peroxidase positive structures, visible in the light microscope, were found to be distributed segmentally along the fibre length, similar to the protamine induced vacuoles mentioned above. Horseradish peroxidase positive primary uptake vesicles were identified either as coated vesicles from the sarcolemma or as vesicles of the same size derived from the transverse tubules. Thus, endocytosis can occur from both the sarcolemma and the transverse tubules, however, in the present study no attempt was made to differentiate quantitatively between the two.

Probably as the result of fusion between several primary uptake vesicles larger peroxidase positive bodies with a single limiting membrane were formed. These were mainly found in the I-band level close to the A-I junction often in close relation to labelled transverse tubules. In regions containing these peroxidase positive structures, we often observed disintegration of myofibrils in the I-band and overdevelopment of tubular and vesicular profiles in the interfibrillar space. An alternative explanation is that primary uptake vesicles may fuse with lysosomes at different stages of development forming heterophagic lysosomes with variable content of horseradish peroxidase and therefore different staining intensities. Autophagic vacuoles containing horseradish peroxidase were also encountered, showing that hetero- and autophagic structures were interconnected.

The activities of the lysosomal enzymes cathepsin D and N-acetylglucosaminidase were both increased in the tibialis anterior and gastrocnemius muscle from dystrophic mice as compared to littermate controls. From previous studies (Jirmanova *et al.*, 1977; Libelius and Lundquist, 1977) stimulation of endocytosis has been shown to be accompanied by lysosomal activation and fibre degeneration in normal skeletal muscle. Data presented here show that both endocytosis and lysosomal enzyme activities in skeletal muscle are increased in murine dystrophy. The hypothesis, that augmented endocytosis in dystrophic skeletal muscle might result in activation of the lysosomal system and thereby in muscle fibre degeneration, is put forward.

Acknowledgements

We are greatly indebted to Dr. J.B. Harris, Muscular Dystrophy Group Research Laboratories, Newcastle upon Tyne General Hospital for the gift of the dystrophic mice used in this study.

References

Engel, A.G. and Macdonald, R.D. (1970). *In:* Muscle Diseases. Proceedings of an International Congress, Milan, 19-20 May 1969 pp.99-108 (J.N. Walton, N. Carol and G. Scarlato, eds.). Amsterdam, Exerpta-Medica.

Graham, R.J. Jr. and Karnovsky, M.J. (1970). *J. Histochem. Cytochem.*, **14**, 291-302.

Jacques, P.J. (1969). *In:* Lysosomes in biology and pathology, vol.2. 395-420 (J.T. Dingle and H.B. Fell, eds.). Amsterdam: North-Holland Publishing Company.

Jirmanová, I., Libelius, R., Lundquist, I. and Thesleff, S. (1977). *Cell Tiss. Res.*, **176**, 463-473.

Libelius, R. (1974). *J. Neural Transm.*, **35**, 137-149.

Libelius, R. (1975). *J. Neural Transm.*, **37**, 61-71.

Libelius, R. and Lundquist, I. (1977). *Cell Tiss. Res.*, in press.

Lundquist, I. and Josefsson J.-O. (1971). *Analyt. Biochem.*, **41**, 567-577.

Malouf, N.N. and Sommer, J.R. (1976). *Am. J. Pathol.*, **84**, 299-316.

Schotland, D.L. (1970). *J. Neuropathol. Exp. Neurol.*, **29**, 241-253.

Schutta, H.S., Kelly, A.M. and Zacks, S.I. (1969). *Brain*, **92**, 191-202.

Weinstock, I.M. and Iodice, A.A. (1969). *In:* Lysosomes in biology and pathology. Vol. 1, 450-468. (J.T. Dingle and H.B. Fell, eds.). Amsterdam: North-Holland Publishing Company.

Warburton, M.J. and Wynn, C.H. (1976). *Biochem. Biophys. Res. Commun.*, **70**, 94-100.

31 Motor endplate disease: functions exhibited in culture by myotubes from med/med mice

W. BURKART · H. JOCKUSCH · M.M. BURGER

Biozentrum der Universität Basel, Klingelbergstr. 70, CH-4056 Basel

Motor endplate disease is an autosomal recessive neuromuscular disorder leading to paralysis from day 12 onwards and to death around day 20 (Duchen, 1970). The disease is due to an abnormality in the function of motor nerve terminals. Although peripheral nerve conduction is normal and direct stimulation of muscles causes twitch responses, muscles fail to contract in response to nerve stimulation or give only a weak twitch (Duchen and Stefani, 1971; Harris and Ward, 1974). Miniature endplate potentials are normal. With longer survival of the animal, fibrillation, hypersensitivity to acetylcholine, and resistance of the muscle action potential to tetrodotoxin, presumably in consequence to 'physiological denervation', are observed (Duchen and Stefani, 1971; Harris and Ward, 1974).

Since homozygous animals die around day 20, the gene (med) has to be kept in a heterozygous stock. In a litter the expected quarter of homozygous animals can be identified by the closely linked (1% recombination frequency) caracul marker (Searle, 1970). Because of this tissue can be obtained from med/med animals more than 10 days before the onset of clinical symptoms. In the search of the primary cause of the motor endplate disease we have compared muscle from med/med mice with muscle of their phenotypically normal (+/?) littermates in tissue and organ culture.

Materials and methods

Muscle cultures

$\frac{Ca^{d}+}{+\ med}$ mice were obtained from Harwell. Newborn animals were identified with 99% certainty as being med/med by their noncaracul whiskers. Leg muscles were removed from 1-2 day old med/med mice and their +/? (caracul) littermates. Explants (about 1/3 mm in diameter) were preincubated for 1-2 days in bacterial dishes, and then placed in collagen coated petri-dishes, 1 mm distant from the ventral side of a previously attached spinal cord section. For monolayers, minced muscle was digested 2-3 times for 20 minutes at 37°C in CMF-Earle containing 0.25% trypsin. After filtration through lens tissue the cells were plated onto collagen coated dishes in DME (88%), heat inactivated horse serum (10%), chick embryo (1%) with penicillin and streptomycin and were cultured for up to 2 months, with changes of 50% of the medium twice a week (Yaffe, 1973; Bowden-Essien, 1972).

Spinal cord cultures

Spinal cords were dissected from embryos on day 13 of gestation and cut into slices (Peterson and Crain, 1970). They were allowed to attach onto collagen coated 35 mm petri-dishes under 0.7 ml of a medium containing 10% fetal calf serum instead of the chick embryo extract.

Staining

Staining for nerve fibres (silver) and acetylcholinesterase activity (thiocholine) was performed by the method of Namba *et al.* (1967).

Results
Myotube-monolayers from dissociated myoblasts

In several experiments the yield of med/med myoblasts per animal was only 30-50% of wildtype but this finding needs confirmation. Cells were plated at a final density of $2\text{-}10 \times 10^6$ cells per 35 mm dish. They fused within 3 days and showed contractility after 6 days in culture. There were no visible differences in the onset of fusion of the myoblasts, the intensity of spontaneous contractions and in the degree of cross-striation between med/med and +/? myotubes. After 3 weeks, a fraction of myotubes degenerated but survival of med/med muscle was not reduced as compared to wild type. A fraction of matured cross-striated med/med myotubes survived and actively contracted for at least 55 days. Thus the lifespan of these myotubes exceeded the lifespan of med/med animals by more than a month.

Co-culture of spinal cord and muscle explants

Muscle piece explants from med/med animals were placed 1 mm to the ventral side of wildtype (NMRI or CBA) spinal cord slices. Myotubes formed by fusion of myoblasts around the muscle piece and after 10 days covered an area 20 to 30 times the area of the explant. Bundles of nerve fibres emerging from the spinal cord explant invaded both the muscle explant and the network of newly formed myotubes. Staining for acetylcholinesterase after 3 weeks showed 10-40 endplates on newly formed myotubes in an irregular distribution. A qualitatively similar result was obtained in coupled cultures with wildtype muscle explants. Maximal outgrowth of nerve fibres and myotubes depended on the timing of explants. Outgrowth of muscle explants may be totally inhibited by spinal cord culture that have been in culture for more than 4-6 days. In that case, extensive innervation of the muscle explants was observed.

Discussion

The histological and physiological investigations by Duchen, Stefani and Harris suggest a presynaptic bloc in the motor endplate disease mutation. Our study did not reveal any abnormality of med/med myotubes in culture, either alone or in conjuction with wildtype spinal cord (Jockusch *et al.*, 1976; Burkart *et al.*, 1977). Yet, as argued elsewhere (Jockusch, 1977), these data are not sufficient to decide between a neurogenic, myogenic or other (e.g. humoral) primary cause of the motor endplate disease. Therefore we are now planning to perform culture experiments where the genotype of the spinal cord is varied. The main problem in these experiments is the fact that spinal cord cultures develop optimally from embryos of 13 day gestational age, while the caracul marker is not recognizable before birth. Furthermore, our cultures may not necessarily acquire the stage of maturation which in the animal is the critical step for the onset of the motor endplate disease, or they may take a much longer time than *in vivo* to do so.

References

Bowden-Essien, F. (1967). *Developmental Biology,* **27,** 351.
Burkart, W., Burger, M.M. and Jockusch, H. (1977). *Mouse News Letters,* **56,** 31.
Duchen, L.W. (1970). *J. Neurol. Neurosurg. Psychiat.,* **33,** 238-249.
Duchen, L.W. and Stefani, E. (1971). *J. Physiol.,* **212,** 535-548.
Harris, J.B. and Ward, M.R. (1974). *Experimental Neurology,* **42,** 169-180.
Jockusch, H. (1977). *Naturwissenschaften,* **63,** (1977) **64,** 260-265.
Jockusch, H., Burger, M.M. and Burkart, W. (1976). *Mouse News Letters,* **55,** 8-9.
Namba, T., Nakamura, T. and Grob, D. (1967). *The American J. of Clinical Pathology,* **47,** 74-77.
Peterson, E.R. and Crain, S.M. (1970). *Z. Zellforsch.,* **106,** 1-21.
Searle, A., (1970). J. Neurol. Neurosurg. Psychiat., **33,** 249-250.
Yaffe, D. (1973). *Tissue culture, Methods and Applications,* p. 106-114. Academic Press.

32 Chemical potentiation of muscle regeneration

R. PARSONS · M.R. WEST

Muscular Dystrophy Research Laboratory, Regional Neurological Centre, Newcastle upon Tyne NE4 6BE

The regeneration of normal muscle has been studied in great depth. Several hypotheses setting out the mechanism for regeneration have been proposed and it remains a matter of choice whether one particular hypothesis is favoured. We chose to investigate regeneration without any bias toward specific mechanisms and with the express purpose of comparing the regenerative capacities of normal and dystrophic mouse muscle. Transplantation experiments reported by Carlson (1972) and by Rolston (1972) indicate a close correlation between blood supply and muscle regeneration. This was clearly demonstrated in Carlson's work, where myotubes could be seen closely aligned with the capillaries. Rolston has examined the regeneration of normal and dystrophic mouse muscle when isotransplanted from one animal to another. In all cases revascularization was evident. However dystrophic muscle was not improved by a normal host environment and continued to degenerate. Normal muscle was not influenced by the dystrophic environment and regenerated to form normal muscle. Our findings from tissue culture experiments indicate most strongly that muscle may regenerate from an inherent genetic capability and that circumstances dictate the course of regeneration. We have also found dystrophic muscle from the mouse to be consistently and grossly defective in attempted regeneration.

Methods and materials

Animals from our own colony of 129 ReJ mice were used throughout. Homozygous dystrophic *dy/dy* and heterozygous normal adult mice provided the source of muscle. Embryonic mice of 14 days gestation were produced by dated mating following hormonal induction of oestrus. The tissues were grown in a Maximow double coverslip assembly. It was modified for some of the experiments by etching a groove across the small round inner coverslip using hydrofluoric acid. The culture medium was either:

(a) Human placental cord serum 33%, chicken embryo extract 10%, Eagles MEM with Earle's salts 57%, 0.85 gl⁻¹ NaHCO₃ (Flow Labs.), glucose 6 mg/ml⁻¹;

or (b) Horse serum (Flow Labs.) 10%, chicken embryo extract 10%, Eagles MEM with Earle's salts 80%, 0.85 gl⁻¹ NaHCO₃ + 20 mM HEPES.

Medium (a) was used in all cultures where spinal cord was grown, and a group of muscle cultures on collagen (Table 1). Medium (b) was used in the evaluation of the plasma clot cultures (Table 2). Muscle samples were teased into explants of 2-6 fibres, 2-7 mm long in Ca^{++} Mg^{++} free Phosphate Buffered Saline. Spinal cord sections were cut to include both dorsal root ganglia of each segment, avoiding any damage to the meningeal membrane (Peterson and Crain, 1970). The sections were then placed on collagen-coated coverslips (Bornstein, 1958) and allowed to become established for 7 days before the addition of muscle explants. When barrier coverslips with a groove were used the barrier was not filled or covered with collagen and was maintained free of cells. Cord sections and muscle explants were placed on opposite sides of the barrier but approximately the same distance apart as in the other cord + muscle cultures. All cultures were fed every 2 or 3 days and examined regularly. Cultures of muscle alone set up on collagen were used as control cultures (a) for the influence of the plasma clot on muscle growth, (b) for the influence of the spinal cord tissue on muscle growth. The tissue combinations and culture types are set out in Tables 1 and 2.

TABLE 1

Culture type medium (a) collagen substrate	Nos. of cultures assessed	Development of pseudostraps	Development of myotubes	% Regeneration
Cord + Normal muscle	63	1	60	95.2
Cord + Dystrophic muscle	37	17	11	29.7
Cord // Normal muscle	10	3	7	70
Cord // Dystrophic muscle	8	3	1	12.5
Normal muscle only	47	0	1	2.1
Dystrophic muscle only	37	0	0	0

Results

Tables 1 and 2 give the numerical analysis of those cultures which were successful. Approximately half of the total number of cultures were rejected for abnormal spinal cord growth patterns or accidental loss or damage. Clearly, regeneration of muscle, which is defined as the formation of multinucleate myotubes, is influenced by the immediate environment.

TABLE 2

Culture Type medium (b)	No. of cultures assessed	No. of cultures with no cell outgrowth %		Pseudostraps	Myotubes	% Regeneration
Normal muscle in Plasma	94	52	55.3	0	13	13.8
Dystrophic muscle in plasma	67	24	35.8	3	0	0
Normal muscle in fibrin	43	28	65.1	0	1 Tetranucleate	2.3
Dystrophic muscle in fibrin	41	24	58.5	1	0	0
Normal muscle on collagen	47	32	68.1	0	2	4.3
Dystrophic muscle on collagen	35	21	60	3	0	0

Muscle on collagen medium (a), (Table 1), and muscle on collagen in medium (b), (Table 2), which represent the baseline controls show that neither culture media will support regeneration. However muscle in a plasma clot in medium (b) (Figs. 1 and 2) does regenerate indicating a plasma influence. That this influence is not merely structural is shown by the almost complete lack of regeneration in a fibrin clot (Figs. 3 and 4).

Muscle will also regenerate on collagen when paired with a spinal cord section, (Table 1). Regeneration is greatly increased over the plasma clot cultures and is due entirely to the presence of the spinal cord tissues (Figs. 5 and 6). That the regeneration is not brought about only by contact between the spinal cord tissue outgrowth and the muscle fibres is proved by the barrier system (Figs. 7 and 8) where regeneration is seen, although diminished by comparison (Table 1). The spinal cord tissue, therefore, has a significant influence on the regeneration of muscle.

Muscle from dystrophic mice exhibits much less regeneration, as these experiments show. It is significantly less when paired with the spinal cord tissue and absent in all other situations. Many cultures show characteristic pseudostraps, which are groups of closely apposed myoblasts resembling a myotube, but they are not syncitial (Moore, 1975).

Discussion

The simple conclusive statement from these results is that muscle can regenerate *in vitro* when the environment or culture conditions will permit. The environment also appears to dictate the degree of regeneration. Therefore we can deduce that muscle will regenerate through an inherent genetic ability, and that a failure to regenerate reflects a lack in the environment. It has been shown (West, 1976) that muscle fibres lose all their nuclei *in vitro* within 5 days. Consequently no regeneration can occur. Therefore whatever the overall influence of the plasma or the spinal cord tissue may be, one of the primary functions of the culture environment must be to maintain viable muscle capable of regeneration.

Our experiments point to a chemical 'factor' present in blood plasma and produced by spinal cord tissue, which potentiates muscle regeneration. Its identity is unknown. Other work (Peterson and Crain, 1972) has shown

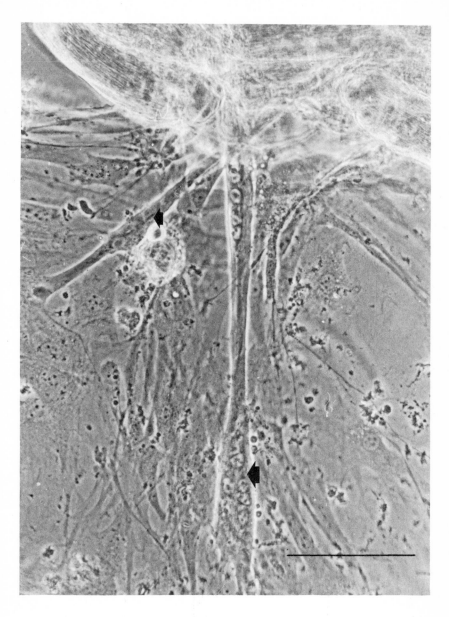

Fig. 1. Normal muscle in a plasma clot. Several myotubes can be seen (→) with groups of nuclei. Bar 0.1 mm.

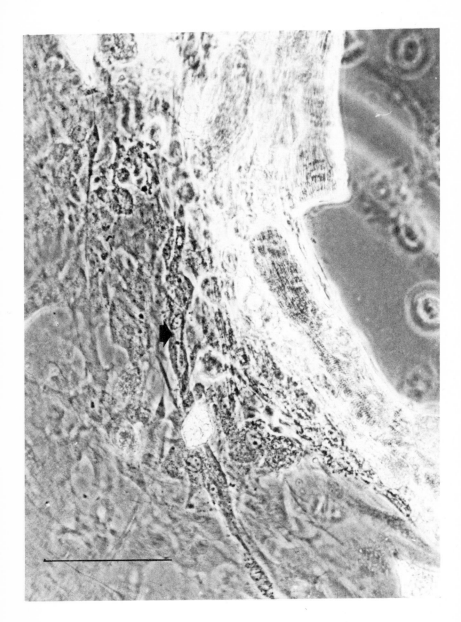

Fig. 2. Dystrophic muscle in plasma clot. This illustrates substantial cellular outgrowth and a pseudostrap (an arrangement of unfused myoblasts)➤. Bar 0.1 mm.

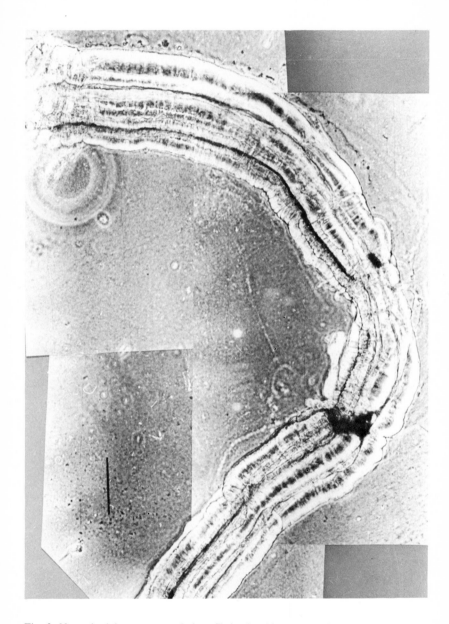

Fig. 3. Normal adult mouse muscle in a fibrin clot. No regeneration or cellular outgrowth can be seen. Bar 0.1 mm.

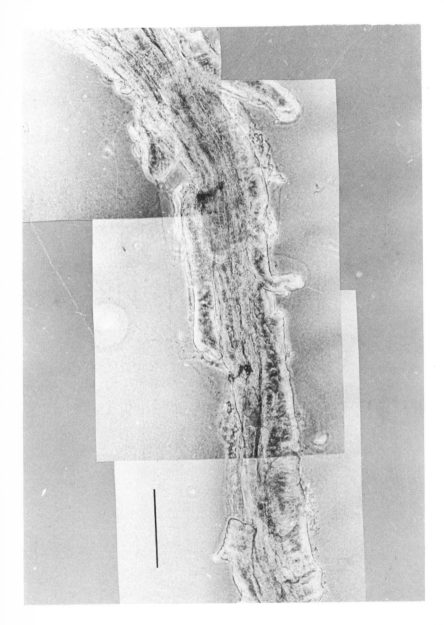

Fig. 4. Dystrophic (dy) mouse muscle in a fibrin clot. No regeneration or cellular outgrowth. Bar 0.1 mm.

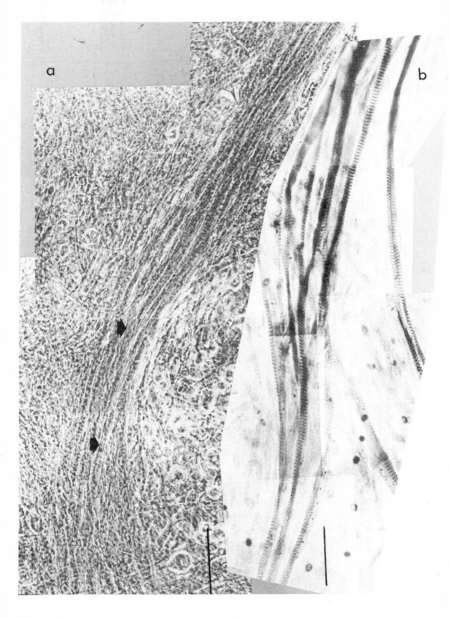

Fig. 5. Normal muscle growth in combination with a spinal cord section. There is extensive regeneration with many striated muscle fibres➤. Bar 0.1 mm. (a) Living culture. (b) Stained culture to show advanced development of striated muscle fibres.

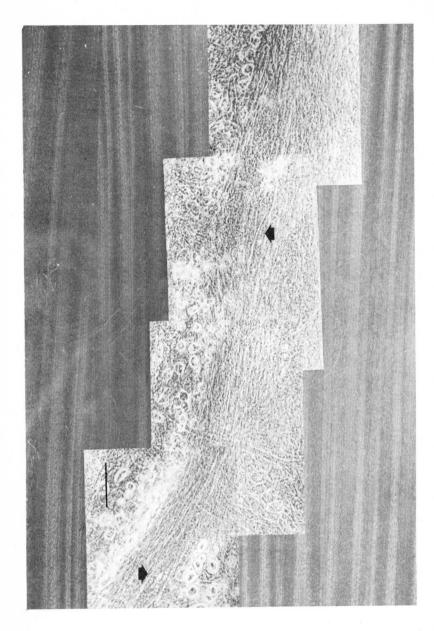

Fig. 6. Dystrophic muscle combination with a spinal cord section. Some myotubes can be seen (⟶) but fewer and less mature. Bar 0.1 mm.

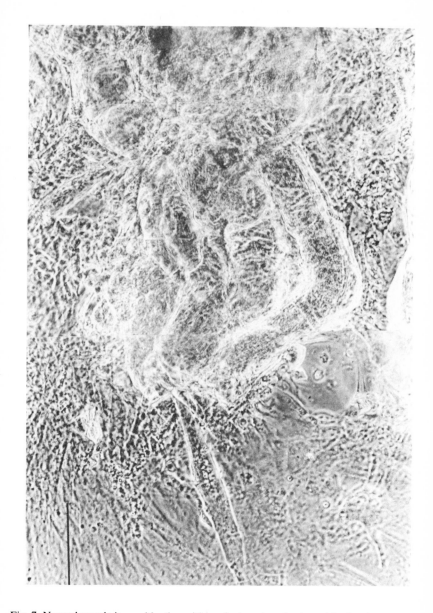

Fig. 7. Normal muscle in combination with a spinal cord section but with a barrier to prevent contact between the cellular outgrowth of the cord section and the muscle. The barrier is a groove or trough etched in the inner round coverslip of the Maximow assembly. Regeneration is much slower and proceeds only to myotube stages. Bar 0.1 mm.

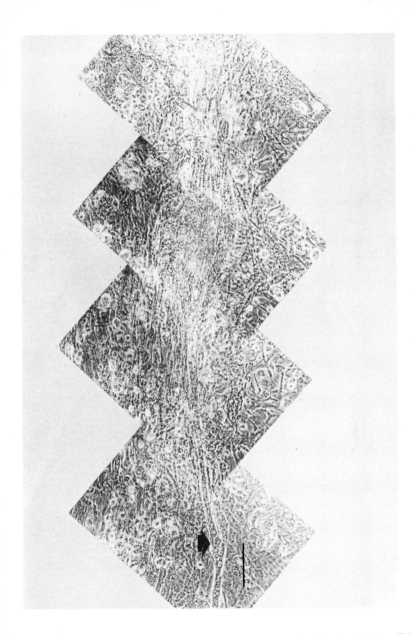

Fig. 8. Dystrophic muscle in combination with a spinal cord section in a barrier situation. This was the only culture to show a myotube ➤. Bar 0.1 mm.

that alternative embryonic tissues, e.g. liver or lung can also support regeneration. Therefore the blood factor could originate from any or many tissues. Our experiments also show that the unknown factor produced by the cord section diffuses into the culture medium, since there is no other way that it could have effected muscle regeneration across the barrier. It is interesting to note here that without a barrier, regeneration is more successful and very much more rapid. This again demonstrates that the nearer the source to the target, the closest being direct cell contact, the more concentrated is the diffusible factor. It is also interesting that in the case of the cord and muscle cultures the factor must be replaced in the culture medium every two or three days because of the necessary feeding schedule. It must therefore be extremely potent in small quantities, or produced very rapidly in large quantities.

Dystrophic muscle regeneration was shown to be significantly less successful in these cultures. This may be due to low satellite cell numbers or an overall low nuclear number. Alternatively one could view the regeneration in these cultures as highly successful, since previous reports (Moore, 1975; Parsons, 1974) have described the absence of myotube formation in dystrophic muscle cultures. Perhaps there is a genuine inability of dystrophic myoblasts to fuse unless the circumstances are optimal. This, together with a decreased satellite cell population would certainly result in slower and less regeneration. Many problems and points of interest have been raised by this work with regard to normal and dystrophic mouse muscle regeneration and we look forward to a progressive elucidation of these problems in the future.

References

Bornstein, M.B. (1958). *Lab. Invest.*, **7**, 134-140.
Carlson, B.M. (1972). The Regeneration of Minced Muscles. S. Karger, Basel.
Moore, M.J. (1975). *J. neurol. Sci.*, **24**, 77-93.
Parsons, R. (1974). *Nature*, **251**, 621-622.
Peterson, E.R. and Crain, S.M. (1970). *Z. Zellforsch.*, **106**, 1-21.
Rolston, J.L.L. (1972). *Arch. Neurol.*, **26**, 258-264.
West, M.R. (1976). Ph.D. Thesis. University of Newcastle upon Tyne.

33 The influence of neuroleptic drugs on the development of muscular rigidity in halothane sensitive pigs

J.V. McLOUGHLIN · C.J. SOMERS · C.P. AHERN · P. WILSON

Department of Pre-Clinical Veterinary Sciences and Department of Biochemistry, Trinity College, Dublin 2, Ireland.

Malignant hyperthermia occurs in man and the pig when susceptible individuals are exposed to the anaesthetic halothane (2-bromo-2-chloro-1,1,1-trifluoroethane) or the depolarising myorelaxant succinylcholine. The syndrome is characterized by extreme muscular rigidity, hyperthermia, tachycardia and cardiac arrythmia, a rise in both lactate formation and oxygen consumption in skeletal muscle and an increase in the concentration of K^+, lactate, glucose, free-fatty acids and catecholamines in blood. The muscular rigidity which is an early and prominent feature of porcine malignant hyperthermia is thought to be due to a rise in the sarcoplasmic concentration of ionized calcium due to a myotoxic action of halothane. It is not known whether the general systemic manifestations of the condition are secondary to this myotoxic effect or result from a direct action of the anaesthetic on other tissues, in particular those of the peripheral and central nervous systems. Although the aetiology of malignant hyperthermia is not fully understood, a variety of procedures has been employed to prevent or alleviate the syndrome. The myorelaxant dantrolene, which either blocks electrical transmission along the internal membrane system or interferes with the release of Ca^{2+} from intracellular storage sites, has been reported to prevent the development of rigidity and to relax already rigid muscle (Harrison, 1975). The administration of high doses of α- but not β-adrenergic blocking agents alleviates the symptoms but does not abolish the initial response of the muscle (Hall *et al.*, 1975). Anaesthesia with barbiturates (Gronert and Theye, 1976; Somers *et al.*, 1977a) and the intramuscular injection of the neuroleptic drugs azaperone, haloperidol and spiperone (Ahern *et al.*, 1977) prior to the administration of halothane delay the onset and attenuate the severity of the syndrome.

Piétrain pigs susceptible to malignant hyperthermia were used in the work reported in this paper. These pigs developed a rigid extension of the limbs and a rise in body temperature after breathing halothane (5%) in O_2 for less than 5 min; and unless anaesthesia was discontinued as soon as the symptoms appeared the progress of the syndrome became irreversible and the animals died 20 to 30 min later (McLoughlin and Mothersill, 1976). The effect of premedication with neuroleptic drugs on this adverse reaction to halothane was studied. The concentrations of creatine phosphate (CP) and adenosine triphosphate (ATP) in skeletal muscle were examined since depletion of high energy phosphate is a feature of the condition. The semitendinosus muscle was used in the investigation because this muscle in the pig had distinct areas of predominantly red and white myofibres (Tarrant et al., 1973) and it was therefore possible to make a comparative study of high energy phosphate changes in mainly oxidatively (red) and anaerobically metabolizing (white) myofibres from the same muscle. The neuroleptics used were azaperone (4-fluoro-[4-2(pyridyl)-piperazinyl]-1-butyrophenone) and spiperone (8-[3-(p-fluorobenzoyl)-propyl]-1,3,8-triazospiro-(4,5)-decan-4-one).

Eight susceptible pigs were given neuroleptic drugs intramuscularly approximately 30 min before anaesthesia with halothane. Five were given azaperone (8mg/Kg) and three spiperone (2mg/Kg). Two azaperone-treated pigs were also infused with the neuroleptic in saline (0.2mg/Kg/min) during a period of 40 min under anaesthesia. The semitendinosus muscles were removed after periods of anaesthesia indicated in the text. Specimens of the red and white myofibre areas of the muscles were frozen in liquid N_2 and subsequently extracted with perchloric acid. The concentration of CP and ATP in the tissue was assayed using glucose-6-phosphate dehydrogenase, hexokinase and creatine kinase in a sequence of $NADP^+$ linked reactions according to a procedure already described (McLoughlin and Mothersill, 1976). Lactate was determined using lactic dehydrogenase and NAD^+. The reactions were followed at 340 nm in a Pye Unicam S.P. 1700 spectrophotometer.

Pretreatment with azaperone delayed the onset of muscular rigidity. The characteristic rigid extension of the limbs occured after 45 to 55 min anaesthesia, in contrast to a delay phase of less than 5 min when the animals had not been premedicated. The infusion of azaperone did not further delay and the development of rigidity. The concentration of high energy phosphate in the semitendinosus muscle is given in Table 1. The CP content of the red myofibres was virtually depleted after 30 min anaesthesia, i.e., before rigidity had yet developed, while after 70 min and following the onset of rigidity the CP content of both myofibre types was depleted. At 30 min, the concentration of CP in the white myofibres was approximately 50% of the value which might be expected from the results of Somers et al. (1977b). These authors found that red myofibres contained 13 μmol CP/g, white 23 μmol CP/g when the semitendinosus muscle was removed from Piétrain pigs under pentobarbitone anaesthesia following premedication

TABLE 1

Effect of azaperone on muscle energy phosphates in halothane-initiated malignant hyperthermia

Period of anaesthesia	Myofibre type	CP+	ATP+
30 min	Red	1.6 ± 0.2	2.2 ± 0.2
(before rigidity)	White	10.7 ± 2.0	5.6 ± 0.3
70 min	Red	1.3 ± 0.3	1.2 ± 0.3
(rigidity)	White	1.5 ± 0.2	2.0 ± 0.6

+ μmol/g wet tissue. Mean values for 5 animals ± S.E.M.

with azaperone. The data are useful as baseline or control values for comparative purposes. The concentrations of ATP in muscle removed after 30 min were appreciably lower than those (red myofibres 7.6 μmol/g, white 8.6 μmol/g) reported by Somers *et al.* (1977b) although rigidity had not developed. The ATP content of the red myofibres had already fallen to the low levels associated with the onset of rigor mortis in skeletal muscle. The ATP content of both myofibre types was depleted after 70 min.

Spiperone had a more marked influence on the reaction of susceptible pigs to halothane than had azaperone. Two pigs premedicated with this neurolpetic did not exhibit muscular rigidity after 90 min anaesthesia (the experiments were terminated at this time). Rigidity developed in the third pig after approximately 65 min. The concentration of high energy phosphate in the semitendinosus muscle is given in Table 2. The CP and ATP content of white myofibres of muscle removed after 40 min was similar to the value reported for normal muscle (Somers *et al.*, 1977b) although the concentration of CP in the red myofibres was probably somewhat low. The muscles from the two pigs which did not develop ridigity up to 90 min were placed at 37°C under N_2. The 1/2 life of ATP in the white myofibres under these conditions was 45 to 65 min. Such rates of ATP loss *in vitro* are high and especially so in view of the high initial levels of CP and ATP in the tissue. These concentrations of high energy phosphate should have given a 1/2

TABLE 2

Effect of spiperone on muscle energy phosphates in halothane-initiated malignant hyperthermia.

Period of anaesthesia	Myofibre type	CP*	ATP*
40 min	Red	6.7 ± 1.2	6.6 ± 0.5
(before rigidity)	White	23.1 ± 1.5	8.5 ± 0.5
75/90 min †	Red	1.5 ± 0.4	3.3 ± 0.9
	White	8.3 ± 4.7	4.6 ± 1.5

* μmol/g wet tissue. † One of 3 animals developed rigidity (75 min). Mean values for 3 pigs ± S.E.M.

life of about 240 min in the presence of adequate levels of glycogen in the muscles at the time of excision (Somers*et al.*, 1977b). Had the glycogen content been low, then the resynthesis of ATP under anaerobic conditions *in vitro* would have depended almost entirely on the initial concentration of CP alone and the rate of ATP loss from the muscle would have been high as a consequence. The accelerated fall in the ATP content of the muscle *in vitro*, however, was not due to initially low levels of glycogen since approximately 100 μmol lactate/g muscle was formed during a 2h incubation at 37°C. This observation suggested that the rate of ATP splitting had been high *in vivo* but nevertheless had been just balanced by resynthesis via the Lohmann reaction, glycolysis and oxidative phosphorylation during the 40 min period of anaesthesia. The mean high energy phosphate content of muscle removed after 75 and 90 min indicated that there had been a progressive loss of CP and ATP with continuing anaesthesia and although the muscle had not yet become rigid at this time it would have become so had the period of anaesthesia been extended. The results reported in this paper showed that when malignant hyperthermia was modified by neuroleptic drugs a loss of high energy phosphate from muscle occurred which preceded the onset of rigidity. The loss of ATP and CP was detected earlier in the red rather than white myofibres but whether this observation indicates a primary involvement of the red myofibres is not clear. Nevertheless, it is relevant to the findings of other workers. Ellis *et al.* (1973) detected myopathic changes in human patients susceptible to malignant hyperthermia and although the manner in which the myopathy presented varied between patients a common feature was an involvement of Type 1 (red) myofibres. Heffron and Isaacs (1976) reported the occurence of abnormal grouping of Type 1 myofibres in individuals susceptible to hyperthermia.

Halothane appears to have a direct action on skeletal muscle from susceptible humans and pigs. Sections of muscle from such individuals contract on exposure to the anaesthetic *in vitro*. Neuromuscular block with tubocurarine does not prevent the development of halothane-initiated rigidity, but the muscle relaxant dantrolene which acts postsynaptically will do so. The way in which neuroleptic drugs delay the onset of rigidity is a matter for speculation. While they may influence calcium binding by cell membranes of muscle and nerve it is perhaps more likely that they exert their effects through a central mechanism. Many neuroleptics not only modulate behaviour but also may have extrapyramidal side effects. Spiperone has weak anti-cholinergic activity and such neuroleptics are most often associated with dyskinesias and Parkinson-like symptoms in man.

References

Ahern, C.P., Somers, C.J., Wilson, P. and McLoughlin, J.V. (1977). Proceedings of the Third International Conference on Production Diseases in Farm Animals, Wageningen, The Netherlands, pp. 169-171.

Ellis, F.R., Keaney, N.P. and Harriman, D.G.F. (1973). *Proceedings of the Royal Society of Medicine,* **66,** 12-23.

Gronert, G.A. and Theye, R.A. (1976). *Anaesthesiology,* **44,** 36-44.

Hall, G.M., Lucke, J.N. and Lister, D. (1975). *Anaesthesia,* **30,** 308-317.

Harrison, C.G. (1975). *British Journal of Anaesthesia,* **47,** 62-65.

Heffron, J.J.A. and Isaacs, H. (1976). *Klinische Wochenschrift,* **34,** 865-867.

McLoughlin, J.V. and Mothersill, C. (1976). *Journal of Comparative Pathology,* **86,** 465-476.

Somers, C.J., Wilson, P., Ahern, C.P. and McLoughlin, J.V. (1977a). Proceedings of the Third International Conferences on Production Diseases in Farm Animals, Wageningen, The Netherlands, pp.167-168.

Somers, C.J., Wilson, P., Ahern, C.P. and McLoughlin, J.V. (1977b). *Journal of Comparative Pathology.* **87,** 177-183

Tarrant, P.J.V., McLoughlin, J.V. and Harrington, M.C.G. (1972). *Proc. Royal Irish Acad.,* **72,** 55-73.

Index